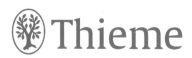

Adult Audiology Casebook

Second Edition

Michael Valente, PhD
Professor of Clinical Otolaryngology
Director of Adult Audiology
Washington University School of Medicine
St. Louis, Missouri

L. Maureen Valente, PhD
Former Associate Professor
Program in Audiology and Communication Sciences
Department of Otolaryngology
Washington University School of Medicine
St. Louis, Missouri

Thieme
New York • Stuttgart • Delhi • Rio de Janeiro

Library of Congress Cataloging-in-Publication Data

Library of Congress Control Number:2019953848

© 2020 Thieme Medical Publishers, Inc.

Thieme Publishers New York
333 Seventh Avenue, New York, NY 10001 USA
+1 800 782 3488, customerservice@thieme.com

Thieme Publishers Stuttgart
Rüdigerstrasse 14, 70469 Stuttgart, Germany
+49 [0]711 8931 421, customerservice@thieme.de

Thieme Publishers Delhi
A-12, Second Floor, Sector-2, Noida-201301
Uttar Pradesh, India
+91 120 45 566 00, customerservice@thieme.in

Thieme Publishers Rio de Janeiro, Thieme Publicações Ltda.
Edifício Rodolpho de Paoli, 25º andar
Av. Nilo Peçanha, 50 – Sala 2508,
Rio de Janeiro 20020-906 Brasil
+55 21 3172-2297 | +55 21 3172-1896
www.thiemerevinter.com.br

Cover design: Thieme Publishing Group
Typesetting by Thomson Digital, India

Printed in The United States of America by
King Printing Co., Inc.   5 4 3 2 1

ISBN 978-1-62623-729-2

Also available as an e-book:
eISBN 978-1-62623-730-8

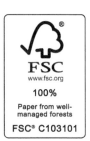

FSC
www.fsc.org
100%
Paper from well-managed forests
FSC® C103101

Contents

Contents

Contributors

Amyn M. Amlani, PhD
Professor and Chair
Consortium Program
University of Arkansas for Medical Sciences
University of Arkansas at Little Rock
Little Rock, Arkansas

David M. Baguley, BSc, MSc, MBA, PhD
Professor in Hearing Sciences
National Institute for Health Research
Nottingham Hearing Biomedical Research Centre
Nottingham, United Kingdom

Katie Barnhouse, AuD
Clinical Audiologist
Puget Sound Veteran's Administration Health Care system
American Lake Division
Tacoma, Washington

Alison M. Brockmeyer-Lauer, AuD
Clinical Audiologist
Washington University School of Medicine
St. Louis, Missouri

Craig A. Buchman, MD
Lindburg Professor of Otolaryngology
Department of Otolaryngology
Washington University School of Medicine
St. Louis, Missouri

Pamela Burch-Sims, PhD, CCCA
Assistant Vice President
Department of Institutional Effectiveness
Tennessee State University
Nashville, Tennessee

Hannah Burrick, BA
Audiology Doctoral Student
Washington University School of Medicine
St. Louis, Missouri

Jacqueline Busen, AuD
Clinical Assistant Professor
Arizona State University
Tempe, Arizona

Oscar M. Cañete, PhD
Postdoctoral Research Fellow
Speech Science, School of Psychology
Tamaki Campus
The University of Auckland
Auckland, New Zealand

Vanessa Chan, BA, MSc
Scientific Officer
Queen Elizabeth Hospital
Kowloon, Hong Kong

Marshall Chasin, AuD
Audiologist and Director of Research
Musicians' Clinics of Canada
Toronto, Ontario, Canada

Kris Chesky, PhD
Professor
College of Music
University of North Texas
Director
Texas Center for Performing Arts Health
Denton, Texas

Richard A. Chole, MD
Professor
Department of Otolaryngology
Washington University School of Medicine
St. Louis, Missouri

Frederick E. Cobb, PhD, CCC-A
Audiologist and Vestibular Assessment Subject Matter
 Expert
C.W. "Bill" Young VA Healthcare System
Bay Pines, Florida

Cathryn Collopy, AuD
Clinical Audiologist
Washington University School of Medicine
St. Louis, Missouri

Gemma Crundwell, BSc (Hons) Audiology, MA
Specialist Audiologist
Cambridge University Hospitals
NHS Foundation Trust
Addenbrooke's Hospital
Cambridge Biomedical Campus
Cambridge, United Kingdom

D. Bradley Davis, AuD, CCC-A
Assistant Professor
Louisiana State University Health Sciences Center
New Orleans, Louisiana

Aniruddha K. Deshpande, PhD, CCC-A
Assistant Professor and Director
The Hear-Ring Lab
Department of Speech-Language Hearing Sciences
Hofstra University
Hempstead, New York

Shruti Balvalli Deshpande, PhD, CCC-A
Assistant Professor
Department of Communication Sciences and Disorders
St. John's University
Queens, New York

Sumitrajit (Sumit) Dhar, PhD
Hugh Knowles Professor
Department of Communication Disorders
Northwestern University
Evanston, Illinois

Kristin Dilaj, AuD, PhD, CCC-A
Director/Audiologist
New England Center for Hearing Rehabilitation, LLC
Hampton, Connecticut

Steven M. Doettl, AuD
Associate Professor
Department of Audiology and Speech Pathology
College of Health Professions
University of Tennessee Health Science Center
Knoxville, Tennessee

Diane Duddy, AuD
Clinical Audiologist
Washington University School of Medicine
St. Louis, Missouri

Kate Dupuis, PhD, CPsych
Schlegel Innovation Leader
Sheridan Centre for Elder Research
Oakville, Ontario, Canada

Katharine Fitzharris, AuD, PhD
Doctoral Fellow
Callier Center for Communication Disorders
University of Texas at Dallas
Dallas, Texas

Nsangou Ghogomu, MD, MA
Surgeon
Department of Otolaryngology, Head & Neck Surgery
Colorado Permanente Medical Group
Denver, Colorado

Andrea Gohmert AuD, ABAC, CCC-A
Director of Audiology Clinical Operations
Clinical Assistant Professor
Callier Center for Communication Disorders
University of Texas at Dallas
Dallas, Texas

Ken E. Hancock, PhD
Instructor
Department of Otology and Laryngology
Harvard Medical School
Boston, Massachusetts

Lauren Harvey, MA (Audiology), MAudSA
Director and Audiologist
Lauren Harvey Audiology
Brisbane, Australia

Gary P. Jacobson, PhD
Professor and Director
Division of Audiology
Department of Hearing and Speech Sciences
Vanderbilt Bill Wilkerson Center
Nashville, Tennessee

Mary Beth Jennings, PhD
Associate Professor
School of Communication Sciences and Disorders
Associate Professor
National Centre for Audiology
Elborn College
Western University
London, Canada

Jack Katz, PhD
Private Practice
Auditory Processing Service, LLC
Prairie Village, Kansas

Suzanne H. Kimball, AuD
Associate Professor
University of Oklahoma Health and Sciences Center
Oklahoma City, Oklahoma

Abin Kuruvilla-Mathew, PhD
Postdoctoral Research Fellow
Speech Science, School of Psychology
Tamaki Campus
The University of Auckland
Auckland, New Zealand

Joe Walter Kutz, Jr., MD, FACS
Professor
Department of Otolaryngology Head and Neck Surgery
University of Texas Southwestern Medical Center
Dallas, Texas

Lainey Lake, AuD
Owner and Audiologist
Hearing and Balance Specialists of Kansas City, LLC
Lee's Summit, Missouri

Ron Leavitt, AuD
Director of Audiology
Corvallis Hearing Center
Corvallis, Oregon

Choongheon Lee, PhD
Research Associate
Washington University School of Medicine
Saint Louis, Missouri

Jeffery T. Lichtenhan, PhD
Assistant Professor
Department of Otolaryngology
Washington University School of Medicine
St. Louis, Missouri

Glenis R. Long, PhD
Speech-Language-Hearing Sciences
City University of New York
New York, New York

Jay R. Lucker, EdD
Professor
Department of Communication Sciences and Disorders
Howard University
Washington, DC

Kathryn F. Makowiec, AuD
Senior Staff Audiologist
Division of Audiology
Department of Otolaryngology
Henry Ford Medical Group
Detroit, Michigan

Valeria Roberts Matlock, EdD, CCCA
Professor
Department of Speech Pathology and Audiology
Tennessee State University
Nashville, Tennessee

Patricia McCarthy, PhD
Professor
Doctor of Audiology (AuD) Program
Department of Communication Disorders & Sciences
Rush University
Chicago, Illinois

Devin L. McCaslin, PhD
Director, Vestibular and Balance Laboratory
Associate Professor, Mayo Clinic College of Medicine
Department of Otorhinolaryngology
Rochester, Minnesota

Jennifer McCullagh, AuD, PhD, CCC-A
Associate Professor
Southern Connecticut State University
New Haven, Connecticut

Jonathan McJunkin, MD
Associate Professor
Department of Otolaryngology Head-Neck Surgery
Washington University School of Medicine
St. Louis, Missouri

Christine Meston, MSc
Audiologist
School of Communication Sciences and Disorders
Elborn College
Western University
London, Canada

Heather Monroe, AuD
Audiologist
St. Louis Children's Hospital
St. Louis, Missouri

Kristi Oeding, AuD
Washington University School of Medicine
St. Louis, Missouri

Amanda J. Ortmann, PhD
Director of Audiology Studies
Washington University School of Medicine
St. Louis, Missouri

Judy Peterein, AuD
Audiologist
Washington University School of Medicine
St. Louis, Missouri

M. Kathleen Pichora-Fuller, PhD
Professor
Department of Psychology
University of Toronto Mississauga
Mississauga, Ontario, Canada

Lori Rakita, AuD
Clinical Research Manager
Phonak Audiology Research Center
Warrenville, Illinois

Marilyn Reed, MSc
Audiology Practice Advisor
Department of Audiology
Baycrest Health Sciences
Toronto, Ontario, Canada

Alicia Restrepo, AuD, FAAA
Assistant Professor
Division of Audiology
University of Miami – Ear Institute
Miami, Florida

Alejandro Rivas, MD
Associate Service Chief, Otology & Neurotology
Associate Professor of Otolaryngology-Head & Neck Surgery
Associate Professor of Neurological Surgery
The Otology Group of Vanderbilt
Vanderbilt University Medical Center
Nashville, Tennessee

Richard A. Roberts, PhD
Vice Chair for Clinical Operations
Assistant Professor
Department of Hearing and Speech Sciences
Vanderbilt University Medical Center
Nashville, Tennessee

Ross J. Roeser, PhD, FAAA
Lois and Howard Wolf Professor in Pediatric Hearing
Callier Center for Communication Disorders
University of Texas at Dallas
Dallas, Texas

Brianna Schmitt, BS
Doctoral Student
Program in Audiology and Communication Sciences
Washington University School of Medicine
St. Louis, Missouri

Andrew Schuette, AuD, CCC-A
Clinical Audiologist
Washington University School of Medicine
St. Louis, Missouri

Diane M. Scott, PhD, CCCA
Professor
Communication Disorders Program
School of Education
North Carolina Central University
Durham, North Carolina

Emily Sharp, AuD, CCC-A
Clinical Audiologist
American Hearing Aid Center & Audiology Services
Oklahoma City, Oklahoma

Kelly A. Sharpe, BS
Fourth Year AuD Extern
Nova Southeastern University
Fort Lauderdale, Florida

Belinda C. Sinks, AuD, CCC-A
Clinical Audiologist Dizziness and Balance Center
Washington University School of Medicine
St. Louis, Missouri

Spencer B. Smith, AuD, PhD
Assistant Professor
Department of Communication Sciences and Disorders
Moody College of Communication
The University of Texas at Austin
Austin, Texas

Steven Smith, AuD, CCC-A
Clinical Audiologist
Washington University School of Medicine
St. Louis, Missouri

Laura Street, AuD
Research Audiologist
Earlens Corporation
Menlo Park, California

Deepa Suneel, BS
Audiologist
Moody College of Communication
University of Texas at Austin
Austin, Texas

Rich Tyler, PhD
Director of Audiology
Department of Otolaryngology - Head and Neck Surgery
Department of Communication Sciences and Disorders
University of Iowa
Iowa City, Iowa

Michael Valente, PhD
Professor of Clinical Otolaryngology
Director of Adult Audiology
Washington University School of Medicine
St. Louis, Missouri

Adam H. Voss, AuD, CCC-A
Clinical Audiologist
Division of Adult Audiology
Washington University School of Medicine
St. Louis, Missouri

Therese C. Walden, AuD
Audiologist
Potomac Audiology, LLC
Rockville, Maryland

Bryan K. Ward, MD
Assistant Professor
Otolaryngology-Head and Neck Surgery
Johns Hopkins Medicine
Baltimore, Maryland

Trent Westrick, AuD
Assistant Professor
Pacific University School of Audiology
Hillsboro, Oregon

Gail M. Whitelaw, PhD
Clinic Director
The Ohio State University Speech-Language-Hearing Clinic
Columbus, Ohio

Wayne J. Wilson, PhD, MAudSA
Associate Professor and Head of Audiology
School of Health and Rehabilitation Sciences
The University of Queensland
St. Lucia, Australia

Amy K. Winston, AuD
Assistant Professor
Department of Communication Disorders and Sciences
Rush University Medical Center
Chicago, Illinois

Eddie Wong, MSc (Audiology)
Scientific Officer (Medical)
Queen Elizabeth Hospital
Kowloon, Hong Kong

Lena LN Wong, PhD
Professor
University of Ho ng Kong
Pok Fu Lam, Hong Kong

HC Yu, MBBS (HK), FRCSEd, FCSHK, FHKCORL, FHKAM (Otorhinolaryngology)
Senior Consultant in Otorhinolaryngology
Union Hospital
Kowloon, Hong Kong

Part I

Hearing Disorders

I

1 Meniere's Disease and Aided Distortion

Lori Rakita

1.1 Clinical History and Description

NA is a 61-year-old male diagnosed with Meniere's disease 10 years ago. He reports previous fluctuating hearing loss that has stabilized for approximately 1 year. Additional symptoms include intermittent bilateral low-frequency roaring tinnitus, but no recent episodes of vertigo or imbalance. NA states the primary symptoms of his Meniere's disease include fluctuating hearing and dizziness, and both have subsided following dietary changes (e.g., lower salt intake and no caffeine). He also reports a history of occupational noise exposure and his mother had hearing loss at a young age from an unknown cause. NA denies recent ear infections, aural fullness, or drainage.

1.2 Audiological Testing

Comprehensive audiometric testing was completed. The audiogram (▶ Fig. 1.1) revealed a bilateral symmetrical moderately severe sensorineural hearing loss. The Speech Recognition Threshold (SRT) was 75 dB hearing level (HL) for the right ear and 65 dB HL for the left ear, in good agreement with pure-tone averages (PTA) for each ear, and revealed a severe loss and a moderately severe loss in the ability to receive speech in the right and the left ears, respectively. Word recognition testing was conducted bilaterally via recorded CD version of the NU-6 (Northwestern University Auditory Test Number 6) using a male talker presented at 85 dB HL. Word Recognition Scores (WRS) obtained were 50% for the right ear and 66% for the left ear. These results indicate very poor ability to recognize speech in the right ear and moderate difficulty in the left ear. Immittance audiometry revealed middle ear pressure (daPa), static compliance (mL), and ear canal volume (mL) to be within the normal range bilaterally. Ipsilateral and contralateral Acoustic Reflex Thresholds (ARTs) at 500 to 4,000 Hz were absent bilaterally.

1.3 Questions to the Reader

1. **How would the scores of NA's word recognition testing guide an audiologist's counseling during a hearing aid evaluation?**
2. **What options for amplification would be most appropriate for NA's hearing loss and history?**
3. **Are there any causes for concern or unexpected inconsistencies in the audiologic testing?**

1.4 Discussion of Questions

1. **How would the scores of NA's word recognition testing guide an audiologist's counseling during a hearing aid evaluation?**

The scores indicate poor word recognition for the right ear and moderate difficulty for the left ear. This suggests that NA may also have difficulty understanding speech with amplification. It is essential for NA to be counseled so he does not have unrealistic expectations relative to his performance with amplification. Explaining the increased difficulty of aided performance in background noise when compared to quiet listening would be an important discussion. Also, NA should understand the methodology behind the WRS as the test was completed at comfortable loudness levels and in a sound-treated room. Therefore, these results may suggest (1) continued difficulty with speech clarity that will still be present with amplification and (2) greater difficulty with aided speech understanding with the right ear in comparison to the left ear.

2. **What options for amplification would be most appropriate for NA's hearing loss and history?**

At this point, based on the information gathered from the comprehensive audiologic evaluation, it seems as though conventional amplification would be the most appropriate option. It would be necessary to ensure sufficient gain and output and appropriate coupling of the hearing aids to NA's ears given NA's hearing loss. In this case, the audiologist recommended receiver-in-canal (RIC) hearing aids with custom c-shells. If a standard earmold were pursued, however, a parallel vent with a small vent (e.g., 1 mm) would be recommended to maintain amplification of the low frequencies and prevent feedback. Given the flat configuration of the hearing loss, a 3- or 4-mm Libby horn would also be recommended to provide additional gain in the frequency region above 2,000 Hz that is so critical to speech understanding.

Also, given NA's poor WRS it would be important to counsel on expectations with amplification. NA should be counseled to report any future fluctuations in hearing and the need for re-testing and re-programming changes would be noted.

3. **Are there any causes for concern or unexpected inconsistencies in the audiologic testing?**

NA's WRS, particularly of the right ear, are a cause for concern. The WRS are perhaps less symmetrical than would be expected given the symmetry of the hearing thresholds even though the difference in WRS does not exceed the bimodal distribution according to Carney and Schlauch.[1] This finding indicates that a referral to an otologist is appropriate to possibly uncover the cause for such asymmetry.

1.5 Additional Hearing Aid Fitting Options

RIC hearing aids with custom c-shells and power receivers were recommended for NA. Following medical clearance from NA's physician, the hearing aids were fitted and programmed to National Acoustics Laboratories prescriptive procedure for fitting linear hearing aids, version 2 (NAL-NL2)[2] and verified with real ear measurements (REM) to ensure real-ear insertion gain (REIG) was within 5 dB of prescribed targets at 50, 65, and 80 dB sound pressure level (SPL) input levels. A tinnitus

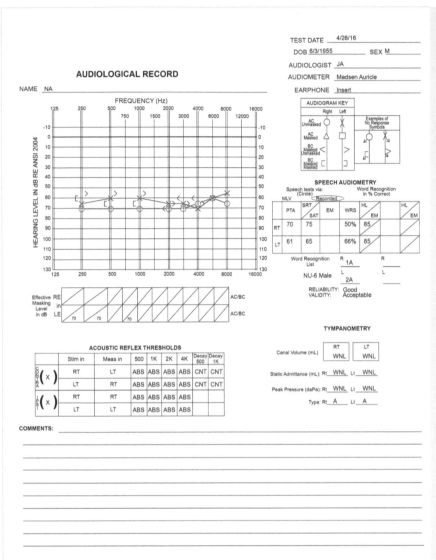

Fig. 1.1 Comprehensive audiological testing for NA.

program was included in the hearing aids to help distract from the roaring tinnitus that NA reported. This noise program utilizes a noise generator with customization of sound type and frequency.

NA returned after a month's trial and stated that the hearing aid for the left ear performed very well, but the hearing aid for the right ear was extremely distorted, even in quiet listening situations. NA said it sounded like "significantly distorted speech" and he could not distinguish any speech with the right hearing aid alone. Further, he felt that with bilateral amplification, speech was distorted and difficult to understand. He asked if he could return the hearing aid for the right ear as he seemed to hear better without it.

1.6 Additional Questions

1. **What are some steps that can be taken to ensure the right hearing aid is working within manufacturer specifications and the problem is not related to a malfunctioning hearing aid?**

2. **What other treatment options might be considered that may be appropriate for NA? What would be the benefits and limitations of these options?**

3. **Why are two hearing aids typically recommended for patients with bilateral hearing loss?**

1.7 Discussion of Additional Questions

1. **What are some steps that can be taken to ensure the right hearing aid is working within manufacturer specifications and the problem is not related to a malfunctioning hearing aid?**

It is essential to first ensure that the right hearing aid is working properly and is functioning within manufacturer specifications. External components should be checked including a wax trap (if the hearing aid has one) and visualization to be sure the hearing aid microphones are clear of debris and changing the microphone filters (if applicable). The receiver should be checked to ensure it is making proper connection with hearing aid and is transmitting sound. Electroacoustic verification should be completed at full-on-gain settings with an input SPL of 50 dB SPL to assess if the hearing aid is meeting manufacturer specifications.[3]

Electroacoustic analysis using a speech-shaped signal at the user settings with a 2-mL coupler should also be completed to serve as a baseline reference to compare against measures obtained at future visits. This should be completed at soft, medium, and loud input levels (e.g. 50, 60, 70, and 80 dB SPL). Additionally, carefully observe the morphology (i.e., shape) of these multiple input frequency response curves as abnormalities (e.g., jagged curves) can be observed in the curves at the higher input levels, which could indicate intermodulation distortion. If this occurs, the hearing aid(s) and printout need to be sent to the manufacturer for repair or replacement. Verification of directional microphone functionality should also be completed using either coupler or REM. In the present case, the directional microphone test was completed in the Verifit2 system and the directional microphone was performing as expected where the frequency response to the signal presented from the back was attenuated relative to the signal arriving from the front.

Finally, a listening check with a listening tube would be useful to determine that the hearing aid and all components are functioning well. If specifications in these tests did not adhere to American National Standards Institute (ANSI)[3] guidelines, it would be necessary to contact the hearing aid manufacturer for a repair or replacement of the hearing aid.

2. **What other treatment options might be considered that may be appropriate for NA? What would be the benefits and limitations of these options?**
If the hearing aid is found to be operating to manufacturer specifications, then perhaps a different type of amplification could be considered as well as follow-up testing. First, it would be necessary to ensure NA's reports of poorer listening with bilateral amplification is present since in most cases binaural amplification typically yields *better* performance than monaural amplification.[4] This could be assessed by evaluating speech understanding with the right and left aids measured monaurally and then bilaterally. If there is an advantage to bilateral listening, counseling on the benefits of binaural hearing would be helpful. If it is the case that NA performs poorer with bilateral listening, then other amplification options may be considered.

A left bilateral contralateral routing of signal (BICROS) hearing aid may be another option with a transmitter on the right ear and receiver/hearing aid on the left ear (i.e., better WRS). The limitation to this suggestion is only using the right ear to send the signal to the left ear instead of the sound input received bilaterally. Because the right ear seemed to have aidable hearing (i.e., WRS of 50%), a BICROS system would not have been a first choice because it would not allow aidable hearing in the right ear. If follow-up testing, however, revealed minimal use of the aided hearing in the right ear and, additionally, greater distortion when the right ear was used when combined with the left ear, a left BICROS may be a better option for awareness of sound on the right side without disrupting audibility and clarity for the left ear.

Another possible option is to pursue a monaural hearing aid fitting for the left ear. In this case, NA would not experience the

bilateral distortion caused by aiding bilaterally and may not experience the drawbacks, as listed above, with the BICROS system. A monaural fitting, however, would result in the better ear being in the shadow of the head when sounds approach from the poorer hearing side. This could lead to difficulty in hearing any signal arriving on the side of the poorer hearing right ear.

3. **Why are two hearing aids typically recommended for patients with bilateral hearing loss?**
There are several reasons why two hearing aids are typically recommended for patients with bilateral hearing loss, particularly related to the central auditory system and the design of this system to take advantage of binaural input. In addition to the qualitative benefit of balance and improved listening effort, patients receive a natural increase in output due to binaural input to the two ears.[4,5,6,7] Further, bilateral hearing improves understanding speech in the presence of background noise (i.e., binaural squelch effect) and localization of sound since these functionalities rely on the information and comparison of interaural differences in time, intensity, and phase on the signals at each ear.[4,5,6,7]

1.8 Recommended Treatment

At this point, the audiologist performed aided word recognition testing monaurally and bilaterally to assess NA's reports of distortion from his right hearing aid. Prior to any sound-field testing, it was necessary to ensure accurate calibration of the sound-field presentation system, in accordance with ANSI S3.6 with sound-field reference to 0 degree.[8] The system was calibrated to binaural listening and 0-degree azimuth. The output level was measured at the reference point (0-degree azimuth) and then compared and subtracted from the expected level (audiometer dial plus reference equivalent sound pressure level, as specified in ANSI S3.6, to ensure this difference was below 2.5 dB.[3] Aided testing was completed at an input level of 65 dB SPL using recorded NU-6 word list with male talker presented at 0-degree azimuth. During all monaural testing, speech-shaped masking noise was presented at 80 dB SPL to the non-test ear via an insert earphone. Results revealed 66% with left monaural, 40% with right monaural, and 50% with bilateral listening.

Since NA expressed discontentment with the hearing aid on his right ear and the reported distortion has been documented through testing, two other fitting options were discussed with NA: either a monaural hearing aid fitting for the left ear or a left BICROS system. NA expressed that he did not use his right ear for aided listening and would try the left BICROS system so he had better sound awareness on his right side. A remote microphone to assist with speech understanding in noise and during meetings was also discussed. This system seemed to be of interest to NA and will be fitted at a future appointment.

1.9 Additional Recommended Testing

It may be assumed that the distortion in NA's auditory system could be due to Meniere's disease. A follow-up with an otologist would be a primary recommendation due to the asymmetry in speech clarity that NA perceives. It is also advisable to recommend additional testing to rule out other causes of the slight asymmetry in speech recognition and distortion. These tests could include radiographic studies such as magnetic resonance imaging and/or computerized axial tomography scan to rule out lesions along the auditory pathway, auditory brainstem response, and otoacoustic emissions to perhaps obtain a clearer picture of the audiologic and/or pathological causes of this distortion. Tests of central processing were also suggested. These tests were recommended during NA's last visit to the clinic, so the results of these tests were unknown at the current time.

1.10 Outcome

The left BICROS was fitted and verified in the test box as well as with REM. Test box verification was completed by first connecting the left receiver hearing aid to the 2-cc coupler and placed in the test box and presenting an ISTS (International Speech Test Signal) speech signal at 50, 65, and 75 dB SPL. Test box verification of the transmitter was completed by placing the transmitter in the test box and removing the 2-mL coupler and connected receiver from the test box and placing them outside the test box. The same signals at 50, 65, and 75 dB SPL were presented to the transmitter aid inside the test box and were verified to be received by the receiver placed on the outside of the test box still coupled to the coupler microphone.

Further verification was also completed via REM using two measures.[9] First, the performance of the receiver aid in the left ear was verified by placing a probe tube in the left ear canal and positioning the reference microphone above the left ear with the transmitter aid turned off. The loudspeaker from the real ear analyzer was positioned at 0 degree and the measured REIG was matched to NAL-NL2.[2] Second, the loudspeaker was now moved to 90 degrees on the receiver side and a measure made using a 65 dB SPL speech-shaped signal. Finally, the loudspeaker was placed at 90 degrees to the transmitter side (right ear), with the transmitter aid turned on, the reference microphone over the right ear turned on, and probe tube still in the left ear. Then, the same 65 dB SPL speech-shaped signal was presented to the transmitter side. The resulting measure should match the measure taken with the loudspeaker at 90 degrees to the left side, indicating that the activation of the transmitter aid eliminated the head shadow effect.

NA was very pleased with his left BICROS system. He found he experienced significantly less distortion from his right ear and improved listening effort. Although research has repeatedly reported that bilateral fitting is the gold standard,[4,5,6,7] the results with NA illustrate that a "one size fits all approach" is not always the best solution.

1.11 Key Points

- WRS testing can be a valuable tool when counseling of hearing aid expectations.
- Not all clinical "standards" are always appropriate for each patient and patient-specific considerations must be included in recommendations.
- BICROS can be an appropriate choice, even for patients with symmetric hearing thresholds but asymmetric WRS.

References

[1] Carney E, Schlauch RS. Critical difference table for word recognition testing derived using computer simulation. J Speech Lang Hear Res. 2007; 50(5): 1203–1209

[2] Dillon H. NAL-NL1: a new procedure for fitting non-linear hearing aids. Hear J. 1999; 52:10–16

[3] American National Standards Institute. American National Standard for Specification of Hearing Aid Characteristics. (ANSI S3.22–2009). New York: ANSI; 2009

[4] Kochkin S. The binaural advantage. Better Hearing Institute. www.betterhearing.org/hearingpedia/hearing-aids/binaural-advantage. Accessed October 24, 2016

[5] Ching TYC, Incerti P, Hill M, van Wanrooy E. An overview of binaural advantages for children and adults who use binaural/bimodal hearing devices. Audiol Neurootol. 2006; 11 Suppl 1:6–11

[6] Day GA, Browning GG, Gatehouse S. Benefit from binaural hearing aids in individuals with a severe hearing impairment. Br J Audiol. 1988; 22(4):273–277

[7] Noble W, Gatehouse S. Effects of bilateral versus unilateral hearing aid fitting on abilities measured by the Speech, Spatial, and Qualities of Hearing Scale (SSQ). Int J Audiol. 2006; 45(3):172–181

[8] American National Standards Institute. Specification for audiometers (ANSI S3.6–2010). New York, NY: ANSI; 2010

[9] Valente M, Valente M, Meister M, et al. Selecting and verifying hearing aid fittings for unilateral hearing loss. In: Valente M, ed. Strategies for Selecting and Verifying Hearing Aid Fittings. New York, NY: Thieme; 1994:228–248

Suggested Reading

[1] Carter AS, Noe CM, Wilson RH. Listeners who prefer monaural to binaural hearing aids. J Am Acad Audiol. 2001; 12(5):261–272

[2] Hawkins DB, Yacullo WS. Signal-to-noise ratio advantage of binaural hearing aids and directional microphones under different levels of reverberation. J Speech Hear Disord. 1984; 49(3):278–286

[3] Taylor B. Contralateral routing of the signal amplification Strategies. Semin Hear. 2010; 31(4):278–392

[4] Courtois J, Johansen PA, Larsen BV, Berlin J. Hearing aid fitting in asymmetrical hearing loss. In: Jensen J, ed. Hearing Aid Fitting: Theoretical and Practical Views. Copenhagen: Stougaard Jenson; 1988:243–256

2 An Unexpected Cause of Sudden Hearing Loss

Kristi Oeding

2.1 Clinical History and Description

A 64-year-old male with bilateral sudden hearing loss presented himself to the audiology clinic after being in the intensive care unit (ICU) for 2.5 weeks.

RH is a 64-year-old man who was scheduled at our audiology clinic for a comprehensive audiologic examination because he reported that 2.5 weeks ago he was hospitalized for 2 weeks with encephalitis. When RH regained consciousness in the ICU, he noticed decreased hearing bilaterally (left ear poorer than the right), bilateral tinnitus (left ear louder than right ear), blurry vision, decreased cognition, weakness, aphasia, and fever. RH denied hearing loss prior to his hospitalization. He had a history of noise exposure from working as a farmer for many years. He reports losing 30 lbs over the last 2.5 weeks. Also, RH had a right parotid Warthin's tumor, but did not have

surgery due to tachycardia. Finally, RH reported he had atrial fibrillation and diabetes.

2.2 Audiologic Testing

The initial audiologic evaluation is presented in ▶ Fig. 2.1. Pure-tone thresholds in the right ear revealed a slight sloping to a severe sensorineural hearing loss (SNHL). Results in the left ear revealed a moderately severe to severe flat SNHL. Speech Recognition Threshold (SRT) revealed a slight loss in the right ear and a moderately severe loss in the left ear in the ability to receive speech. Word Recognition Score (WRS) testing revealed slight difficulty in the right ear and very poor ability to recognize speech in the left ear. Tympanometry was within normal limits bilaterally. Acoustic Reflex Thresholds (ART) were absent bilaterally in response to ipsilateral and contralateral stimulation.

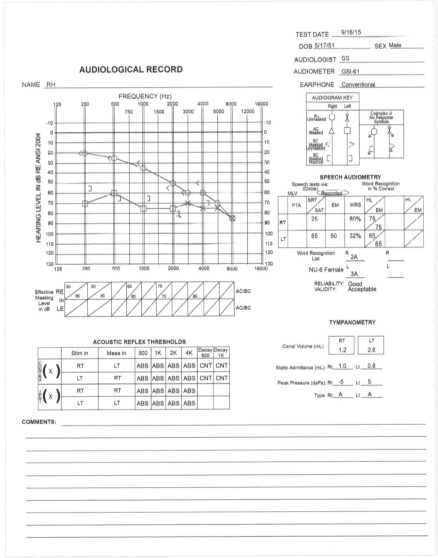

Fig. 2.1 RH's initial comprehensive audiometric evaluation.

2.3 Questions to the Reader

1. What are some potential causes of the sudden hearing loss and symptoms RH reported?
2. What audiologic recommendations could be made for RH?
3. What type of hearing loss occurs with sudden hearing loss?

2.4 Discussion of Questions

1. **What are some potential causes of the sudden hearing loss and symptoms RH reported?**

The potential causes of his hearing loss and symptoms could be a viral infection, vascular lesion, autoimmune disorder, and acoustic neuroma/vestibular schwannoma. Also, many patients with sudden SNHL are idiopathic in nature, which means that after careful testing a cause to explain the hearing loss could not be found.

2. **What audiologic recommendations could be made for RH?**

There are several audiologic recommendations that can be made if the patient's hearing remains stable and similar to the audiologic results reported in ▶ Fig. 2.1. RH could consider obtaining bilateral hearing aids or a monaural hearing aid to the left ear to determine benefit. If RH does not report benefit with monaural or bilateral amplification, a right Bilateral Contralateral Routing of the Signal (BICROS) hearing aid could be considered. In this case, a transmitting microphone would be placed over the left ear and the signal would be routed wirelessly and amplified with a hearing aid coupled to the right ear. Hearing Assistive Technology (HAT) could also be beneficial when background noise is present, such as an FM (frequency modulator) system or a wireless remote microphone. Finally, due to the very poor WRS in the left ear, another option is determining if RH is a candidate for a cochlear implant (CI) in the left ear and he could wear a hearing aid in the right ear (i.e., bimodal fitting).

3. **What type of hearing loss occurs with sudden hearing loss?**

Sudden hearing loss usually manifests itself as a unilateral SNHL and is idiopathic in 85 to 90% of cases.[1] While RH has SNHL, the hearing loss is bilateral, which is not common for sudden hearing loss. In some rare cases, however, bilateral SNHL can occur. Some conditions that may cause sudden bilateral SNHL include meningitis, encephalitis, autoimmune inner ear disease, Lyme's disease, Cogan's syndrome, and Ramsay Hunt's syndrome.[1,2] It is possible that the encephalitis, which was caused by something else, may have caused the hearing loss.

2.5 Diagnosis and Recommended Treatment

An otolaryngologist determined that the cause of his symptoms and hearing loss was West Nile virus (WNV). The physician recommended returning in 3 weeks and repeating the audiogram.

The physician did not prescribe steroids, such as dexamethasone, at the time, possibly due to the patient being diabetic.

The patient returned 2 months later for a follow-up audiologic evaluation, which is presented in ▶ Fig. 2.2. The patient reported improved hearing, and his strength and balance had improved as well. Pure-tone thresholds in the right ear revealed normal hearing sensitivity at 250 to 1,000 Hz sloping to a moderate predominantly SNHL from 2,000 to 3,000 Hz and rising to a mild hearing loss from 6,000 to 8,000 Hz. The left ear revealed a slight sloping to severe SNHL at 250 to 8,000 Hz. Please see the bottom right of ▶ Fig. 2.2 documenting the magnitude of improved hearing relative to the audiometric results reported in ▶ Fig. 2.1. SRTs revealed a slight loss in the ability to receive speech in the right ear. A Speech Awareness Threshold (SAT) was obtained in the left ear and revealed a mild loss in the ability to detect speech. WRS testing revealed slight difficulty in the right ear and very poor speech recognition in the left ear. Tympanometry was within normal limits bilaterally. ART testing for ipsilateral stimulation revealed normal ARTs at 500 and 1,000 Hz and absent ARTs at 2,000 and 4,000 Hz bilaterally. ART testing for contralateral stimulation revealed elevated ARTs at 500 and 1,000 Hz and absent ARTs at 2,000 and 4,000 Hz for right contralateral ART, and within normal limits at 500 and 1,000 Hz and absent ARTs at 2,000 and 4,000 Hz for left contralateral ART. The otolaryngologist recommended a repeat audiologic examination in 6 months and decided to continue to wait to prescribe steroids since hearing had improved.

The patient returned approximately 9 months later for a repeat audiologic examination. At this appointment, the patient reported otalgia in the right ear. His hearing had remained stable, but sound was distorted (diplacusis—sound was different in pitch compared to the other ear and echoed) in the left ear. RH mentioned that it sounded as if he were listening in a "tin can." He reported vertigo when getting out of bed for the past several months. He had constant ringing tinnitus in the left ear that fluctuated in loudness and could be bothersome.

The results of the second follow-up audiologic evaluation are presented in ▶ Fig. 2.3. Pure-tone threshold testing in the right ear revealed normal hearing sensitivity sloping to a moderate SNHL from 250 to 3,000 Hz and rising to a mild hearing loss from 4,000 to 8,000 Hz. Results in the left ear revealed a slight sloping to a severe SNHL (see audiogram for changes). SRT testing revealed normal ability in the right ear and a moderately severe loss in the left ear in the ability to receive speech. WRS testing revealed a normal ability in the right ear and a very poor ability in the left ear to recognize speech. Overall, RH's hearing had remained stable since the last audiologic examination. At this appointment, the otolaryngologist determined RH had right benign paroxysmal positional vertigo after performing the Dix–Hallpike test. The patient was counseled on performing the Epley maneuver and his vertigo resolved.

2.6 Outcome

Amplification options were discussed with RH. These options included a left hearing aid, right hearing aid, bilateral hearing aids, a right BICROS and a CI in the left ear coupled with a

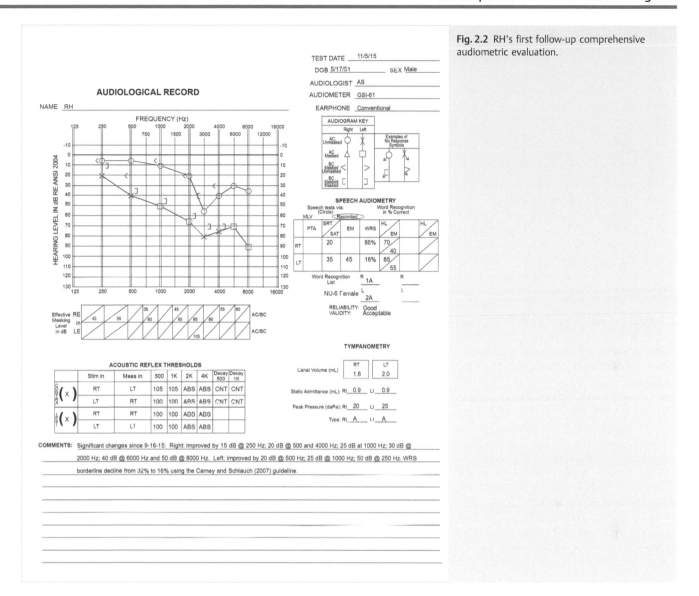

Fig. 2.2 RH's first follow-up comprehensive audiometric evaluation.

possible hearing aid to the right ear. He was most interested in a CI, but unfortunately his insurance would not cover the cost and RH did not qualify for current research studies. The patient decided to wait to determine how well he can compensate for his hearing loss before pursuing amplification.

When a person contracts WNV, 20% are symptomatic with flulike symptoms, such as headache, fever, and nausea.[3,4] One percent experience neurological complications such as meningitis, encephalitis, and acute flaccid paralysis, which can include an altered mental state, weakness, tremor, and problems with gait/balance.[3,4,5] This usually occurs in persons that are elderly and/or immunocompromised. The effects of WNV on hearing are still unknown other than through a few published case studies.[4,6,7,8,9] These case studies reveal that bilateral hearing loss can occur ranging from mild to profound. The hearing loss can be symmetric or asymmetric and occasionally spontaneous

recovery of hearing can occur. The occurrence of hearing loss appears to be rare and is usually present in the elderly or immunocompromised.

2.7 Key Points

- WNV, although rare, could cause a bilateral sudden hearing loss. This is typically found in the elderly and others who are immunocompromised.
- Hearing loss from WNV can sometimes recover spontaneously.
- A variety of amplification options are available to patients with asymmetric hearing loss and the patient should be made aware of the advantages and disadvantages of each option.

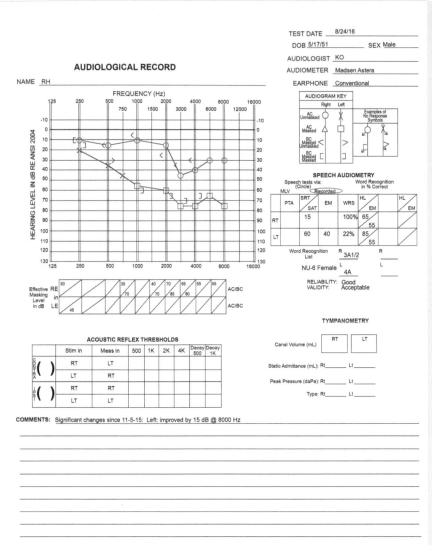

Fig. 2.3 RH's second follow-up comprehensive audiometric evaluation.

References

[1] Stachler RJ, Chandrasekhar SS, Archer SM, et al. American Academy of Otolaryngology-Head and Neck Surgery. Clinical practice guideline: sudden hearing loss. Otolaryngol Head Neck Surg. 2012; 146(3) Suppl:S1–S35

[2] Rauch SD. Clinical practice. Idiopathic sudden sensorineural hearing loss. N Engl J Med. 2008; 359(8):833–840

[3] Sejvar JJ, Haddad MB, Tierney BC, et al. Neurologic manifestations and outcome of West Nile virus infection. JAMA. 2003; 290(4):511–515

[4] Cohen BE, Durstenfeld A, Roehm PC. Viral causes of hearing loss: a review for hearing health professionals. Trends Hear. 2014; 18:1–17

[5] Hayes EB, Sejvar JJ, Zaki SR, Lanciotti RS, Bode AV, Campbell GL. Virology, pathology, and clinical manifestations of West Nile virus disease. Emerg Infect Dis. 2005; 11(8):1174–1179

[6] Marciniak C, Sorosky S, Hynes C. Acute flaccid paralysis associated with West Nile virus: motor and functional improvement in 4 patients. Arch Phys Med Rehabil. 2004; 85(12):1933–1938

[7] McBride W, Gill KR, Wiviott L. West Nile virus infection with hearing loss. J Infect. 2006; 53(5):e203–e205

[8] Jamison SC, Michaels SR, Ratard R, Sweet JM, Deboisblanc BP. A 41-year-old HIV-positive man with acute onset of quadriplegia after West Nile virus infection. South Med J. 2007; 100(10):1051–1053

[9] Casetta I, Ciorba A, Cesnik E, Trevisi P, Tugnoli V, Bovo R. West Nile virus neuroinvasive disease presenting with acute flaccid paralysis and bilateral sensorineural hearing loss. J Neurol. 2011; 258(10):1880–1881

3 Audiologic Management of an African American Patient with Sickle Cell Disease

Valeria Roberts Matlock, Pamela Burch-Sims, and Diane M. Scott

3.1 Clinical History and Description

This is a case report of a 20-year-old male who presented with initial complaint of hearing loss and pain in his right ear. The onset of the hearing loss was reportedly within the last 6 months.

At the time of audiologic testing, JB was a 20-year-old male attending college on a full scholarship seeking a bachelor's degree in elementary education. JB experienced difficulty hearing his instructors and experienced pain in his right ear. He was seen by a nurse practitioner (NP) in the university's student health clinic. A physical examination was completed and JB was prescribed an antibiotic for an ear infection. JB returned to the clinic as directed upon completion of his medication. JB reported his hearing improved, but his hearing had not returned to normal. At that point, JB was referred to the university's audiology clinic.

3.2 Audiologic Testing

During the case history interview with the audiologist, JB reported experiencing fluctuating hearing loss for the past 6 months. Prenatal and family histories were unremarkable. Medical history was negative for tinnitus, sensation of movement, and head trauma, but positive for chronic upper respiratory infections (URI).

An audiologic evaluation (▶ Fig. 3.1) revealed a mild-to-moderately severe sensorineural hearing loss (SNHL) in the right ear and normal pure-tone thresholds in the left ear. Speech Recognition Thresholds (SRTs) were in agreement with the Pure-Tone Average (PTA) and revealed a mild loss in the ability to receive speech in the right ear and normal ability in the left ear. Word Recognition Scores (WRS) indicated moderate difficulty for the right ear and normal ability to recognize speech in the left ear when stimuli were presented at 80 dB hearing level (HL). When the intensity level was reduced to 70 dB HL, the WRS for the right ear improved (i.e., 64–88%) with slight difficulty in recognizing speech. This finding resulted in a Phonetically Balanced Performance Intensity (PB-PI) function Rollover Index (RI) of 0.27 (i.e., 88–64%/88%), which is suggestive of cochlear pathology.

Tympanometry revealed normal ear canal volume, normal static admittance, normal middle ear pressure in the left ear, and normal ear canal volume, normal static admittance, and negative middle ear pressure in the right ear. Ipsilateral and contralateral Acoustic Reflex Thresholds (ART) were consistent with cochlear hearing loss in the right ear because ARTs were obtained at reduced sensation levels. Normal sensation levels were reported when stimulating the left ear for ipsilateral and contralateral ARTs. Acoustic reflex decay was not observed in either ear.

3.3 Questions to the Reader

1. **Given JB's medical history and initial audiologic findings, what impressions can be drawn with respect to potential causes(s) of his hearing loss?**
2. **At this point, would further diagnostic testing be recommended? If yes, what additional tests would be recommended?**
3. **What indications from the initial audiologic evaluation would warrant Auditory Brainstem Response (ABR) and Otoacoustic Emission (OAE) testing?**

3.4 Discussion of Questions

1. **Given JB's medical history and initial audiologic findings, what impressions can be drawn with respect to potential causes(s) of his hearing loss?**

Given the asymmetrical nature of JB's pure-tone thresholds, retrocochlear pathology should be ruled out. Due to the reduced sensation levels of the ARTs in the right ear; however, cochlear pathology must also be considered.

2. **At this point, would further diagnostic testing be recommended? If yes, what additional tests would be recommended?**

Further diagnostic testing would be recommended given the test results. Determining site of lesion is necessary given the possibility of retrocochlear pathology. ABR and OAE testing could aid in the differential diagnosis of site of lesion.

3. **What indications from the initial audiologic evaluation would warrant Auditory Brainstem Response (ABR) and Otoacoustic Emission (OAE) testing?**

Significant asymmetry in pure-tone thresholds and/or WRS is an important indicator for ABR testing. Given a disagreement between the ARTs and OAE results, ABR could indicate whether or not cochlear pathology is present.

3.5 Additional Testing

ABR testing was performed bilaterally the following day using a click stimulus (80 dB HL). Absolute and interwave latencies were obtained and were found to be consistent with normative values for each ear. Interaural latency comparison of wave V was normal. The latency-intensity functions were normal for each ear. Wave V was repeatable to 25 dB HL in the left ear and to 45 dB HL in the right ear. Waveform morphology was judged to be good for each ear (▶ Fig. 3.2). Distortion Product Otoacoustic Emissions (DPOAEs) were absent through 2,000 Hz in the right ear and present and repeatable at normal amplitudes in the left ear from 2,000 through 6,000 Hz.

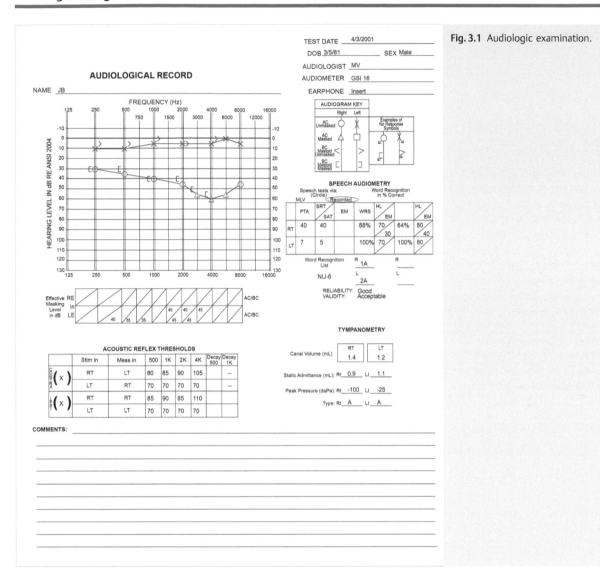

Fig. 3.1 Audiologic examination.

AUDIOLOGICAL RECORD

TEST DATE __4/3/2001__
DOB __3/5/81__   SEX __Male__
AUDIOLOGIST __MV__
AUDIOMETER __GSI 16__
EARPHONE __Insert__

NAME __JB__

SPEECH AUDIOMETRY

Speech tests via: (Circle) MLV / Recorded   Word Recognition in % Correct

	PTA	SRT / SAT	EM	WRS	HL / EM		HL / EM
RT	40	40		88%	70 / 30	64%	80 / 40
LT	7	5		100%	70	100%	80

Word Recognition List   R __1A__   R
NU-6   L __2A__   L

RELIABILITY: Good
VALIDITY: Acceptable

TYMPANOMETRY

	RT	LT
Canal Volume (mL)	1.4	1.2

Static Admittance (mL): Rt __0.9__ Lt __1.1__

Peak Pressure (daPa): Rt __-100__ Lt __-25__

Type: Rt __A__ Lt __A__

ACOUSTIC REFLEX THRESHOLDS

	Stim in	Meas in	500	1K	2K	4K	Decay 500	Decay 1K
(x) CONTRA	RT	LT	80	85	90	105	--	
	LT	RT	70	70	70	70	--	
(x) IPSI	RT	RT	85	90	85	110		
	LT	LT	70	70	70	70		

COMMENTS: _____

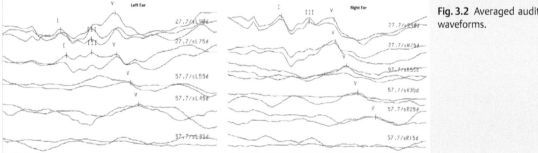

Fig. 3.2 Averaged auditory brainstem response waveforms.

JB was referred to an otologist to determine the possible etiology of the SNHL in his right ear and to obtain medical clearance for possible hearing aid usage. JB was asked to return to the audiology clinic in 1 month for an audiometric reevaluation to monitor the stability of his audiologic results. JB was also referred to the university's Office for Students with Disabilities to obtain a Frequency Modulation (FM) system for use in the classroom and other accommodations including preferential seating and real-time closed captioning services.

The otologist reported no remarkable findings during a physical examination. Additional medical history, however, was obtained during the visit. JB admitted to experiencing chronic swelling of his feet, fatigue, and achy joints since childhood. The otologist referred JB to a rheumatologist who completed blood work. Results of the blood work revealed 28% hemoglobin S, indicating an abnormal component of hemoglobin that is consistent with sickle cell disease (SCD). JB was then referred to a physician specializing in the treatment of SCD.

3.6 Additional Questions for the Reader

1. **Based on the ABR and DPOAE results, along with the results of the blood work, what conclusions can be made with regard to the cause of JB's hearing loss?**
2. **What type of treatment, intervention, and/or rehabilitation options would be recommended based on the findings of impaired cochlear function?**
3. **What medical complications and symptoms of SCD should be considered in the determining appropriate recommendations?**
4. **What are the implications of SCD on auditory function?**

3.7 Discussion of Additional Questions

1. **Based on the ABR and DPOAE results, along with the results of the blood work, what conclusions can be made with regard to the cause of JB's hearing loss?**

Auditory dysfunction in patients with SCD has been documented; however, there are a limited number of research studies investigating the relationship between SCD and hearing loss. One study identified hearing loss in 22% of a group of 83 individuals with SCD.[1] Another study concluded that the site of lesion of auditory dysfunction among a group of 113 subjects with SCD was cochlear in nature.[2] Several other studies also observed abnormal cochlear findings.[3,4,5,6,7] Yet, one study conducted in 2015 found statistically no significant differences between OAE test results among 35 children with SCD and 115 control subjects.[7]

2. **What type of treatment, intervention, and/or rehabilitation options would be recommended based on the findings of impaired cochlear function?**

A hearing aid evaluation and fitting would be recommended for an individual with impaired cochlear function. Given JB's fluctuating hearing impairment, a hearing aid with flexible programming would be recommended.

3. **What medical complications and symptoms of SCD should be considered in the determining appropriate recommendations?**

Appropriate medical management of individuals with SCD requires care by specialists and comprehensive primary care. Most individuals, however, do not receive comprehensive care due to limited financial resources and limited availability of comprehensive sickle cell centers.[8] Although blood transfusions and pain medications are used to treat patients with SCD, hydroxyurea is the standard of care for the management of SCD. Hydroxyurea is an oral chemotherapy causing serious complications in some patients.[9] Stem cell and bone marrow transplantation are two therapeutic options for children with SCD. This intervention, however, requires finding a disease-free, human lymphocyte antigen (HLA) matched donor sibling or relative, which can be challenging. Suitable stem cell donors also face the same risk factors associated with any type of transplantation.[10]

Common health-related problems related to SCD include infection, anemia, visual disorders, renal disease, and stroke. Adults with end-stage renal disease due to SCD are three times more likely to pass away.[11] Acute chest syndrome, a vasoocclusive event within the pulmonary vascular system, is the most common cause of death and hospitalization in patients with SCD. Stroke is another common and serious consequence of the disruption of blood flow caused by the sickling of red blood cells (RBC) or the formation of stiff rods within the RBC and altering it to a crescent or sickle shape. Strokes are managed with general support and transfusion. The goal in managing strokes is to lower the concentration of HbSS to less than 30% and an exchange blood transfusion may be required.[12]

The most common and painful complication related to SCD is a vasoocclusive crisis. Sickled blood cells create blockage of blood flow in a blood vessel and deprive tissue of oxygen, causing severe pain. Control of acute pain crises is often managed in emergency rooms by using opioids and transfusion therapy to increase hemoglobin levels.[9]

4. **What are the implications of SCD on auditory function?**

In light of the inconsistencies in audiologic results of individuals with SCD and speculative etiology presented in the literature, the correlation between SCD, hearing sensitivity, and auditory function requires additional testing. Audiologists need to be aware that SCD may lead to temporary or permanent SNHL and may have effects on other parts of the auditory system including the central nervous system.

3.8 Diagnosis and Recommended Treatment

JB was seen for an audiologic reevaluation (▶ Fig. 3.3). He reported experiencing severe pain in some joints. His body temperature was 101.2 °F. It was recommended that JB contact his SCD specialist immediately and reschedule his appointment. He preferred to complete the testing due to recently observed changes in hearing sensitivity. Pure-tone thresholds revealed a slight mid-frequency SNHL in the left ear and a significant decrease in pure-tone air and bone conduction thresholds at 2,000 to 8,000 Hz in the right ear as seen in ▶ Fig. 3.3. SRTs were commensurate with the PTA and revealed a mild to moderately severe loss in the ability to receive speech in the right ear and normal ability in the left ear. WRS was normal for the left ear at 80 dB HL and revealed slight difficulty in the right ear at 90 dB HL. Tympanometry revealed normal ear canal volume, middle ear pressure, and static compliance bilaterally. ARTs were consistent with previous sensation levels in each ear. DPOAEs were absent at high frequencies in the left ear and at the mid-frequencies in the right ear (▶ Fig. 3.4). ABR could not be completed due to patient discomfort. It was recommended that JB seek immediate medical attention regarding his pain crisis, consult with his physician regarding the changes in his hearing sensitivity, and return for an audiologic reevaluation and possible hearing aid consultation in 1 month.

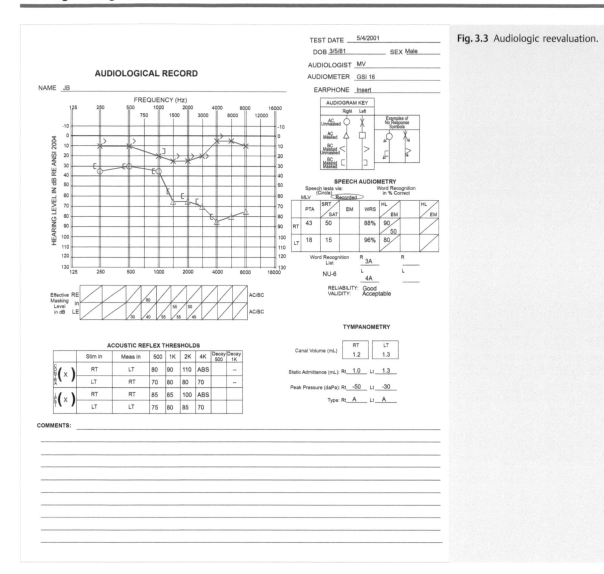

Fig. 3.3 Audiologic reevaluation.

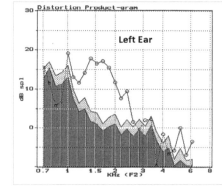

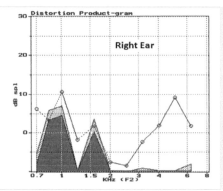

Fig. 3.4 Distortion Product Otoacoustic Emissions present at the mid-frequencies for the left ear and in only at the high frequencies for the right ear.

3.9 Outcome

JB received medical clearance following a negative MRI (magnetic resonance imaging) and received a hearing aid for the right ear. He received his hearing aid evaluation and orientation at the Vanderbilt Bill Wilkerson Center (VBWC) because the university audiology clinic where he received his audiologic evaluations could not dispense hearing aids. He was seen frequently at the VBWC for reprogramming the hearing aid due to the fluctuant nature of his hearing sensitivity, particularly in the right ear.

3.10 Key Points

- SCD is a group of disorders characterized by the sickling of RBCs. It is an autosomal recessive genetic disorder. This condition was first identified in an African-American dental student in 1912. This irregularity is associated with the exchange of valine, an amino acid, for glutamine in the β-globin chain of the hemoglobin molecule. Abnormal hemoglobin combinations cause RBCs to become firm and friable as they develop into a sickle shape. The distorted shape of the RBCs block blood vessels that often leads to tissue hypoxia and other medical complications.[9] There are six different classifications of SCD: HbSS, HbSC, HbS beta thalassemia, HbSD, HbSE, and HbSO.[13]

- The number of individuals with SCD is unknown; however, the Centers for Disease Control and Prevention (CDC) estimates that approximately 100,000 Americans have SCD. An incidence rate of approximately 1 out of 14 African American infants with the recessive trait for SCD is projected. The CDC also estimates that 1 out of 365 African-American births and 1 out of 16,300 Hispanic births present with SCD.[13] SCD and the recessive trait for SCD are most commonly identified now through routine newborn health screening tests.
- The presence of SCD can lead to temporary or permanent hearing impairment.

3.11 Acknowledgments

The case described is based on a compilation of audiological results obtained from two patients studied as a part of an NIH Grant P 60-HL38737 provided to Earnest A. Turner, MD, Principal Investigator, Comprehensive Sickle Cell Center, Meharry Medical College, 1989–1999.

References

[1] Todd GB, Serjeant GR, Larson MR. Sensori-neural hearing loss in Jamaicans with SS disease. Acta Otolaryngol. 1973; 76(4):268–272

[2] Burch-Sims GP, Matlock V. Auditory dysfunction in sickle cell disease. J Nat Soc Allied Health 2004;2(3):17–24

[3] Downs CR, Stuart A, Holbert D. Distortion product otoacoustic emissions in normal-hearing children with homozygous sickle cell disease. J Commun Disord. 2000; 33(2):111–127, quiz 128–129

[4] Mgbor N, Emodi I. Sensorineural hearing loss in Nigerian children with sickle cell disease. Int J Pediatr Otorhinolaryngol. 2004; 68(11):1413–1416

[5] Burch-Sims GP, Matlock VR. Hearing loss and auditory function in sickle cell disease. J Commun Disord. 2005; 38(4):321–329

[6] de Castro Silva IM, Magalhães IQ, Toscano RA, Gandolfi L, Pratesi R. Auditory-evoked response analysis in Brazilian patients with sickle cell disease. Int J Audiol. 2010; 49(4):272–276

[7] Kegele J, Hurth H, Lackner P, et al. Otoacoustic emission testing in Ghanaian children with sickle-cell disease. Trop Med Int Health. 2015; 20(9):1209–1212

[8] Grosse SD, Schechter MS, Kulkarni R, Lloyd-Puryear MA, Strickland B, Trevathan E. Models of comprehensive multidisciplinary care for individuals in the United States with genetic disorders. Pediatrics. 2009; 123(1):407–412

[9] Segal JB, Strouse JJ, Beach MC, et al. Hydroxyurea for the Treatment of Sickle Cell Disease. Evidence Reports/Technology Assessments, No. 165. Rockville, MD: Agency for Healthcare Research and Quality (US); 2008

[10] Thompson LM, Ceja ME, Yang SP. Stem cell transplantation for treatment of sickle cell disease: bone marrow versus cord blood transplants. Am J Health Syst Pharm. 2012; 69(15):1295–1302

[11] Agency for Healthcare Research and Quality. Statistical Brief #21. Healthcare Cost and Utilization Project (HCUP). Rockville, MD: Agency for Healthcare Research and Quality; 2006

[12] Distenfeld A. Sickle cell anemia. Available at: http://www.emedicine.com/MED/topic2126.htm. Published 2007. Accessed January 30, 2008

[13] Centers for Disease Control and Prevention. Sickle Cell Disease (SCD): Data and Statistics. Atlanta, GA: Centers for Disease Control and Prevention; 2016

Suggested Readings

[1] Ashley-Koch A, Yang Q, Olney RS. Sickle hemoglobin (HbS) allele and sickle cell disease: a HuGE review. Am J Epidemiol. 2000; 151(9):839–845

[2] Scott DM. Auditory and neurocognitive impact of sickle cell disease in early childhood. In: Chabon SS, Cohn ER, eds. The Communication Disorders Casebook: Learning by Example. Boston, MA: Pearson/Allyn & Bacon; 2011:46–51

4 Diagnostic and Treatment Outcomes for an Adolescent with Left Functional Hemispherectomy

Jennifer McCullagh and Kristin Dilaj

4.1 Clinical History and Description

Research related to the effectiveness and efficacy of Aural Rehabilitation (AR) in patients with neurological impairment is limited, and audiologists are left to draw on the existing literature and theoretical basis to develop intervention plans for these patients. The following case highlights the importance of treating the audiological and central auditory processing symptoms utilizing the limited literature as well as sound theoretical basis for a patient with a left functional hemispherectomy.

KP is an 18-year-old male seen for audiologic and central auditory processing evaluations due to concerns regarding difficulty hearing in background noise. KP was diagnosed with infantile spasms at 4 weeks of age, which were treated with adrenocorticotropic hormone. At 9 months of age, KP was diagnosed with epilepsy. As a result of intractable seizures, KP underwent brain resections of the left hemisphere at 2.5 and 3.5 years of age. Seizures continued and at 6 years of age, he had a left functional hemispherectomy. Following the surgery, KP developed a left gaze preference, right hemiparesis, and right homonymous hemianopsia (loss of half of the visual field on the same side in both eyes). Fortunately, KP has not experienced seizures since this surgery.

An audiologic evaluation conducted by an audiologist when KP was 8 years of age indicated normal peripheral hearing and Otoacoustic Emissions (OAE), bilaterally. No additional audiologic or central auditory processing testing was conducted until KP was almost 18 years old. At that point, KP was believed to have normal functional hearing; however, he was easily bothered by background noise and experienced difficulty localizing sound. In order to hear at a comfortable listening level, KP increased the volume when watching television and utilized a speakerphone when communicating on the phone. KP enjoyed singing and listening to music, but he did so at a volume setting others found to be too loud. KP denied experiencing ear pain or tinnitus and had no significant history of otitis media.

4.2 Clinical Testing

Otoscopy revealed normal-appearing external ear canals and tympanic membranes bilaterally. ▶ Fig. 4.1 reveals the results from KP's most recent audiometric evaluation. Pure-tone audiometry revealed hearing to be within normal limits bilaterally at 250 to 8,000 Hz. Speech Recognition Thresholds (SRT) were 5 and 0 dB HL in the left and right ears respectively, and were in good agreement with the pure tone averages bilaterally. Word Recognition Scores (WRS) revealed slight difficulty to recognize speech in the right ear and normal ability to recognize speech in the left ear. WRS were assessed using the PBK-50 word list at the initial evaluation in order to control for the potential impact of vocabulary. Tympanometry indicated normal ear canal volume, static admittance, and middle ear pressure bilaterally. Distortion product otoacoustic emissions (DPOAEs) were present at 1,500 to 3,500 Hz and at 1,500 to 4,000 Hz in the left and right ears, respectively. DPOAEs were weak in the right ear at 1,000 Hz and in the left ear at 1,000 and 4,000 Hz.

The Words-in-Noise (WIN) test[1,2] is used to assess the ability to hear in noise. The WIN test uses the NU-6 (Northwestern University Auditory Test No. 6) word lists embedded in speech babble. A signal-to-noise ratio (SNR in dB HL) threshold is measured and a value of ≤ 6 dB is considered normal. KP's WIN SNR thresholds indicated mild difficulty for the left ear (SNR threshold = 7.6 dB), severe difficulty for the right ear (SNR threshold = 16.4 dB), and moderate difficulty binaurally (SNR threshold = 10.8 dB). These results indicated that KP had significant difficulty hearing in background noise and asymmetrical performance (right and binaural poorer than left ear alone). This was expected since KP's contralateral pathway is dominant and auditory information presented to the right ear cannot be perceived accurately by the left hemisphere because the left hemisphere has been surgically resected. Binaural interference is also indicated since binaural performance is poorer than the left ear-only performance.

Auditory Brainstem Responses (ABRs), Middle Latency Responses (MLRs), and late auditory evoked potentials were recorded for each ear. ABR waves I, III, and V were present bilaterally. Absolute wave latencies and interwave intervals were within normal limits bilaterally. The interaural latency delay was within normal limits. These results indicated normal processing of click stimuli from the auditory nerve through the lower brainstem.

The negative (Na) and positive (Pa) waveforms of the MLR were present bilaterally. When testing the right ear, a postauricular muscle artifact was present. This is a common artifact and its presence may not allow for accurate interpretation of the Na waveform. Thus, the following information should be interpreted with caution. The Na–Pa amplitude was approximately 1 μV larger at each electrode site for the right ear compared to the left ear. Pa latencies were approximately 6 ms longer in the right ear compared to the left ear. Again, due to muscle artifact and the documented anatomical differences in KP's cortex, the MLR waveforms cannot be interpreted with confidence.

The late auditory evoked potentials (N1 and P2) were present when the left ear was stimulated and waveforms were characterized by normal latencies and reduced amplitudes across electrode sites. The right ear N1 and P2 waveforms were absent at the Cz, C4, and C3 electrode sites. These results suggested that auditory information presented to the left ear was processed by the auditory cortex, but fewer auditory cortical neurons were responding synchronously. Auditory cortical processing was impaired when auditory information was presented to the right ear. These findings are consistent with KP's history of a left hemispherectomy (i.e., auditory information presented to the right ear is typically processed by the left temporal lobe).

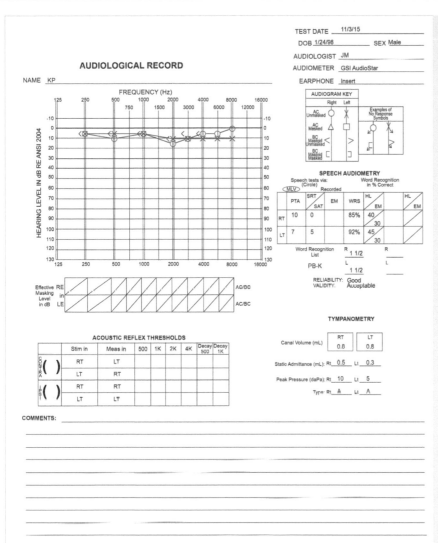

Fig. 4.1 KP's audiometric test results including pure tone air and bone conduction testing, speech testing, and tympanometry.

In addition to the electrophysiologic measures, auditory processing tests were administered (▶ Table 4.1). Dichotic listening was assessed using the **dichotic digits test** as well as the **dichotic rhyme test**. The dichotic digits test is designed to assess the central auditory process of binaural integration (divided attention) as well as interhemispheric transfer of acoustic information with a reduced linguistic load. In this test, four numbers between 1 and 10 (except 7) are presented simultaneously to the patient, two numbers in each ear. The patient is asked to repeat all four numbers in any order. Scores were 90 and 50% in the left and right ears, respectively. The normative values for KP's age are 90% for each ear. Thus, performance for the right ear was not within normal limits. Single digits were then presented (one digit to each ear, simultaneously) to determine if performance might improve when the linguistic and cognitive loads were reduced. Scores were 90 and 70% in the left and right ears, respectively, indicating improved performance for the right ear, but still below normal performance. The dichotic rhyme test is designed to assess binaural integration as well as interhemispheric transfer of acoustic information. This test is not impacted by attention. Two rhyming consonant–

Table 4.1 Initial central auditory processing evaluation results. Words-In-Noise (WIN) test is scored in signal-to-noise ratio (SNR in dB). Therefore, a lower SNR is considered better performance.

	Left ear	Right ear	Binaural
Dichotic digits: single	90%	70%	
Dichotic digits: double	90%	50%	
Dichotic rhyme	53.3%	23%	
Frequency patterns: labeled response			22%
Frequency patterns: hummed response			100%
WIN	7.6 dB	16.4 dB	10.8 dB

vowel–consonant (i.e., ten, pen) are presented to the listener at the same time (one word/ear) and the listener must repeat the word, or words. Scores were 53.3% in the left ear and 23% in the right ear. Norms for KP's age are 30 to 60% and 32 to 78% in the left and right ears, respectively. As a result of these two tests, dichotic listening performance (single- and double-digits and rhyme) indicated a weakness in the right ear, but normal performance in the left ear. These results were expected since the right ear pathway crosses contralaterally to the surgically resected left hemisphere and the left ear pathway crosses contralaterally to the intact right hemisphere.

The **frequency patterns test** is designed to assess aspects of auditory temporal processing including frequency discrimination, temporal ordering, interhemispheric transfer of nonverbal auditory information, auditory memory, and linguistic labeling. The patient is asked to report the pattern of three consecutive tones, which include two of one frequency and one of another (e.g., high, low, high). KP's binaural score was 22.2% and a normative value is 75%. When instructed to hum, rather than label the response, KP's binaural score improved to 100%. Although KP had difficulty labeling the patterns, he was able to hum the patterns with a high degree of accuracy. This finding was consistent with his history of left hemispherectomy as the left temporal lobe is responsible for linguistic labeling and the right temporal lobe is responsible for pattern perception and musical skills.

KP's ability to perceive sounds in words was assessed using Arthur Boothroyd's (AB) isophonemic monosyllabic word lists.[3] Prior to beginning this test, KP's articulation was assessed using one AB list in a live-voice, face-to-face condition with visual cues to determine a baseline for speech production. KP had difficulty producing /r/, /s/, /p/, /sh/, and /ch/ in the final position and consistently overexploded consonant sounds. Concerns regarding the overall loudness of his voice and excessive voicing of sounds existed as well. These "baseline" sound production errors were taken into consideration when scoring the results. Following this baseline measure, KP was tested in various listening conditions without access to visual cues. KP was asked to repeat what he heard. Testing was completed using monitored live-voice (MLV) presentation at soft (30 dB HL), normal (50 dB HL), and loud (65 dB HL) input levels as well as in quiet versus background noise (+ 10 SNR with speech-weighted and babble

background noise presented at 0-degree azimuth). Testing was repeated while using a hearing aid and frequency modulation (FM) system. KP was fitted binaurally with "in-house" Oticon Sensei Pro Behind-The-Ear (BTE) hearing aids using the Desired Sensation Level (DSL) i/oV5 (adult) target for a flat 25 dB hearing loss. In addition, a Phonak Roger Inspiro microphone was utilized to trial a direct microphone (DM) system with the hearing aids. A Phonak Roger X receiver was coupled to the hearing aids using an FM 9 audio shoe. See ▶ Table 4.2 and ▶ Table 4.3 for results. Unaided word recognition testing did not reveal significant difficulty in quiet or noise as KP performed similarly for each ear at all input levels and performed similarly in both types of background noise. Aided testing resulted in significant improvement for WRS only in the soft condition and the DM system resulted in improved listening in background noise. The use of the hearing aids and the FM system resulted in benefits that were observable to the testers. It should be noted that testing was completed with one and two hearing aids. The test results presented in ▶ Table 4.3 were the best aided condition scores. The best aided condition was when the hearing aid was fitted only to the right ear. The best DM condition was when the FM was only in the right ear. With access to amplification, KP's voice level was immediately reduced to an appropriate level suggesting better self-monitoring ability. Without hearing aids, KP frequently "over-articulated" and provided consonant sounds that were forced or had a large burst. Hearing aid use resulted in speech production that did not sound as forced or as harsh. This was confirmed by two professionals and his parents.

KP's ability to perceive words in sentences was assessed using Hearing-in-Noise Test for Children (HINT-C)[4] sentences presented via MLV through a loudspeaker in quiet and in noise. The HINT-C sentences were chosen as they are simple sentences containing between four to six words per sentence. KP was evaluated in various listening conditions without visual cues. KP was asked to repeat what he heard. KP completed this task at 30 and 50 dB HL in quiet at 0 degree azimuth and at 50 dB HL

Table 4.2 Results on the Arthur Boothroyd (AB) lists for the right and left ears at three presentation levels using insert earphones

	Right ear Soft (30 dB HL)	Left ear Soft (30 dB HL)	Right ear Normal (50 dB HL)	Left ear Normal (50 dB HL)	Right ear Loud (65 dB HL)	Left ear Loud (65 dB HL)
Total phonemes	93%	93%	97%	93%	97%	100%
Total consonants	90%	90%	95%	90%	95%	100%
Initial consonants	100%	100%	90%	80%	100%	100%
Final consonants	80%	80%	100%	100%	90%	100%
Vowels	100%	100%	100%	100%	100%	100%
Total words	80%	80%	90%	80%	90%	100%

Table 4.3 Results on the Arthur Boothroyd (AB) lists in binaural unaided and aided (hearing aid and FM) listening tasks presented in sound field in quiet (soft and normal) and using two noise sources (steady-state and multitalker babble)

	Unaided Quiet normal	Unaided Quiet soft	Aided Quiet soft	Unaided noise steady	Unaided noise talker	Aided noise FM right ear
Total phonemes	93%	83%	90%	80%	87%	100%
Total consonants	90%	75%	85%	75%	80%	100%
Initial consonants	90%	80%	80%	70%	90%	100%
Final Consonants	90%	70%	90%	80%	70%	100%
Vowels	100%	100%	100%	90%	100%	100%
Total words	80%	50%	80%	70%	60%	100%

Table 4.4 Words correct score using the Hearing-in-Noise Test for Children (HINT-C) in quiet (30 dB HL) and noise (50 dB HL in a + 10 dB S/N ratio)

	Unaided	Aided HA only	Aided HA + FM
Speech at 30 dB HL in quiet	76%	81%	DNT
Speech at 50 dB HL in a + 10 S/N ratio	74%	DNT	96%

Abbreviations: DNT, did not test; HA, hearing aid; FM, frequency modulation; HINT-C, Hearing-in-Noise Test for Children.

in multitalker background noise at a + 10 SNR with the noise and talker at 0 degrees azimuth. See ▶ Table 4.4 for unaided and aided results. Unaided sentence recognition revealed that KP had difficulty processing words in sentences. This was evidenced in both quiet and noise by his difficulty using correct grammar and language when repeating the sentences. These results are consistent with a diagnosis of Central Auditory Processing Disorder (CAPD). Use of a DM system resulted in noticeable differences in his ability to use correct grammar and appropriate language when repeating the sentences. KP also exhibited quicker and more confident responses. Language error patterns that were present in the unaided conditions were minimized when KP had access to the DM system. KP appropriately used "ing," correct verb tense, and pronouns with access to the DM system.

4.3 Questions to the Reader

1. **The audiologic evaluation conducted when KP was 8 years of age indicated normal bilateral peripheral hearing sensitivity. Was this expected? When would a central auditory processing evaluation referral have been appropriate?**
2. **Given what is known about the central auditory nervous system pathways, were the central auditory processing findings expected for KP?**
3. **In completing the functional auditory evaluation, would word recognition testing alone have been sufficient to reveal a deficit?**

4.4 Discussion of Questions

1. **The audiologic evaluation conducted when KP was 8 years of age indicated normal bilateral peripheral hearing sensitivity. Was this expected? When would a central auditory processing evaluation referral have been appropriate?**

Yes, normal peripheral hearing for pure tones is often expected for patients with neurological involvement. While it is important to first determine the peripheral hearing sensitivity in patients with neurological histories, it is also important to investigate beyond the audiogram for auditory weaknesses. If a patient or members of his or her family have auditory concerns and normal peripheral hearing sensitivity has been established, a referral for a central auditory processing evaluation is prudent in order to determine an appropriate rehabilitation plan.

2. **Given what is known about the central auditory nervous system pathways, were the central auditory processing findings expected for KP?**

These findings were expected given KP's history of a left functional hemispherectomy. Given that the contralateral pathway is dominant, a right ear deficit was expected on these tests. The left temporal lobe is typically responsible for processing acoustic information such as speech. Patients with weak auditory processing abilities experience difficulties understanding speech, especially in background noise.

3. **In completing the functional auditory evaluation, would word recognition testing alone have been sufficient to reveal a deficit?**

Individual ear word recognition in quiet would not have indicated that KP was experiencing listening difficulties. Listening tasks assessed in quiet and noise as well as the sentence listening tasks are where deficits were demonstrated. Evaluating several speech input levels as well as the differences in performance with the addition of background noise is critical in assessing functional difficulties for patients whose reported symptoms do not agree with the audiogram or suprathreshold WRS.

4.5 Description of Disorder and Recommended Treatment

It was recommended that KP utilize a mild gain hearing aid during all waking moments in addition to having access to a personal FM/DM system coupled to the hearing aid for school. A hearing aid with mild gain amplification was thought to provide KP with a more robust signal that resulted in increased ease and confidence when listening to sound as well as a reduction in his vocal volume. Since testing demonstrated equal or better performance with the right hearing aid alone versus two hearing aids and due to the right ear being the weaker ear as indicated by KP's central auditory processing testing, a trial with a right hearing aid was recommended. An Oticon Sensei Pro BTE hearing aid was ordered and programmed as described earlier during the in-office trial. Settings were verified by using real ear measures with an Otometrics Aurical FreeFit analyzer at 55, 65, and 80 dB SPL. An FM/DM recommendation was provided to his school system. An Oticon Amigo T30 microphone and an Oticon R12 receiver were ordered for KP. The FM system was fitted by the audiologist and transparency between the hearing aid and FM system was verified in the Aurical Hearing Instrument Test (HIT) box. KP's family and school team received in-services regarding the use of the hearing aid and FM system.

In addition to recommending amplification, compensatory strategies, direct skills remediation, and environmental modifications were recommended. **Direct skills remediation** emphasized the improvement of central auditory processing, specifically dichotic listening, skills. The **Dichotic Interaural Intensity Difference training (DIID)**[5,6] was offered to the family as part of participation in a research study since the evidence base for this program is still emerging. The training did not occur until approximately 10 months after the initial central auditory processing evaluation and approximately 5 months

Table 4.5 Pre- and post-DIID training results for KP

	Left ear		Right ear		Binaural	
	Pre-DIID	Post-DIID	Pre-DIID	Post-DIID	Pre-DIID	Post-DIID
DD-double	90%	95%	35%	37.5%		
DD-single	95%	95%	25%	25%		
DR	66.7%	66.7%	16.6%	16.7%		
CS	82%	92%	0%	0%		
FP-label					26.7%	20%
FP-hum					86.7%	86.7%
WIN	3.6 dB	5.2 dB	14 dB	8.4 dB	4.4 dB	9.2 dB

Abbreviations: DD-double, dichotic digits, double digits; DD-single, dichotic digits, single digits; DIID, Dichotic Interaural Intensity Difference training; DR, dichotic rhyme; CS, competing sentences; FP-label, frequency patterns, labeled response; FP-hum, frequency patterns, hummed response; WIN, words in noise.
Note: WIN is scored in S/N in dB.

Table 4.6 Results on the Arthur Boothroyd (AB) word lists at 7 months after the initial functional auditory evaluation and fitting of the hearing aid and frequency modulation (FM) system

	Quiet normal Unaided (50 dB HL)	Quiet normal Aided (50 dB HL)	Quiet soft Unaided (30 dB HL)	Quiet soft Aided (30 dB HL)	Noise Unaided	Noise Aided
Total phonemes	100%	100%	90%	97%	87%	100%
Initial consonants	100%	100%	80%	90%	70%	100%
Final consonants	100%	100%	90%	100%	100%	100%
Vowels	100%	100%	100%	100%	90%	100%
Total words	100%	100%	70%	90%	70%	100%

Table 4.7 Results on the Hearing-in-Noise Test for Children (HINT-C) sentences at 30 and 50 dB HL in quiet and at + 10 dB SNR at 7 months after the initial functional auditory evaluation and fitting of the hearing aid frequency modulation (FM) system

	Unaided Initial evaluation	Unaided Second evaluation	Aided Initial evaluation	Aided Second evaluation
Speech at 50 dB HL in quiet	74%	76%	81%	94%
Speech at 30 dB HL in quiet	76%	88%	92%	90%
Speech at 50 dB HL in + 10 dB S/N ratio	74%	82%	96%	86%

after KP was fitted with amplification and the FM technology to the right ear. KP participated in 30-min sessions, two to three times per week for 5 weeks of formal DIID training (12 sessions in total). The goal of the training was to improve dichotic listening abilities in the right ear (weaker ear) in order to enhance auditory processing and hearing in background noise.

4.6 Outcome

Diagnostically, KP had normal peripheral hearing sensitivity, but he had significant central auditory processing weaknesses. Outcomes for the DIID training presented in ▶ Table 4.5

indicated that KP did not demonstrate any change in his central auditory processing abilities. Many reasons exist for this result, but are likely related to KP's age (18 years) and the time elapsed since his hemispherectomy (approximately 12 years). Brain plasticity is greatest in younger children and when therapy begins closer to the onset of neurological injury.

KP's functional listening was re-assessed 7 months after he was fitted with amplification and the FM system and approximately 2 weeks after he completed DIID training. His mother reported KP was using the hearing aid consistently. There was a noticeable reduction in his voice level and he was faster to respond to soft sounds in his environment. KP regularly requested the hearing aid and preferred wearing it.

Unaided word recognition testing (▶ Table 4.6) did not reveal significant difficulty in quiet or noise and WRS were similar between the first and second evaluations. It should be noted, however, that KP demonstrated overall slightly better word recognition performance in both the unaided and aided conditions at the second evaluation. KP was subjectively faster to respond and more confident and clear in his production of speech sounds as rated by the two initial testers. It should be noted that the slight differences in scores observed between the first and second evaluations were not statistically significant and could be within test–retest or due to the use of shortened word lists. As a result, KP's requests to use the hearing aid, the improved performance at the soft conversational level, the subjective reports of reduced levels of the TV/phone and his own voice by his family, and the subjective observations of the testers supported continued use of the hearing aid.

Unaided sentence recognition (▶ Table 4.7) continued to indicate difficulty processing words in sentences. This was evidenced in quiet and noise by KP's difficulty using correct grammatical markers such as pronouns and word endings when repeating the sentences. The use of the hearing aid continued to result in benefits for use of correct grammar when repeating sentences, a decrease in overall voice level, and, as noted earlier, overall improvement in the clarity of speech quality. Voice and speech quality levels were subjectively assessed with and without the hearing aid by the speech language pathologist. Interestingly, for sentence perception there was a slight improvement in unaided scores between the first and second evaluations. KP's scores continued to show improvement between unaided and aided conditions on the sentence recognition tasks at the second session. Once again, the changes in scores were not statistically significant. While only slight improvements were noted objectively, results suggested that the hearing aid continued to benefit his ability to self-monitor his voice, utilize correct grammar and language in his sentences, and listen with more confidence (as evidenced by his quicker responses with the hearing aid on vs. off).

4.7 Key Points

- A neurological history impacting the central auditory nervous system should warrant a referral for a central auditory processing evaluation.
- Deficit-based intervention such as dichotic listening training to improve dichotic listening should be conducted on a trial basis to determine if changes can be made in central auditory processing. The potential for improvement is unknown in patients with neurological histories. This is especially true for patients for whom onset was several years ago. It is, however, important to try to capitalize on cortical plasticity to assess if improvements can be made. Colleagues in other rehabilitative professions such as physical therapy, speech-language pathology, and occupational therapy do it and audiologists should consider it as a treatment option as well.
- Auditory testing at multiple input levels, in quiet and noise, and using sentence as well as word recognition tasks provide functional information that can lead to recommendations that might not have been considered based on a conventional audiological evaluation.
- An aided in-office trial for patients with a functional deficit assists in determining if amplification is an appropriate recommendation and whether an in-home/in-school trial is warranted.
- Close monitoring of the effects of training is important to determine if changes are elicited. If not, the clinician should consider other options. If the treatment is providing positive changes, then continue. In this case, DIID did not elicit measurable change after 5 weeks, so it was decided to pursue other interventions. Amplification, however, resulted in continued benefit that was demonstrated in testing in the office as well as in KP's unwavering desire to use the hearing aid at home and the hearing aid and FM at school.
- It should not be assumed that individuals with neurological histories will lack benefit from auditory intervention. Oftentimes the presence of normal peripheral hearing does not correlate with functional listening and functional listening should be addressed through observations, functional listening evaluations, and rehabilitation trials.

References

[1] Wilson RH. Development of a speech-in-multitalker-babble paradigm to assess word-recognition performance. J Am Acad Audiol. 2003; 14(9):453–470

[2] Wilson RH, Burks CA. Use of 35 words for evaluation of hearing loss in signal-to-babble ratio: a clinic protocol. J Rehabil Res Dev. 2005; 42(6):839–852

[3] Boothroyd A. Developments in speech audiometry. British J Audiol. 1968; 2 (1):3–10

[4] Nilsson MJ, Soli SD, Gelnett DJ. Development of the Sharing in Noise Test for Children (HINT-C). Los Angeles, CA: House Ear Institute; 1996

[5] McCullagh J, Palmer S. The effects of auditory training on dichotic listening: A neurological case study. Hear Balance Commun. 2017; 15(1):30–37

[6] Musiek F, Weihing J, Lau C. Dichotic interaural intensity difference (DIID) training: a review of existing research and future directions. J Acad Rehabil Audiol. 2008; 41:51–65

5 Tympanic Membrane Perforation as a Result of a Japanese Beetle

Kristi Oeding and Jonathan McJunkin

5.1 Clinical History and Description

NH is a 73-year-old woman who was scheduled at the audiology clinic for a comprehensive audiologic examination. One month prior, a Japanese beetle flew into her left ear canal while she was mowing her lawn. She experienced extreme otalgia and could feel the beetle digging into her ear canal. She poured peroxide in her ear canal and the beetle exited. She noted hearing loss, bothersome tinnitus, and intermittent shooting otalgia in the left ear. She had tinnitus prior to the incident, but the tinnitus increased in intensity. She also reported having some imbalance after the incident. In the past, NH has had left ear infections with otorrhea, but no episodes were reported recently. She was evaluated by a local otolaryngologist, who noted a left tympanic membrane perforation and performed a paper patch myringoplasty, which was unsuccessful.

5.2 Audiologic Testing

The initial audiologic evaluation is reported in ▶ Fig. 5.1. Pure-tone thresholds in the right ear revealed a normal to slight Sensorineural Hearing Loss (SNHL). Results in the left ear revealed a mild sloping to moderately severe mixed hearing loss from 250 to 2,000 Hz, rising to a slight to mild mixed hearing loss from 3,000 to 8,000 Hz. Speech Recognition Threshold (SRTs) revealed a normal ability to receive speech in the right ear and a mild loss in the ability to receive speech in the left ear. Word Recognition Scores (WRS) revealed a normal ability to recognize speech in each ear. Tympanometry revealed normal ear

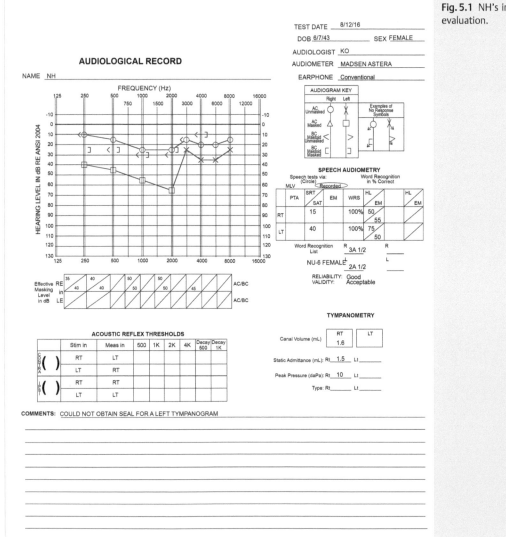

Fig. 5.1 NH's initial comprehensive audiometric evaluation.

canal volume, static compliance, and middle ear pressure in the right ear. An appropriate seal could not be maintained for immittance audiometry for the left ear, likely due to the perforation.

5.3 Questions for the Reader

1. **Can a Japanese beetle cause a tympanic membrane perforation?**
2. **What is the success rate for tympanoplasty?**

5.4 Discussion of Questions

1. **Can a Japanese beetle cause a tympanic membrane perforation?**

There has been one published case study[1] that reported a 37-year-old man who noted a foreign object had entered his right ear canal. Upon inspection, a Japanese beetle was in his ear canal and after removing the wings and part of the body, the beetle's legs or possibly its head was embedded in his

tympanic membrane and a large perforation was noted. While uncommon, it is possible for a Japanese beetle to damage the tympanic membrane.

2. **What is the success rate for tympanoplasty?**

There are several factors contributing to the success rate for a tympanoplasty. These include the size of the perforation, age of the patient, eustachian tube function, smoking status, etc.[2,3,4,5] In general, the range of success rate for tympanoplasty is 75 to 87%.[2,3,4,5] The average range of closure of the air–bone gap is 6 to 11 dB.[2,3,4]

5.5 Final Diagnosis and Recommended Treatment

After discussion of the risks and benefits of surgery, the patient elected to undergo a second tympanoplasty. The tympanic membrane was repaired with a temporalis fascia underlay graft. Postoperatively, a follow-up audiologic evaluation was scheduled. If the tympanoplasty was not successful, a left hearing aid,

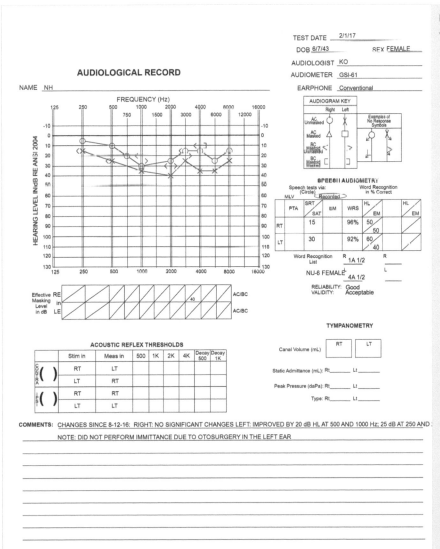

Fig. 5.2 NH's postoperative comprehensive audiometric evaluation.

bone-anchored hearing aid, or Hearing Assistive Technology (HAT) could be considered.

5.6 Outcome

At the first postoperative visit 3 weeks after surgery, the tympanic membrane was examined and noted to be healing well. NH reported her hearing was still muffled, but improved. She reported mild persistent imbalance.

Upon follow-up 3 months after surgery, the patient reported further improvement in hearing despite persistent tinnitus. The postoperative comprehensive audiologic evaluation is presented in ▶ Fig. 5.2. Pure-tone thresholds in the right ear revealed normal to slight SNHL, with a mild hearing loss at 1,000 Hz. Results in the left ear revealed normal hearing sloping to a slight to mild mixed hearing loss. Pure-tone thresholds in the right ear remained stable, but hearing improved by 20 dB HL at 500 and 1,000 Hz and by 25 dB HL at 250 and 2,000 Hz in the left ear since her last audiologic evaluation. SRTs revealed a normal ability to receive speech in the right ear and a mild loss in the ability to receive speech in the left ear. WRS a revealed normal ability to recognize speech in each ear. Tympanometry was not performed due to otosurgery in the left ear.

NH was counseled on the results of the audiologic evaluation. She was not interested in pursuing a hearing aid or HAT for the left ear and may return to attend a class offered by the audiology clinic on management options for tinnitus.

5.7 Key Points

- Japanese beetles can cause soft-tissue trauma in the ear canal including a tympanic membrane perforation.
- The success rate for tympanoplasty ranges from 75 to 87%.

References

[1] Kimbrig M. Tympanic membrane destroyed by Japanese beetle. JAMA. 1939; 113(7):589

[2] Saha AK, Munsi DM, Ghosh SN. Evaluation of improvement of hearing in type I tympanoplasty & its influencing factors. Indian J Otolaryngol Head Neck Surg. 2006; 58(3):253–257

[3] Deosthale N, Khadakkar S, Kumar P, et al. Effectiveness of type I tympanoplasty in wet and dry ear in safe chronic suppurative otitis media. Indian J Otolaryngol Head Neck Surg. 2017:1–6

[4] Demirpehlivan IA, Onal K, Arslanoglu S, Songu M, Ciger E, Can N. Comparison of different tympanic membrane reconstruction techniques in type I tympanoplasty. Eur Arch Otorhinolaryngol. 2011; 268(3):471–474

[5] Mohamad SH, Khan I, Hussain SS. Is cartilage tympanoplasty more effective than fascia tympanoplasty? A systematic review. Otol Neurotol. 2012; 33(5): 699–705

6 Middle Ear Effects from Playing a Brass Musical Instrument

Ross J. Roeser, Kris Chesky, Katharine Fitzharris, and Joe Walter Kutz Jr.

6.1 Clinical History and Description

LD is 58-year-old male professional trumpet player who presented with progressive, fluctuating hearing loss in his right ear for approximately 18 years. He denied tinnitus, dizziness, or autophony (when patients hear themselves talk at an uncomfortably high intensity and sometimes hear themselves breathe and chew). Other than his occupational experiences with music, he denied any additional history of excessive noise exposure. He reported aural fullness and hearing loss in his right ear that was temporarily relieved with auto-insufflation (Valsalva) and certain jaw movements. He denied a history of otologic surgery or infections.

6.2 Audiologic Testing

Initial diagnostic audiological evaluation that included immittance audiometry was performed at the initial visit and during a follow-up visit 3 years later (▶ Fig. 6.1 and ▶ Fig. 6.2). Left ear pure-tone thresholds were within normal limits through at 250- to 2,000-Hz sloping to a mild-to-moderate sensorineural hearing at 3,000 to 8,000 Hz. Right ear pure-tone thresholds revealed a moderate hearing loss rising to within normal limits at 3,000 Hz and then falling to a mild conductive hearing loss at 4,000 to 8,000 Hz. Significant air–bone gaps were revealed at 250 to 2,000 Hz in ▶ Fig. 6.1 and 3,000 Hz in ▶ Fig. 6.2. Speech Recognition Thresholds (SRTs) were in agreement with pure-tone average, indicating a mild loss in the ability to receive speech in the right ear in the initial examination (▶ Fig. 6.1) and

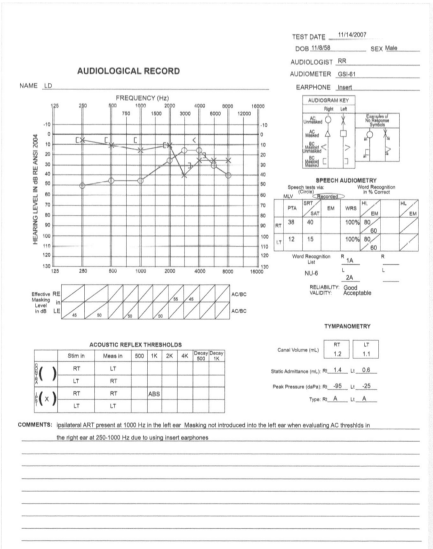

Fig. 6.1 Initial diagnostic audiological evaluation.

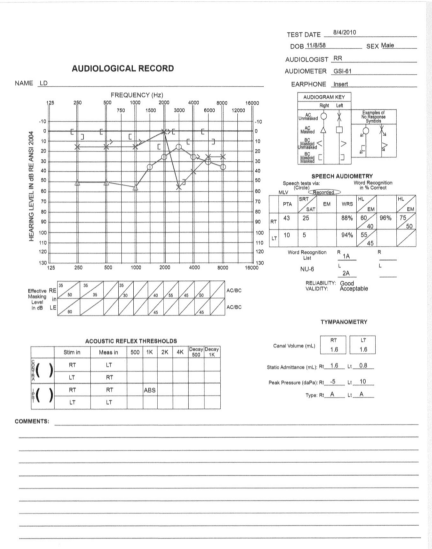

Fig. 6.2 Initial follow-up diagnostic audiological evaluation.

improving to a slight loss in the ability to receive speech in the second examination (▶ Fig. 6.2). Results for the left ear in both examinations indicated normal ability to receive speech. Masked Word Recognition Scores (WRS) in ▶ Fig. 6.1 revealed normal ability to recognize speech in each ear. In ▶ Fig. 6.2, the WRS decreased to slight difficulty in the ability to recognize speech, while results for the left ear still indicated normal ability to recognize speech. Tympanometry in ▶ Fig. 6.1 and ▶ Fig. 6.2 revealed normal ear canal volume, static admittance, and middle ear pressure; however, the static admittance for the right ear was double that of the left and excessively high at 1.4 and 1.6 mL in ▶ Fig. 6.1 and ▶ Fig. 6.2. In ▶ Fig. 6.1, an ipsilateral Acoustic Reflex Threshold (ART) at 1,000 Hz was present for the left ear, but absent for the right ear. Results from admittance audiometry support the finding of a possible conductive component in the right ear.

6.3 Additional Audiologic Testing

The patient was seen once again 10 years following his initial examination (▶ Fig. 6.3). Findings for the left ear were essentially unchanged, but the right ear low-frequency thresholds showed an additional 5- to 10-dB decrease. Video otoscopy was performed while the patient performed the Valsalva maneuver and results can be viewed in Video 28.1. Remarkably, the positive middle ear pressure generated during the Valsalva maneuver resulted in a significant distension of the tympanic membrane into the ear canal. Other tests of eustachian tube function (see below) were not performed. The patient reported that during the process of playing his trumpet, he routinely performed a Valsalva maneuver to improve his hearing sensitivity and his ability to hear himself play.

6.4 Questions for the Reader

1. **Are the findings for this patient what is expected for a professional musician?**
2. **What is the prevalence of conductive hearing loss resulting from playing brass musical instruments?**
3. **What symptoms would differentiate eustachian tube dysfunction (ETD) from a patulous eustachian tube dysfunction (pET)?**

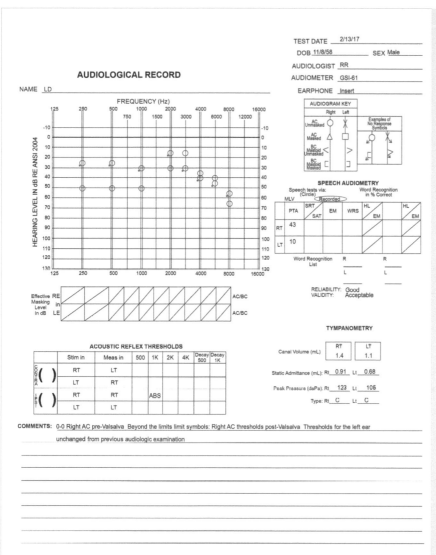

Fig. 6.3 Second follow-up diagnostic audiological re-evaluation.

4. **Did the patient have pET and/or what could be the cause of the pET in this patient?**
5. **What are tests of eustachian tube function that can be performed in a clinical audiology setting?**
6. **What other tests of eustachian tube function are available?**

6.5 Discussion of Questions

1. Are the findings for this patient what is expected for a professional musician?

Hearing loss from musical instruments typically results from excessive intensity, which results in noise-induced permanent threshold shift (NIPTS). In this case, there is possible evidence of exposure to high noise levels due to the left ear high-frequency sensorineural hearing loss (▶ Fig. 6.1, ▶ Fig. 6.2, ▶ Fig. 6.3). The left ear hearing loss, however, does not display the stereotypical 4,000- to 6,000-Hz notch found in most NIPTS. The finding of a conductive hearing loss in the right ear was not expected.

2. What is the prevalence of conductive hearing loss resulting from playing brass musical instruments?

To the knowledge of the authors, this is the first case study reporting conductive hearing loss from long-standing playing of a brass musical instrument, which likely resulted from insufficient eustachian tube function that permitted excessive pressure to be forced into the middle ear during the time the instrument was played. An attempt was made to find additional brass musical instrument players by posting a notice at a local university that has a nationally recognized music program. Several musicians responded to the notification, but were unwilling to follow through with audiometric testing because they were concerned that the knowledge or presence of a potential hearing loss might have influence on their musical careers or performance and did not elect to follow through with testing.

3. What symptoms would differentiate ETD from a patulous eustachian tube dysfunction (pET)?

Patients with pET report autophony (hearing themselves talk or sometimes breathe) and hyperacusis, while patients with ETD report sensations of pain, either intermittent or sustained, as well as of fluid in the ear. Aural fullness, "popping," distorted sounds, hearing loss, tinnitus, and/or imbalance are common complaints of both conditions. The ET is chronically closed or blocked in patients with ETD, leading to negative middle ear pressure, since there is no mechanism to equate pressures of the atmosphere and middle ear. The ET is open for longer periods of time than normal in patients with pET, leading to persistent communication between the middle ear space and the nasopharynx and the constant transfer of pressure changes between the atmosphere and middle ear.

4. Did the patient have pET and/or what could be the cause of the pET in this patient?

The most common causes of pET are weight loss, hormonal alterations, and changes in tissue (e.g., scarring). Surrounding the medial cartilaginous portion of the ET is fatty tissue, known as Ostmann's fat pads, the lateral of which exerts static pressure on the ET keeping it closed. The lateral pad also limits the opening of the ET by transferring pressure from the tensor muscles, acting like a fulcrum.[1] With weight loss and aging, there is a decrease in the amount of tissue in Ostmann's fat pads, which may lead to pET. In women who are pregnant or taking hormone-based birth control, changing levels of estrogen have been shown to affect the cartilaginous compliance and mucosal viscosity of the ET, leading to pET. Patients who have undergone nasopharyngeal surgery or radiation therapy can have scarring in the surrounding tissues of the ET, reducing the elasticity of the ET and inhibiting normal closure. Also, patients with recurrent chronic otitis media have been shown to have an increased prevalence of pET, thought to be due to alterations in ET tissue elasticity and changes in the mucosal surface tension from the chronic inflammation of the middle ear.[1] Less common causes of pET include neuromuscular disorders, which could lead to alteration in the timing of ET closure, as well as other neurological disorders such as multiple sclerosis, trauma, polio, and Parkinson's disease.[1]

LD denied weight change, was male (thus negating pregnancy and birth control), and had no history of surgery, radiation, or middle ear disease. The outstanding aspect of LD's history was his lifetime of trumpet playing.

Wind instruments can be qualified in terms of their resistance: high-resistance instruments (e.g., trumpet, French horn) require a great amount of air flow through a smaller surface area (bore size), whereas low-resistance instruments (e.g., tuba, trombone) require less air flow and utilize a larger surface area (bore size).[2] In audiological terms, impedance can be used interchangeably with resistance, so that, like in tympanometry, more force (e.g., sound pressure) is necessary in a high-resistance instrument and less force is needed in a low-resistance instrument in order to produce tones of similar frequency and intensity. This necessary force has been measured in terms of intraoral pressure in several studies of trumpet players. First reported by Bouhuys,[3] the threshold of intraoral pressure to produce a note was measured to be approximately 30 mm Hg and the maximal pressure was measured to be approximately 105 mm Hg. A study[4] found that some professional trumpet players could produce intraoral pressures as high as 187 mm Hg. Furthermore, there was a nonlinear relationship found

between pressure and resultant sound pressure levels. Over a specific range, doubling of pressure resulted in a 15-dBA increase in intensity; however, after a threshold that was variable by frequency, a doubling of pressure resulted in only a 3-dBA gain in intensity.[4] Furthermore, the authors found a linear relationship between increases in pressure and frequency. Other studies have reported a range of maximum intraoral pressures (60–110 mm Hg) across frequencies and intensities.[5,6,7] A final study examined the hypopharyngeal (area above the larynx, where the larynx and esophagus meet) pressure, which was found to have a mean pressure of 88 mm Hg across several trumpet players.[8] Overall, these studies have found pressures created by trumpet playing are significant enough to induce the Valsalva maneuver (40–50 mm Hg).[7] Forceful and repeated Valsalva maneuvers (as in trumpet playing) can result in the weakening of the tensor veli palatini muscle, leading to an abnormally open, or patulous, eustachian tube.[9]

5. What are tests of eustachian tube function that can be performed in a clinical audiology setting?

Otoscopy: Typically the first procedure completed in a visit, otoscopy can sometimes reveal a middle ear effusion or a tympanic membrane with retracted pockets in the presence of ETD, due to the negative pressure in the middle ear space. The TM typically appears normal in individuals with pET; however, TM movement can sometimes be observed in synchrony with respiration. Pneumatic otoscopy, where TM movement is directly observed in response to manually changing the relative pressure in the ear canal, can also indicate the presence of ETD: if the TM fails to move with pressure changes, this is considered indicative of middle ear effusion or ETD. Normal TM movement would be observed in the presence of pET. Finally, TM movement can be observed with the patient performing a sniff (forcefully and rapidly inhaling air through the nose), Valsalva maneuver (holding the nose with the mouth closed and "blowing"), or Toynbee maneuver (holding the nose and swallowing with the mouth closed). ETD is indicated if there is little to no observable movement with these patient-induced pressure changes.

Immittance measures can be the most informative when evaluating ET function. Significant negative pressure ($\geq$ –200 daPa) during tympanometry is indicative of ETD at the time of testing, but does not necessarily indicate chronic disorder. In many immittance analyzers, there is a specific ET function test protocol built into the software. Typically for an intact TM, these procedures involve completing a tympanogram while the patient is at rest and then having the patient perform a Valsalva and/or a Toynbee maneuver and repeating the tympanogram following each maneuver. Similar procedures can be completed if an ET function protocol is not available with the immittance analyzer. With normal ET function and with pET, the peak pressure of the tympanogram should change at least 15 to 20 daPa in the positive direction following a Valsalva and in the negative direction following a Toynbee maneuver.

Inflation–deflation test is also used to evaluate ET function. A positive (or negative) pressure, such as $\pm$ 200 daPa, is introduced into the patient's ear canal. The patient is instructed to swallow repeatedly, until the recorded pressure stops changing. Both the number of swallows and the resulting pressure are recorded.

If the TM is not intact, due to a perforation or tympanostomy tube, ET function can still be evaluated with immittance. Again, many current immittance analyzers have this protocol built into the software so that the clinician can follow onscreen prompts with the patient. Alternately, the clinician can introduce pressure into the canal, such as ± 200 daPa, and if ET function is normal, the ET should open and the recorded pressure should move back toward the 0-daPa baseline.

Contralateral reflex decay: With ipsilateral probe placement, either the contralateral ear is unoccluded or an external/nonauditory stimulus can be selected in the immittance software. The patient is instructed to breathe deeply through their mouth, nose, or ipsilateral nostril (occluding the nostril contralateral to the probe ear) and fluctuations in compliance are recorded in a ≥ 10-second recording window. Changes in compliance (> 0.07 mL) are observed to be synchronous with the patient's breathing to indicate pET on the probe side.

Traditional audiometry can indicate the presence of hearing loss, which is often present in ETD. In the differential diagnosis of pET, however, either nasally conducted audiometry or nasally presented masking has been introduced as potentially useful clinical measures.[10,11] For the latter procedure, conventional air-conducted thresholds are established. Then, thresholds are again obtained while a constant level of narrowband masking noise is presented to an ipsilateral nostril and the patient blocks the contralateral nostril. The noise is delivered using a specialized probe tip typically used in sonotubometry. Large threshold shifts, especially in the lower frequencies, have been observed in patients with pET in the masked condition due to the open communication between the nasopharynx and the middle ear. Although these measures are not currently part of traditional clinical measures, they offer additional options in the diagnosis of pET.

6. **What other tests of eustachian tube function are available?**

Endoscopic examination, sonotubometry, tubomanometry, electromyography, and imaging (MRI [magnetic resonance imaging] and CT [computed tomography]) can all be used to assess the ET, but are outside the audiological scope of practice. For more detail, please refer to Smith and Tysome.[12]

6.6 Diagnosis and Recommended Treatments

There is a paucity of studies in the medical literature addressing treatment for atrophic tympanic membranes in patients with pET. Occasionally, patients will develop a mobile portion of the tympanic membrane. The most common primary complaints in patients with pET is aural fullness and mild hearing loss. Treatment options include reassurance, reinforcing the tympanic membrane with cartilage,[13] laser myringoplasty,[14] placement of a shim to partially occlude the ET,[15] or closure of the ET and placement of a tympanostomy tube.[16]

In this case report, LD has severe atelectasis of the tympanic membrane resulting in significant conductive hearing loss that improved temporarily with auto-insufflation. A simple solution is to mass load the tympanic membrane with a substance such as blue tack or cigarette paper.[17,18] This intervention is low risk,

but temporary. If mass loading the tympanic membrane provides hearing improvement, a cartilage-graft tympanoplasty reinforcing the tympanic membrane would possibly provide a long-term solution. A tympanostomy tube alone would not improve hearing since the tympanic membrane would remain flaccid.

Of course, the possibility of improved hearing through traditional hearing instrument fitting or a bone-anchored device is an option. The challenge of a traditional fitting is the rising configuration of the hearing loss and the mild threshold sensitivity loss in the mid frequencies.

6.7 Outcome

An otological referral was recommended and, after the third appointment, obtained. The physical examination was consistent with the audiometric and immittance results and the treatment options were discussed with LD. At this point, LD is considering the treatment options. He is not enthusiastic about possible surgical options, but may consider hearing instruments, with a soft band bone-conduction aid for a trial.

6.8 Key Points

- This patient, a professional brass instrument musician, presented with an unusual case of conductive hearing loss resulting from a long-standing history of playing the trumpet.
- Conductive hearing loss from brass musical instrument playing has not been reported previously in the audiological literature, and further investigation is needed to document the possible prevalence.
- Audiological tests of ET function are available to audiologists and should be employed when indicated. Unfortunately, for a number of circumstantial reasons, they were not performed on this patient.

References

[1] Dornhoffer JL, Leuwer R, Schwager K, Wenzel S, Pahnke J. A Practical Guide to the Eustachian Tube. Berlin: Springer; 2014

[2] Schuman JS, Massicotte EC, Connolly S, Hertzmark E, Mukherji B, Kunen MZ. Increased intraocular pressure and visual field defects in high resistance wind instrument players. Ophthalmology. 2000; 107(1):127–133

[3] Bouhuys A. Sound-power production in wind instruments. J Acoust Soc Am. 1965; 37(3):453–456

[4] Fletcher NH, Tarnopolsky A. Blowing pressure, power, and spectrum in trumpet playing. J Acoust Soc Am. 1999; 105(2, Pt 1):874–881

[5] Bianco T, Fréour V, Cossette I, Bevilacqua F, Caussé R. Measures of facial muscle activation, intra-oral pressure, and mouthpiece force in trumpet playing. J New Music Res. 2012; 41(1):49–65

[6] Fréour V, Caussé R, Cossette I. Simultaneous measurements of pressure, flow and sound during trumpet playing. Proceedings of the 10ème Congrès Français d'Acoustique, April 12, 2010; Lyon, France

[7] Faulkner M, Sharpey-Schafer EP. Circulatory effects of trumpet playing. BMJ. 1959; 1(5123):685–686

[8] Stansey CR, Beaver ME, Rodriguez M. Hypopharyngeal pressure in brass musicians. Med Probl Perform Art. 2003; 18(4):153–155

[9] Levine HL. Functional disorders of the upper airway associated with playing wind instruments. Cleve Clin Q. 1986; 53(1):11–13

[10] Hori Y, Kawase T, Hasegawa J, et al. Audiometry with nasally presented masking noise: novel diagnostic method for patulous eustachian tube. Otol Neurotol. 2006; 27(5):596–599

[11] Paradis J, Bance M. Assessment of nasal-noise masking audiometry as a diagnostic test for patulous Eustachian tube. Otol Neurotol. 2015; 36(2): e36–e41

[12] Smith ME, Tysome JR. Tests of Eustachian tube function: a review. Clin Otolaryngol. 2015; 40(4):300–311

[13] Brace MD, Horwich P, Kirkpatrick D, Bance M. Tympanic membrane manipulation to treat symptoms of patulous eustachian tube. Otol Neurotol. 2014; 35 (7):1201–1206

[14] Kurokawa H, Goode RL. Treatment of tympanic membrane retraction with the holmium laser. Otolaryngol Head Neck Surg. 1995; 112(4):512–519

[15] Rotenberg B, Davidson B. Endoscopic transnasal shim technique for treatment of patulous Eustachian tube. Laryngoscope. 2014; 124(11):2466–2469

[16] Orlandi RR, Shelton C. Endoscopic closure of the eustachian tube. Am J Rhinol. 2004; 18(6):363–365

[17] Boedts M. Paper patching of the tympanic membrane as a symptomatic treatment for patulous eustachian tube syndrome. J Laryngol Otol. 2014; 128(3): 228–235

[18] Bartlett C, Pennings R, Ho A, Kirkpatrick D, van Wijhe R, Bance M. Simple mass loading of the tympanic membrane to alleviate symptoms of patulous eustachian tube. J Otolaryngol Head Neck Surg. 2010; 39(3):259–268

7 Maximum Conductive Hearing Loss Secondary to Surgical Closure of the External Auditory Canal

Alicia Restrepo

7.1 Clinical History and Description

DS is a 48-year-old female who scheduled an appointment with otolaryngology in February 2017. DS's medical history is significant for recurrent cholesteatoma in the left ear, fibromyalgia, meningoencephalocele, and a transient ischemic attack (TIA) that occurred 3 years ago. DS has undergone two surgeries in her home country of Colombia due to recurrent cholesteatoma. Surgical records were not available; however, DS reported the left external auditory canal was surgically closed during the second procedure.

DS scheduled an appointment with otolaryngology due to reported significant subjective hearing handicap, bothersome tinnitus in the left ear, and pain in the left mastoid region. She also reported aural fullness on the left side and intermittent headaches. The pain in the left mastoid area and headaches began 3 months before DS scheduled an appointment with otolaryngology. The otolaryngologist referred DS to a neurotologist at a major university hospital due to her complex medical history and then referred to audiology for a comprehensive audiologic evaluation.

7.2 Audiologic Testing

The results of the comprehensive audiologic evaluation revealed normal hearing in the right ear and a severe rising to moderately severe conductive hearing loss in the left ear with significant air-bone gaps present at 250 to 4,000 Hz (▶ Fig. 7.1). There was an interaural asymmetry of 45 to 65 dB Healing Level (HL) for air conduction thresholds, with the left ear being poorer than the right ear. Bone conduction thresholds were symmetric and within normal limits bilaterally with the exception of a slight loss at 500 Hz in the right ear. Speech Recognition Threshold (SRT) revealed normal ability to receive speech in the right ear and a moderately severe loss in the ability to receive speech in the left ear. Word Recognition Scores (WRS) were performed using a full Northwestern University Auditory Test No. 6 (NU-6) word list and administered via monitored live voice (MLV) using a female talker. Results revealed normal ability to recognize speech bilaterally. Tympanometry indicated normal middle ear pressure, ear canal volume, and static compliance in the right ear. Distortion Product Otoacoustic Emissions (DPOAEs) were present and robust at 1,600 to 8,000 Hz in the right ear, which is consistent with the audiometric thresholds. Tympanometry and DPOAEs could not be performed in the left ear due to a surgically closed external auditory canal.

7.3 Questions for the Reader

1. **Explain why a WRS of 100% would be expected with a hearing loss of this severity in the left ear.**
2. **Explain the difference between a conductive and mixed hearing loss.**
3. **What is crossover? How does masking help prevent crossover?**

7.4 Discussion of the Questions

1. **Explain why a WRS of 100% would be expected with a hearing loss of this severity in the left ear.**

A WRS revealing normal ability to recognize speech is expected when the bone conduction thresholds are within normal limits, regardless of the severity of air conduction thresholds.[1] A patient with a mixed or sensorineural hearing loss will demonstrate a decrease in WRS depending on the severity of the sensorineural component of the hearing loss due to distortion at the level of the cochlea, auditory nerve, or higher structures.[1,2]

2. **Explain the difference between a conductive and mixed hearing loss.**

A conductive hearing loss occurs when bone conduction thresholds are within normal limits (i.e., 0–15 dB HL), air conduction thresholds are either within normal limits or outside of normal limits, and there is an air–bone gap of 15 dB HL or greater between the bone conduction and the air conduction thresholds of the same ear. A mixed hearing loss occurs when the bone conduction thresholds are outside the normal range and there is an air–bone gap of 15 dB HL or greater between the bone conduction and air conduction thresholds of the same ear.[3]

3. **What is crossover? How does masking help prevent crossover?**

Crossover occurs when a stimulus presented to the test ear (TE) simultaneously stimulates the cochlea of the non-test ear (NTE). This can occur when the stimulus to the TE is sufficiently loud to leak out of the transducer (headphones or inserts) and travel around the head to the cochlea of the NTE or if the stimulus travels through the skull and stimulates the contralateral cochlea. The stimulus is able to leak out of headphones and stimulate the contralateral cochlea at a lower intensity level than if the audiologist were to use insert earphones. When using traditional headsets, masking is required for air conduction testing (i.e., audiometric threshold, SRT, or WRS) when there is a 40 dB HL difference between the presentation level and the bone conduction threshold of the contralateral ear (i.e., *contralateral comparison between air and bone conduction thresholds*). When using an insert earphone, because of its increased interaural attenuation, masking is required for air conduction testing (i.e., audiometric threshold, SRT or WRS) when there is a 60 dB HL difference between the presentation level and the bone conduction threshold of the contralateral ear. Masking is required with bone conduction testing when a

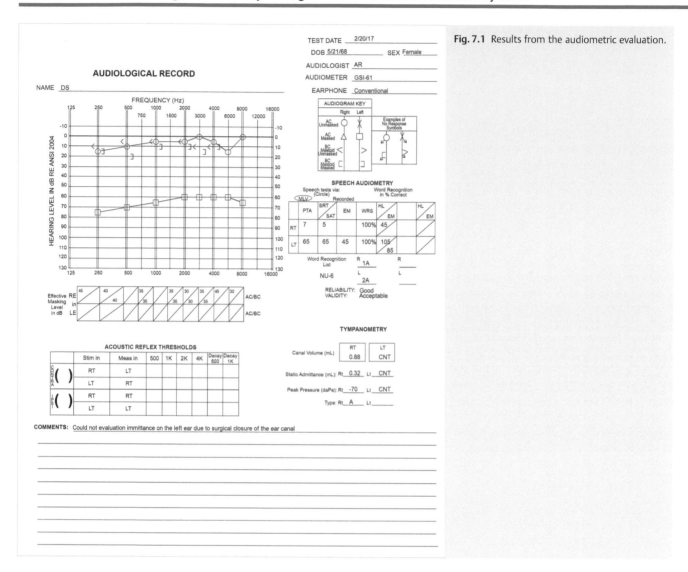

Fig. 7.1 Results from the audiometric evaluation.

15 dB or greater difference is noted between the air conduction threshold and bone conduction threshold of the TE (i.e., *ipsilateral comparison between air and bone conduction thresholds*).[4]

7.5 Diagnosis and Recommended Treatment

DS was diagnosed with recurrent cholesteatoma while living in Colombia. Cholesteatoma often occurs when a patient has chronic eustachian tube dysfunction, chronic middle ear infection, or a perforation of the tympanic membrane. The negative pressure in the middle ear space caused by chronic eustachian tube dysfunction or middle ear infection may cause the tympanic membrane to be stretched or sucked inward. This area allows for squamous epithelium to collect within this pouch. A cholesteatoma has the potential to be harmful if not discovered and treated early. It can erode surrounding tissue and bony structures including the ossicles and the cochlea. If the growth reaches the cochlea, permanent hearing loss or balance disorders may occur. In addition, cholesteatoma may be infected with bacteria. In severe cases, the cholesteatoma may exit the middle ear space and reach the brain, which can lead to severe complications such as meningitis or an abscess of the brain, which may result in death.[5]

Cholesteatomas are most often acquired; however, congenital cholesteatomas occur as well. The most common symptoms that occur with cholesteatoma are discharge from the impacted ear and hearing loss. Occasionally, patients with cholesteatoma report otalgia, tinnitus, balance issues, headaches, bleeding from the ear, and facial nerve weakness. These symptoms are most often associated with advanced cholesteatoma.[5] Once a patient is diagnosed with cholesteatoma, he or she will most likely undergo surgery to remove the growth. The most common surgical treatment for cholesteatoma is a canal-wall-down mastoidectomy, where the posterior canal wall and mastoid are removed.[6] It is conventional for the surgeon to order magnetic resonance imaging (MRI) or perform a "second look" surgery 6 to 18 months following the first surgery to ensure that the entire cholesteatoma was removed and to assess for regrowth.[7] The surgeon may also reconstruct any structures that were damaged by the cholesteatoma such as the tympanic membrane or the ossicles during the second surgery if the patient shows no signs of cholesteatoma regrowth.[6]

A patient who demonstrates chronic middle ear disease such as recurrent cholesteatoma or chronic otitis media may be a candidate for a blind sac closure, also known as middle ear obliteration. This procedure is not considered until other surgical and medical strategies have been exhausted. During a blind sac closure, the surgeon removes the tympanic membrane, malleus, and incus, and seals the eustachian tube. The middle ear space is filled with abdominal fat. The purpose of the middle ear obliteration is to eliminate the possibility of infection in the middle ear space or temporal bone by keeping the middle ear space dry and removing any structures prone to chronic infection. This procedure results in a maximum conductive hearing loss; however, the cochlea is preserved.[8]

7.6 Outcome

DS was referred to a neurotologist at a major university hospital due to her complicated medical history and reported pain in the left mastoid. DS will receive audiologic services at the same university hospital. This patient would be an excellent candidate for a Bone-Anchored Hearing Aid (BAHA) because her bone conduction thresholds are within normal limits. In this case, a BAHA would provide stimulation to both cochleas and allow DS better sound awareness from the left side, localization, and speech understanding in background noise.[9] A right CROS (Contralateral Routing of Signal) hearing aid is also available as a nonsurgical option for DS.

7.7 Key Points

- Proper masking is essential for determining accurate air conduction and bone conduction thresholds, SRT, and WRS. Accurate test results are necessary for deciding the best course of treatment for the patient. Masking must be utilized when obtaining SRT if a difference of 40 dB is noted between the presentation level of the TE and the best bone conduction threshold at 500, 1,000, or 2,000 Hz of the NTE. Masking must be utilized when measuring WRS if there is a difference of 40 dB between the presentation level to the TE and the best bone conduction threshold at 500, 1,000, or 2,000 Hz of the NTE. Masking should always be utilized when evaluating

WRS to prevent crossover because the presentation level to evaluate WRS is generally 40 dB or greater than the presentation level of the SRT.[4]
- Cholesteatoma has the potential to be a devastating, even fatal disease if it is not detected and treated in a timely manner.[5]

References

[1] Hood J, Poole J. Speech audiometry in conductive and sensorineural hearing loss. Br J Audiol. 1971; 5(2):30–38

[2] Roeser R, Valente M, Hosford-Dunn H. Diagnostic procedures in audiology. In: Roeser R, Valente M, Hosford-Dunn H, eds. Audiology Diagnosis. 2nd ed. New York, NY: Thieme Medical Publishers; 2007:1–16

[3] Roeser R, Clark J. Pure-tone tests. In: Roeser R, Valente M, Hosford-Dunn H, eds. Audiology Diagnosis. 2nd ed. New York, NY: Thieme Medical Publishers; 2007:238–260

[4] Roeser R, Clark J. Clinical masking. In: Roeser R, Valente M, Hosford-Dunn H, eds. Audiology Diagnosis. 2nd ed. New York, NY: Thieme Medical Publishers; 2007:261–287

[5] Kuo CL, Shiao AS, Yung M, et al. Updates and knowledge gaps in cholesteatoma research. BioMed Res Int. 2015; 2015:854024

[6] Gantz BJ, Wilkinson EP, Hansen MR. Canal wall reconstruction tympanomastoidectomy with mastoid obliteration. Laryngoscope. 2005; 115(10):1734–1740

[7] Williams MT, Ayache D, Alberti C, et al. Detection of postoperative residual cholesteatoma with delayed contrast-enhanced MR imaging: initial findings. Eur Radiol. 2003; 13(1):169–174

[8] Muzaffar SJ, Dawes S, Nassimizadeh AK, Coulson CJ, Irving RM. Blind sac closure: a safe and effective management option for the chronically discharging ear. Clin Otolaryngol. 2017; 42(2):473–477

[9] Hol MK, Snik AF, Mylanus EA, Cremers CW. Does the bone-anchored hearing aid have a complementary effect on audiological and subjective outcomes in patients with unilateral conductive hearing loss? Audiol Neurootol. 2005; 10(3):159–168

Suggested Readings

[1] Gaillardin L, Lescanne E, Morinière S, Cottier JP, Robier A. Residual cholesteatoma: prevalence and location. Follow-up strategy in adults. Eur Ann Otorhinolaryngol Head Neck Dis. 2012; 129(3):136–140

[2] Sanna M, Dispenza F, Flanagan S, De Stefano A, Falcioni M. Management of chronic otitis by middle ear obliteration with blind sac closure of the external auditory canal. Otol Neurotol. 2008; 29(1):19–22

[3] Snik AF, Mylanus EA, Cremers CW. The bone-anchored hearing aid in patients with a unilateral air-bone gap. Otol Neurotol. 2002; 23(1):61–66

8 When Mild Hearing Loss Accompanies Mild Cognitive Impairment

Marilyn Reed, Kate Dupuis, and M. Kathleen Pichora-Fuller

8.1 Clinical History and Description

BC is a 73-year-old male referred by his geriatrician to the audiology clinic following assessment 1 month earlier in the geriatric assessment clinic. The geriatrician had diagnosed BC with mild cognitive impairment (MCI) and was aware of recent evidence linking hearing loss with cognitive decline.[1,2,3,4] As a part of the recommendations, the geriatrician stated, "Hearing impairment is a known risk factor for development of cognitive decline. Although the patient's audiology assessment 6 months ago was normal, it would not be unwise to repeat this assessment at this time." This case study is particularly relevant to current practice in audiology given the rapidly aging population. Age is the greatest risk factor for dementia and, as longevity increases, it is increasingly likely that audiologists will need to understand how to effectively manage hearing loss in patients with cognitive impairment because they will be called upon to provide rehabilitation for older patients with cognitive decline.

In the audiologic case history, BC denied having any significant difficulty with hearing or daily communication. His wife, however, also present, reported BC's hearing seemed to have been gradually decreasing over the past few years and she was required to repeat frequently during conversations. She also noticed he was no longer participating as much as he had in social conversations at Friday night family dinners and other social situations with multiple talkers. Both BC and his wife reported he was a very high functioning individual who still worked as a court interpreter in five languages, acted as cantor for a small congregation, and functioned independently in all activities of daily living. Nevertheless, his wife had noticed over the past few months that he had increasing difficulty with word-finding and remembering names. His mother had been diagnosed with Alzheimer's disease in her 80s, suggesting a possible family history of dementia. This family history added to the concern of BC and his wife because of his diagnosis of MCI and their knowledge that patients with MCI are at increased risk of progressing to dementia.

The remainder of the audiologic case history was unremarkable, with no significant noise exposure, family history of hearing loss, ear pain, ear pathology, ear surgery, or tinnitus. BC reported undergoing neurologic evaluation for vertigo that had been attributed to low blood pressure, but he denied having seen an otolaryngologist. He had cataracts and wore bifocals. He did not report any other medical conditions or taking any current medications. His hearing had been assessed 6 months previously in the office of a large commercial hearing aid chain where it was described as being borderline normal.

8.2 Clinical Testing

▶ Fig. 8.1 reports the results of BC's audiologic examination, performed by an audiologist. Pure-tone air and bone conduc-

tion testing revealed bilateral, slightly asymmetric high-frequency Sensorineural Hearing Loss (SNHL) above 1,000 Hz, sloping to moderate on the right ear and moderately severe on the left ear at 8,000 Hz. Speech Recognition Thresholds (SRT) indicated a mild loss in the ability to receive speech in each ear. Word Recognition Scores (WRs) revealed normal ability to recognize speech in each ear. Loudness Discomfort Levels (LDL) were 110 dB HL or greater, bilaterally. Tympanometry revealed middle ear pressure, static compliance, and ear canal volume to be within normal limits bilaterally. Ipsilateral Acoustic Reflex Thresholds (ART) were present at normal stimulus levels bilaterally. Contralateral ART were also present at normal hearing levels when stimulating the left ear, but absent when stimulating the right ear. However, a referral to otolaryngology to investigate the possibility of retrocochlear pathology was not made since a neurologist had recently investigated BC.

To further investigate BC's reports of greater difficulty understanding speech in noisy environments, speech-in-noise testing was performed to assess his signal-to-noise hearing loss (SNRHL), which refers to the increase in SNR required by a listener to obtain 50% correct recognition of words, sentences, or words in sentences, compared to normal performance. The BKB-SIN Test, using the Bamford–Kowal–Bench sentences,[5] was chosen because the sentences are at approximately a first-grade reading level and easier than most other sentence tests. The high school language level and length of the Institute of Electrical and Electronics Engineers (IEEE) sentences used in the QuickSIN can be too difficult for use with certain populations, including older adults with auditory memory deficits.[5] While still being a valid representation of speech in the real world, the BKB-SIN is relatively simple and less taxing for memory.[5] Testing binaurally under headphones, BC obtained a score of 2.5 dB SNRHL, indicating performance within normal limits.

8.3 Questions to the Reader

1. **Is BC's hearing loss sufficient to require amplification or would it be better to advise BC to return for annual monitoring?**
2. **How should patients, families, and caregivers be counseled regarding seeking help for mild hearing loss?**
3. **What is BC's cognitive status? Is it important to know cognitive status and how it can be measured?**
4. **How should knowledge of cognitive status be taken into account when considering recommendations for rehabilitation?**

8.4 Discussion of the Questions

1. **Is BC's hearing loss sufficient to require amplification or would it be better to advise BC to return for annual monitoring?**

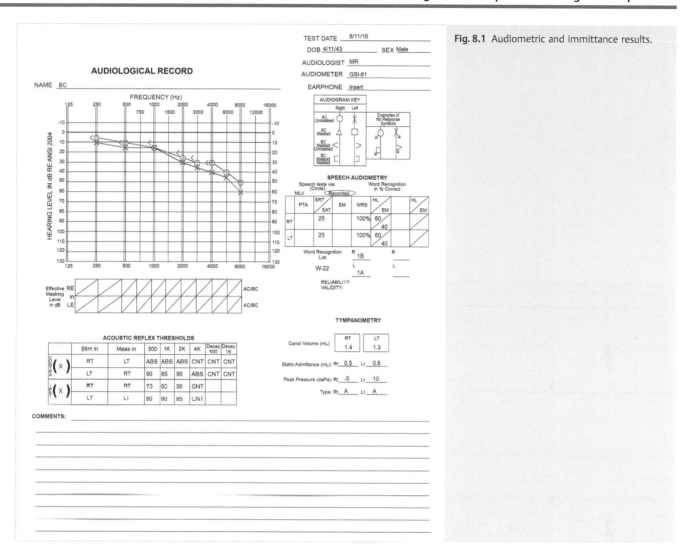

Fig. 8.1 Audiometric and immittance results.

In the past, with a patient such as BC who denied having significant communication difficulty, audiologists might have simply advised BC to return for annual monitoring. Many patients, however, with mild high-frequency SNHL may be fitted successfully with hearing aids if they are motivated and if they believe that their hearing loss has negatively affected their quality of life.[6,7] In addition, in the light of current evidence of a link between hearing loss and dementia, and the possibility that hearing loss may be a risk factor for cognitive decline, the advice of audiologists might now be different. Earlier intervention using a health promotion approach to encourage help-seeking for hearing loss may be particularly advantageous for those with hearing and cognitive loss.[8] There is growing evidence to suggest that communication difficulties due to age-related hearing loss in persons with cognitive impairment can increase stress and fatigue for the patient and their communication partner/caregiver, as well as exacerbate behavioral symptoms related to the cognitive decline.[9] In the context of this evidence, audiologists are advised to take a more proactive approach to the management of mild hearing loss, especially in patients at risk for dementia. Given that BC had been diagnosed with MCI, a major risk factor for dementia, had a family history of Alzheimer's disease, and that his geriatrician had referred

him based on concerns about hearing loss as a possible additional risk factor, the audiologist decided to move forward with discussing amplification.

2. How should patients, families, and caregivers be counseled regarding seeking help for mild hearing loss?

In taking the audiologic case history, it became apparent that BC was denying having any significant difficulty hearing. His wife, on the other hand, reported that BC was participating less socially and repetition was becoming a burden for her, causing her communication with BC to become stressful. Therefore, the audiologist felt that it was important to motivate BC to accept that his mild hearing loss was affecting his communication function and it was important to address this in order for him to maintain his current level of social and occupational activity.

Motivational counseling involved discussing with him that his wife, as his main communication partner, was experiencing the burden of his hearing loss. She would be an important beneficiary of improvements in how he managed his hearing loss. Since they had a close and supportive relationship, BC was able to see that getting help for his hearing loss was a logical course of action that would be helpful for his wife as well as himself. This inclusion of his wife's needs in the audiologist's counseling exemplifies a family-centered approach to adult audiologic care.[10]

BC and his wife were also counseled about the relationship between hearing and cognition in order to explain how his hearing loss could compound his cognitive loss, especially his memory loss, and make it more difficult for him to function effectively in his daily activities. Since his activities as an interpreter and a cantor in challenging environments demanded excellent communication ability, even mild hearing loss could affect his ability to function effectively and increase listening effort,[11] at the expense of his ability to process and remember information. Discussion of the links between hearing loss and other age-related declines in mental and physical health now plays an important role in counseling older adults about the benefits of audiologic rehabilitation (AR) for even mild hearing loss. By framing hearing health care in the context of healthy aging, audiologists can explain to patients how improved hearing might also improve their health, productivity, and quality of life as they age.[12] This is particularly true for BC, who was still involved in demanding occupational and social activities. Both BC and his wife were very eager and motivated to participate in any intervention to optimize his brain health and enable him to maintain his current lifestyle. They were very interested in the connection between hearing loss and memory loss and were willing to try amplification and participate in a research study on this topic that was being conducted in the audiology department in collaboration with psychologists.

3. What is BC's cognitive status? Is it important to know cognitive status and how it can be measured?

In light of the nature of the referral, with the patient's consent, the audiologist reviewed his medical record to learn more about his diagnosis and cognitive status. The report from the geriatrician stated that BC scored 25/30 on the Montreal Cognitive Assessment (MoCA),[13] a screening test for cognitive function. BC lost points in the visual–spatial/executive portion of the cognitive screening test and on the delayed recall item. BC was referred by his geriatrician to a neuropsychologist for more intensive testing and was seen by the neuropsychologist approximately 2 weeks after his initial audiologic assessment. According to the neuropsychologist's report, BC had relative difficulty on tests of memory and language, in the context of an otherwise normal cognitive profile. Specifically, he had difficulty recalling a list of words[14] and recognizing details from a story,[15] with the neuropsychologist noting, "the gist of a story was misremembered." In addition, BC was administered memory tests in the visual modality[16,17] (copying and then later recalling a variety of printed figures) and he showed weak performance on these visual recall tasks. BC had difficulty in language production, for example, on a semantic fluency test,[18] where he was asked to list as many animal names and as many boys' names as he could in 1 minute, and on a test of confrontation naming,[19] where he was asked to provide the names of pictures of common objects printed in a booklet such as a bed, or a tree, as quickly as he could. BC wore reading glasses during the neuropsychological assessment and did not use any form of auditory amplification, as he had not yet received his hearing instruments. Although testing was purportedly carried out in a quiet room, it is possible that background noise could have influenced BC's results on testing.[20] Given the results of testing,

BC's neuropsychologist arrived at a diagnosis of amnestic MCI affecting multiple domains (memory and language). With the pattern of test findings for BC and his family history, the neuropsychologist indicated that neurodegeneration due to Alzheimer's disease was a likely differential diagnosis. The clinical diagnosis of MCI was consistent with current consensus guidelines[21]: (1) BC reported decline in memory function over the past year, and his wife corroborated this report; (2) there was objective evidence of cognitive impairment in one or more cognitive domains; (3) the effect of cognitive impairments on daily functioning did not preclude independence; and (4) BC did not meet criteria for dementia.

MCI is a major risk factor for dementia, with a conversion rate of approximately 10 to 15% of individuals per year. Eighty percent of individuals with MCI will convert to dementia within 6 years of diagnosis.[22] It is important to note, however, that not all individuals with MCI develop dementia. Cognitive and behavioral interventions have been shown to be effective at improving cognitive and functional abilities, as well as mood, in individuals with MCI.[23] This was an important aspect of BC's counseling by the audiologist, as both he and his wife were worried about his risk of developing dementia. It was made very clear that it is impossible to predict his trajectory and currently there is no published evidence to suggest that the provision of amplification for patients with concurrent hearing loss and MCI can serve to slow down cognitive decline. Knowing, however, that hearing loss is a risk factor for dementia and there would be benefits from improved communication, it was suggested that BC pursue a trial with amplification.

The neuropsychological test results provide important information for the audiologist that can inform decisions around managing BC's hearing loss. In addition to the challenges that BC encounters in conversation with his wife because of his combined hearing and cognitive losses, BC's memory loss may also make it difficult for him to follow or understand instructions such as those provided in standard hearing aid manufacturers' user manuals. Furthermore, since his memory loss is likely to be progressive, it may affect his ability to cope with complicated hearing aid features, options, and accessories in the future. In addition, because his wife may need to assist and remind him concerning hearing aid management, care, and maintenance, it is particularly important for her to be included in the rehabilitation process. AR would also be useful in enabling BC and his wife to participate more fully in a group intervention program offered in the psychology department to assist patients with MCI and their family members to manage the effects of cognitive loss.

In an earlier study at this geriatric audiology clinic, where the average age of patients is 85 years, it was found that even audiologists with extensive experience working with older clients tended to underestimate the degree of cognitive loss in their patients.[24] As part of a research project, administration of the MoCA to patients in the audiology clinic revealed that a surprising 80% of these patients did not obtain a passing score.[25] While it may be relatively easy to identify patients with more severe levels of cognitive loss, it is much more difficult to recognize MCI, especially at an initial encounter.

Although it will not always be readily available, audiologists are advised to seek information on cognitive status in the patient's health record when possible. Audiologists could also consider performing cognitive screening in older patients, using tests such as the MoCA,[13] or at the very least integrating questions about memory changes into the case history. Audiologists should certainly be on the alert for any comments raised by patients or significant others that suggest concerns about memory or cognitive difficulties. In particular, it is important to gain insight into how age-related changes in hearing loss and cognition may combine to affect communication.[26]

4. How should knowledge of cognitive status be taken into account when considering recommendations for rehabilitation?

In consideration of the information presented thus far, the audiologist recommended a trial period with hearing aids. Amplification was, however, part of a comprehensive approach to BC's hearing rehabilitation that included a series of four AR group classes for new hearing aid users, which he attended with his wife. The hearing aid evaluation included additional questions about BC's vision and manual dexterity, along with discussion about his memory and cognition insofar as these factors would influence his use of amplification. The Client Oriented Scale of Improvement (COSI)[27] questionnaire was used to identify situations in which his hearing loss caused hearing and communication difficulties. On the COSI, BC identified four situations and prioritized them in the following order:

1. Hearing in court, in his job as a court interpreter in five languages. He reported having difficulty hearing the judges and lawyers at a distance, often in an environment with poor acoustics.
2. In the synagogue, as a cantor, and at social events such as receptions with multiple talkers.
3. At family dinners, where he had difficulty participating in conversation with multiple speakers and relied upon his wife to tell him what was being said.
4. Watching TV, where he needed to increase the volume and ask his wife what was being said.

Hearing aid styles, technology levels, features, and accessories were all discussed with BC and his wife. Lifestyle needs and cosmetic concerns were discussed. Based on the discussion, bilateral premium rechargeable Receiver-In-the-Canal (RIC) aids were prescribed. RIC aids were chosen in order to allow a more open fit that would be suitable for BC's mild high-frequency loss. The coupling method initially recommended was open domes, since his hearing was normal at frequencies up to 1,000 Hz. Rechargeable aids were recommended since they do not require the wearer to remember when or how to change batteries. Although the couple was counseled about wireless Bluetooth accessories, none was recommended initially as the couple did not feel that these accessories were necessary and they preferred to keep BC's technology as simple as possible. Specifically, options such as the use of a remote microphone and Smartphone Apps were not pursued. Other wireless TV devices were discussed, but BC chose to wait and see if the hearing aids addressed his problems hearing the TV before obtaining any additional assistive devices. Other solutions such as closed captioning were also discussed. Counseling for the couple included education around the use of behavioral communication strategies and the selection and modification of communication environments was discussed in the context of

BC's communication challenges in social groups and in his work in court. Use of a telecoil with induction loop would also have been recommended had the courtroom and synagogues that he worked in been equipped with these technologies. These topics were also addressed in more detail in the group AR classes.

Knowledge of BC's cognitive status was useful in informing the audiologist's decisions about tailoring the management of his hearing loss to his needs. For patients with known cognitive impairment, recommendations usually strive to

- Keep technology simple to minimize cognitive demand and stress while optimizing audibility.
- Involve significant others and/or caregivers in all appointments to optimize social support.
- Formulate realistic expectations for the success of interventions while anticipating a relatively rapid progressive decline in cognitive functioning and increase in caregiver burden.
- Provide in-depth and highly structured instruction and counseling to client and family.
- Provide supporting written or video documentation of instructions that can be taken home for later reference or to share with other key communication partners.
- Increase the number of follow-up appointments as needed for counseling about adjustment to hearing loss and to consolidate and reinforce learning about use of devices. In future, it may become easier to provide additional appointments for counseling and hearing aid tuning using tele-audiology.

The neuropsychologist's recommendations also included referral to "Learning the Ropes for Living with MCI," a Baycrest cognitive intervention program for individuals with MCI that uses a health promotion approach to staying physically, mentally, and socially active, with an emphasis on the transfer of newly learned skills to everyday situations. The program has demonstrated benefit in terms of increases in individuals' well-being and their knowledge and use of memory strategies.[28]

8.5 Outcome

At BC's first hearing aid check, which took place 2 weeks after the fitting, BC reported finding the hearing aids very helpful. COSI responses indicated he was hearing "better" or "much better" in three out of the four target situations he had identified (he had not watched much TV during the trial period) and he rated his ability to hear in those situations as "almost always."

Later that same week, he arrived at the clinic reporting his hearing aids were falling out, even though he was apparently inserting the ear tips (generic domes) correctly. In an attempt to improve retention and ease of management, impressions were taken to order custom earmolds.

Two weeks later when the custom earmolds were fitted, he was found to be having great difficulty inserting them and did not appear to be able to follow instructions about handling them. In addition, his rechargeable batteries were found to be dead, indicating that he had not understood instructions regarding charging them. To help prevent this problem from recurring, the right side of the charger was marked with a red dot to cue correct placement of the aids in the charger.

Seeing his difficulty managing the hearing aids, his wife was very distressed and indicated she was concerned about his cognitive function. The audiologist tried to reassure BC's wife, but the audiologist was concerned that she would be functioning outside of her scope of practice. At that point, the audiologist asked for consent to have the psychologist come into the session and speak to the couple about the important possible connections between hearing loss and cognitive function. Given BC's wife's distress, the audiologist also referred them to a specialized program, managed by social workers, to specifically address caregiver burden and offer support to family caregivers. Providing support for BC's wife was deemed to be important given a growing body of literature emphasizing the risk of caregiver burden in individuals caring for someone with either cognitive loss[29,30] or hearing loss[31,32] and the likelihood that the burden experienced by a family member would be even higher when caring for someone with both MCI and mild hearing loss.

Three weeks later, BC returned the hearing aids due to difficulties managing them and his associated frustration. Given the fact that the COSI had indicated that amplification had been very helpful in meeting his functional communication goals, he was strongly encouraged to persevere in his use of amplification. Both BC and his wife, however, were feeling somewhat overwhelmed and needed to "take a break," stating they hoped his apparent cognitive decline was a result of the side effects of new medication.

One month later, BC called to request a new prescription for different custom hearing aids that he thought might be easier to insert and retain in his ears. The audiologist explained the rationale for recommending RIC aids and he agreed to proceed with this style, but with a different style of custom earmolds that could provide better retention. Three months later, he reported finding the new hearing aids provided significant benefit and he was using them successfully with the encouragement and assistance of his wife.

This case illustrates how MCI can cause difficulties comprehending and remembering information, not only during everyday communication, but also at audiology appointments, including the information needed to learn how to successfully use hearing aids. BC's cognitive loss likely increased his frustration in adjusting to amplification and frequent return visits were needed to assist him and his wife through this critical period of adjustment. Although there may be no obvious cognitive impairment at the initial visit to audiology, challenges with cognitive function often become more apparent as the patient struggles with managing hearing aids and other devices.[33] In fact, because audiologists see patients over extended periods of time, they may be the first to suspect cognitive loss and they may need to be prepared to discuss and make appropriate referrals. For those who have been diagnosed with MCI or dementia, audiologists will need to anticipate how the client and family will need to continue to adapt as declines in cognition progress over time.

This case study illustrates how BC and his wife were able to benefit from interprofessional teamwork between the audiologist and psychologist in the provision of care, and from the services provided by social workers. It emphasizes the importance of having multiple disciplines gain access to one another's expertise. Such a model could become more widespread in geriatric audiology, to the benefit of patients and their family members. While it is becoming more common for audiologists to work in interprofessional teams in residential settings for older adults,[34] this case illustrates the value of an interprofessional approach for older adults who are still living in the community.

Hearing aids are an important component of hearing loss management for patients with cognitive impairment. In order for hearing aid use to be successful for this population, however, it should always be part of a comprehensive management plan that includes supportive partners and addresses the unique needs of this population.

While future research is needed to provide strong evidence as to whether or not hearing rehabilitation can contribute to the prevention or slowing of cognitive decline, it is reasonable to expect that appropriate audiologic interventions can help maintain participation in social activities and relationships and preserve quality of life, thereby contributing to health in general, including cognitive health. There is a pressing need for audiologists to better understand how cognitive impairment interacts with hearing impairment so that audiologists can develop best practices and tailor interventions to best meet the needs of our patients with cognitive impairment and their caregivers.

8.6 Key Points

- With the aging of the population, an increasing number of patients with hearing loss will also present with MCI or dementia. It is important for audiologists to gather information about cognitive health by being alert to disclosures about it made by the patient or significant others, including questions about it during history taking, reviewing information in the patient record and referral documents, and/or administering cognitive screening tests.
- Interdisciplinary teamwork can enrich the audiologist's understanding of other health issues such as cognitive decline that may affect hearing care, particularly in a geriatric practice. Likewise, it is important for audiologists to provide information about hearing and assist other disciplines to accommodate the hearing needs of patients in a wide range of care situations. Interprofessional collaboration can also improve patient care, especially when the needs of the patient go beyond the current knowledge, comfort zone, and/or scopes of practice for the collaborating professionals.
- Family-centered care is especially important when audiologists work with patients with cognitive decline. Including a significant other at every stage of the rehabilitation process is essential for success with management, not only so that the significant other can support the patient, but also because their inclusion may help alleviate the caregiver burden that they themselves experience.

References

[1] Lin FR. Hearing loss and cognition among older adults in the United States. J Gerontol A Biol Sci Med Sci. 2011; 66(10):1131–1136

[2] Lin FR, Ferrucci L, Metter EJ, An Y, Zonderman AB, Resnick SM. Hearing loss and cognition in the Baltimore Longitudinal Study of Aging. Neuropsychology. 2011; 25(6):763–770

[3] Lin FR, Metter EJ, O'Brien RJ, Resnick SM, Zonderman AB, Ferrucci L. Hearing loss and incident dementia. Arch Neurol. 2011; 68(2):214–220

[4] Lin FR, Yaffe K, Xia J, et al. Health ABC Study Group. Hearing loss and cognitive decline in older adults. JAMA Intern Med. 2013; 173(4):293–299

[5] Bench J, Kowal A, Bamford J. The BKB (Bamford-Kowal-Bench) sentence lists for partially-hearing children. Br J Audiol. 1979; 13(3):108–112

[6] Knudsen LV, Öberg M, Nielsen C, Naylor G, Kramer SE. Factors influencing help seeking, hearing aid uptake, hearing aid use and satisfaction with hearing aids: a review of the literature. Trends Amplif. 2010; 14(3):127–154

[7] Timmer B. It may be mild, slight, or minimal, but it's not insignificant. Hearing Review. 2014; 21(4):30–33

[8] Pichora-Fuller MK. Cognitive decline and hearing health care for older adults. Am J Audiol. 2015; 24(2):108–111

[9] Mamo SK, Oh ES, Price C, Reed NS, Occhipinti D, Lin FR. Hearing loss treatment in older adults with mild cognitive impairment or dementia: a systematic review. Alzheimers Dement. 2016; 12(7):P:597–P598

[10] Singh G, Hickson L, English K, et al. Family-centered adult audiologic care: a Phonak position statement. Hearing Review. 2016; 23(4):16–20

[11] Phillips NA. The implications of cognitive aging for listening and the Framework for Understanding Effortful Listening (FUEL). Ear Hear. 2016; 37 Suppl 1:44S–51S

[12] Pichora-Fuller MK, Dupuis K, Reed M, Lemke U. Helping older people with cognitive decline communicate: Hearing aids as part of a broader rehabilitation approach. Semin Hear. 2013; 34(4):308–330

[13] Nasreddine ZS, Phillips NA, Bédirian V, et al. The Montreal Cognitive Assessment, MoCA: a brief screening tool for mild cognitive impairment. J Am Geriatr Soc. 2005; 53(4):695–699

[14] Belkonen S. Hopkins verbal learning test. In: Kreutzer J, DeLuca J, Caplan B, eds. Encyclopedia of Clinical Neuropsychology. New York, NY: Springer; 2011:1264–1265

[15] Wechsler D. Wechsler Memory Scale. 4th ed. San Antonio, TX: Pearson; 2009

[16] Osterrieth PA. Le test de copie d'une figure complexe. Arch Psychol. 1944; 30: 206–356

[17] Benedict RH, Schretlen D, Groninger L, Dobraski M, Sphritz B. Revision of the brief visuospatial memory test: studies of normal performance, reliability, and validity. Psychol Assess. 1996; 8(2):145–153

[18] Delis DC, Kaplan E, Kramer JH. Delis-Kaplan Executive Function System (D-KEFS). San Antonio, TX: Psychological Corporation; 2001

[19] Kaplan E, Goodglass H, Weintraub S. Boston Naming Test. Austin, TX: Pro-Ed; 2001

[20] Dupuis K, Marchuk V, Pichora-Fuller MK. Noise affects performance on the Montreal Cognitive Assessment. Can J Aging. 2016; 35(3):298–307

[21] Albert MS, DeKosky ST, Dickson D, et al. The diagnosis of mild cognitive impairment due to Alzheimer's disease: recommendations from the National Institute on Aging-Alzheimer's Association workgroups on diagnostic guidelines for Alzheimer's disease. Alzheimers Dement. 2011; 7(3):270–279

[22] Petersen RC, Doody R, Kurz A, et al. Current concepts in mild cognitive impairment. Arch Neurol. 2001; 58(12):1985–1992

[23] Li H, Li J, Li N, Li B, Wang P, Zhou T. Cognitive intervention for persons with mild cognitive impairment: A meta-analysis. Ageing Res Rev. 2011; 10(2): 285–296

[24] Keymanesh A, Dupuis K, Reed M, Finkelstein H, Ostroff D, Pichora-Fuller MK. Could cognitive screening improve audiologic rehabilitation for older adults? Paper presented at 32nd World Congress of Audiology; Brisbane, Australia; May 2014

[25] Dupuis K, Reed M, Finkelstein H, Keymanesh A, Ostroff D. Perspectives on conducting interdisciplinary research in a geriatric audiology clinic. Canadian Audiol. 2016; 3(4)

[26] Pichora-Fuller MK. Auditory and cognitive processing in audiologic rehabilitation. In: Spitzer J, Montano J, eds. Adult Audiologic Rehabilitation: Advanced Practices. 2nd ed. San Diego, CA: Plural Publishing; 2013:519–536

[27] Dillon H, James A, Ginis J. Client Oriented Scale of Improvement (COSI) and its relationship to several other measures of benefit and satisfaction provided by hearing aids. J Am Acad Audiol. 1997; 8(1):27–43

[28] Troyer AK, Murphy KJ, Anderson ND, Moscovitch M, Craik FI. Changing everyday memory behaviour in amnestic mild cognitive impairment: a randomised controlled trial. Neuropsychol Rehabil. 2008; 18(1):65–88

[29] Etters L, Goodall D, Harrison BE. Caregiver burden among dementia patient caregivers: a review of the literature. J Am Acad Nurse Pract. 2008; 20(8): 423–428

[30] Dunkin JJ, Anderson-Hanley C. Dementia caregiver burden: a review of the literature and guidelines for assessment and intervention. Neurology. 1998; 51(1) Suppl 1:S53–S60, discussion S65–S67

[31] Scarinci N, Worrall L, Hickson L. The ICF and third-party disability: its application to spouses of older people with hearing impairment. Disabil Rehabil. 2009; 31(25):2088–2100

[32] Scarinci N, Worrall L, Hickson L. Factors associated with third-party disability in spouses of older people with hearing impairment. Ear Hear. 2012; 33(6): 698–708

[33] Pichora-Fuller MK, Singh G. Effects of age on auditory and cognitive processing: implications for hearing aid fitting and audiologic rehabilitation. Trends Amplif. 2006; 10(1):29–59

[34] Pichora-Fuller MK, Schow R. Audiologic rehabilitation across the adult life span: assessment and management. In: Schow RL, Nerbonne MA, eds. Introduction to Audiologic Rehabilitation. 7th ed. Columbus, OH: Pearson; 2017. 307–392.

Suggested Reading

[1] Weinstein B. Geriatric Audiology. 2nd ed. New York, NY: Thieme; 2012

9 Audiologic Management of a Patient with Psychogenic Hearing Loss

Valeria Roberts Matlock and Diane M. Scott

9.1 Clinical History and Description

WC is 31-year-old female who works part-time in a large retail store. WC's immediate supervisor expressed concern about her difficulty communicating with customers in person and over the phone during a recent performance evaluation. WC's coworkers also complained for approximately 2 months about her inability to accurately follow instructions. Fearing that her job was in jeopardy, WC was referred by her general practitioner for an audiological evaluation.

9.2 Audiologic Testing

During a case history interview, WC reported that she often asks individuals to repeat portions of their conversations. Medical history was reportedly positive for middle ear pathology as a child and negative for tinnitus, sensation of movement, head trauma, and recent illness. WC reported that she was taking prescription medication for anxiety and high blood pressure.

An audiologic evaluation (▶ Fig. 9.1) revealed a mild to moderate Sensorineural Hearing Loss (SNHL) in the right ear and a slight to mild SNHL in the left ear. Speech Recognition Thresholds (SRT) were commensurate with the pure-tone average (PTA) and revealed a mild loss in the ability to receive speech bilaterally. Word Recognition Scores (WRS) indicated slight difficulty in the ability to recognize speech when stimuli were presented at 80 dB HL.

Immittance audiometry revealed negative middle ear pressure and normal static admittance in the right ear and normal middle ear pressure and static admittance in the left ear. Ipsilateral and contralateral Acoustic Reflex Thresholds (ART) were consistent with cochlear loss. ART were obtained at reduced sensation levels when stimulating each ear bilaterally. No acoustic reflex decay was observed at 1,000 Hz bilaterally.

It was recommended that WC be seen by an otologist to rule out possible retrocochlear pathology and to obtain medical clearance for binaural hearing aids. WC was counseled on the various appropriate styles of hearing aids. Behind-The-Ear (BTE) style hearing aids were selected. Impressions for earmolds were made.

9.3 Questions for the Reader

1. **Given WC's medical history and initial audiological findings, what impressions can be drawn with respect to potential causes(s) of her hearing loss?**
2. **At this point, would further diagnostic testing be recommended, and if so, what additional tests would be recommended?**
3. **What indications from the initial audiological evaluation would warrant Auditory Brainstem Response (ABR) and Otoacoustic Emissions (OAE) testing?**

9.4 Discussion of the Questions

1. **Given WC's medical history and initial audiological findings, what impressions can be drawn with respect to potential causes(s) of her hearing loss?**

Retrocochlear pathology should be ruled out due to a slight asymmetry of pure-tone findings. Cochlear pathology, however, must also be considered based on the reduced sensation levels of the ART.

2. **At this point, would further diagnostic testing be recommended, and if so, what additional tests would be recommended?**

Further diagnostic testing and referral to an otologist would be recommended given the test results. In order to determine the site of lesion, ABR and OAE testing could provide useful information in the differential diagnosis of site of lesion.

3. **What indications from the initial audiological evaluation would warrant Auditory Brainstem Response (ABR) and Otoacoustic Emissions (OAE) testing?**

The recent onset of hearing loss with no direct cause, the asymmetry in pure-tone thresholds, and the reduced ART are important indicators for ABR and OAE testing.

9.4.1 Hearing Aid Evaluation and Additional Testing

WC received medical clearance for binaural hearing aid use 2 months later following a negative physical examination by her otologist and an imaging study. Prior to fitting WC with binaural BTE hearing aids, pure-tone thresholds were reassessed to establish prescriptive targets for Real Ear Measures (REM). Pure-tone audiometry (▶ Fig. 9.2) revealed a mild to moderate SNHL bilaterally, indicating a significant decrease in hearing sensitivity in the left ear when compared to results obtained in ▶ Fig. 9.1. SRT were commensurate with the PTA and revealed a mild to moderate loss in the ability to receive speech bilaterally. SRT revealed a 10 dB HL or greater shift. WRS indicated slight difficulty in the ability to recognize speech when stimuli were presented at 80 dB HL in the left ear and moderate difficulty for speech when presented at 80 dB HL in the right ear, which was a significant decrease for the right ear. Immittance audiometry revealed normal middle ear pressure and static admittance bilaterally. Ipsilateral and contralateral ART were consistent with cochlear loss having been obtained at reduced sensation levels when stimulating each ear. Acoustic reflex decay testing was negative bilaterally.

WC was informed that changes in her hearing levels were observed during the reassessment of previous test results. WC was also informed that additional testing was needed to determine the possible cause of the observed shift in hearing

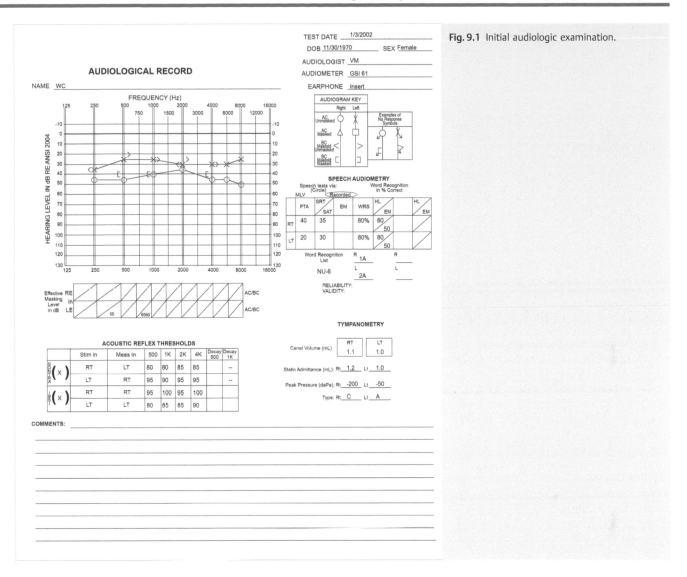

Fig. 9.1 Initial audiologic examination.

sensitivity of the right and left ears prior to initiating the hearing aid evaluation. WC agreed to undergo additional testing. An ABR was performed the same day, using a click stimulus (80 dB HL). Absolute and interwave latencies were obtained and consistent with normative values for each ear. Interaural latency comparison of Wave V was normal. The latency-intensity functions were normal for each ear. wave V was repeatable to 25 dB HL in the left ear and to 15 dB HL in the right ear. Waveform morphology was judged to be good for each ear (► Fig. 9.3). Distortion Product Otoacoustic Emissions (DPOAEs) were present from 1,000 through 6,000 Hz with present and repeatable normal amplitudes at each test frequency with the exception of 1,500 Hz in the left and 2,500 Hz bilaterally (► Fig. 9.4).

9.5 Additional Questions for the Reader

1. **Based on the ABR and DPOAE results, what conclusions can be made with regard to WC's hearing sensitivity?**

2. **What are the implications that audiologists should consider when suspecting a pseudohypacusis or nonorganic hearing loss (NOHL)?**
3. **What conclusions can be made with regard to WC's behavioral results?**
4. **What type of intervention would be recommended based on the findings of the last audiologic evaluation?**

9.6 Discussion of the Additional Questions

1. **Based on the ABR and DPOAE results, what conclusions can be made with regard to WC's hearing sensitivity?**

Based on the ABR findings, WC's hearing sensitivity appeared to be better than admitted behavioral results. DPOAE results provided only general quantitative information about WC's hearing sensitivity. ART are an effective objective tool to support an NOHL when admitted thresholds are greater than 60 dB HL.[1] This, however, is not applicable in WC's case.

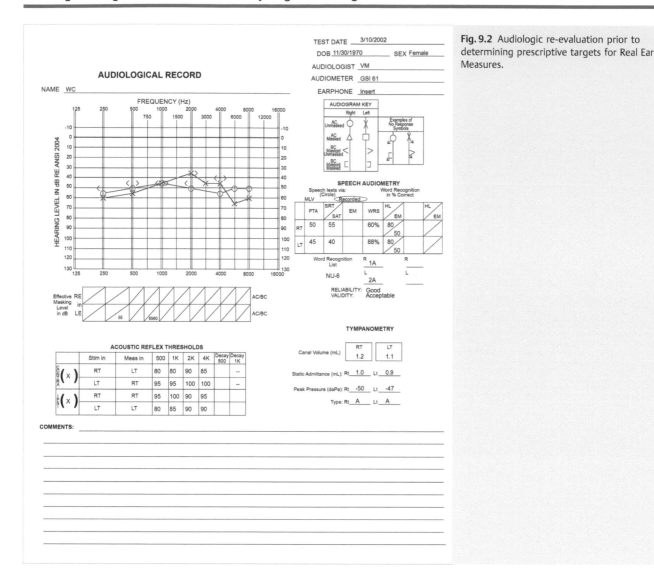

Fig. 9.2 Audiologic re-evaluation prior to determining prescriptive targets for Real Ear Measures.

2. What are the implications that audiologists should consider when suspecting pseudohypacusis or a nonorganic hearing loss (NOHL)?

NOHL can be defined as behavioral responses given by a patient that are inconsistent with that individual's actual organic threshold levels. While some experts suggest that the role of the audiologist should only involve the diagnosis of NOHL,[2] others conclude that it is important that the audiologist consider the patient's underlying motivation or intention in order to make appropriate recommendations for management.

3. What conclusions can be made with regard to WC's behavioral results?

Psychogenic hearing loss, though rare, has been documented in the literature; however, there are a limited number of research studies addressing differential diagnosis of various types of NOHL. One study concluded that individuals who feign hearing loss were more consistent at judging loudness levels of behavioral thresholds within the profound hearing loss range or the mild hearing loss range, compared to threshold levels in between, which is inconsistent with WC's admitted pure-tone

results for the right ear and later for both ears.[3] It is often possible to use the discrepancies between pure-tone threshold average at 500, 1,000, and 2,000 Hz and SRT to check the reliability of pure tones. An agreement of 6 to 10 dB HL between the PTA and the SRT is a standard criterion. Threshold differences between pure tones and spondees are attributed to calibration reference differences between pure tones and speech at 0 dB and to perceptual difference between detection of tones for thresholds and recognition of speech for SRT.[4] Unlike individuals who appear to intentionally provide inaccurate responses, WC's threshold differences for SRTs and PTAs were within 5 dB HL for each test session.

4. What type of intervention would be recommended based on the findings of the last audiologic evaluation?

If a psychogenic hearing loss is suspected, it is recommended that the audiologist simply report the specific outcomes of the evaluation. When a psychological referral is warranted, the audiologist must carefully counsel the patient in a manner that is not offensive and does not directly imply that a psychological disorder exists.

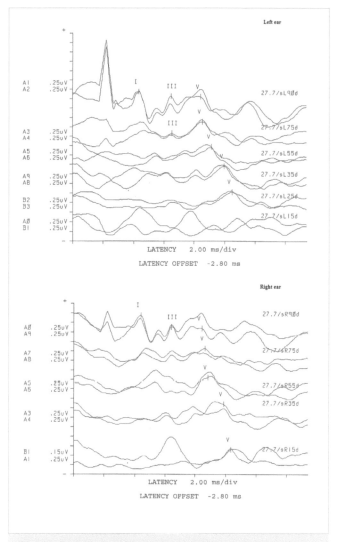

Fig. 9.3 Averaged **Auditory Brainstem Response** waveforms.

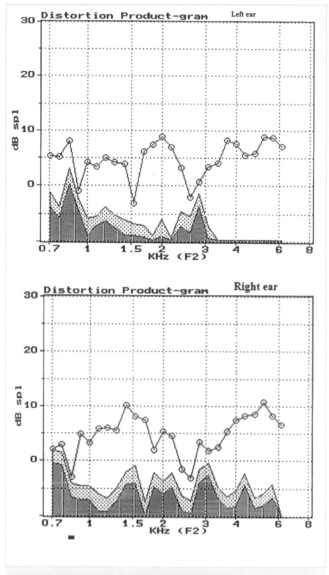

Fig. 9.4 Distortion-product otoacoustic emissions.

9.7 Outcome

WC was counseled on the outcomes and discrepancies between test results. It was recommended that pure tone and speech audiometry be reassessed. She consented to the reassessment. WC was reinstructed on the directions for pure-tone audiometry, SRT, and WRS. SRT were obtained first at 10 dB HL. Using an ascending method, WC's pure-tone thresholds were measured to be within normal limits bilaterally without the necessity for consistent verbal reinforcement. SRT were commensurate with the PTA for each ear. WRS were normal bilaterally. These test results (▶ Fig. 9.5) were discussed with WC; however, she did not appear to realize that her behavioral responses were inconsistent with previous responses.

WC was very cooperative at all times and her responses to test stimuli were consistent during each test session. Typical situations, conditions, and behaviors associated with deliberate malingering were not observed at any time, such as obvious financial motivation, exaggerated efforts to hear or lip-read during the case history and test sessions, excessive false-negative or positive responses, or a "saucer-shaped" audiogram configuration.

With WC's written consent, the audiometric results and interpretation were discussed with her psychologist. WC's psychologist reported that WC was a survivor of a violent home invasion the previous fall. Her psychologist referred WC for psychiatric consultation.

9.8 Key Points

- In addition to analyzing inconsistencies among audiologic test outcomes, the reader should observe the patient's listening behaviors during the case history interview and throughout the test session when ruling out the possibility of NOHL.

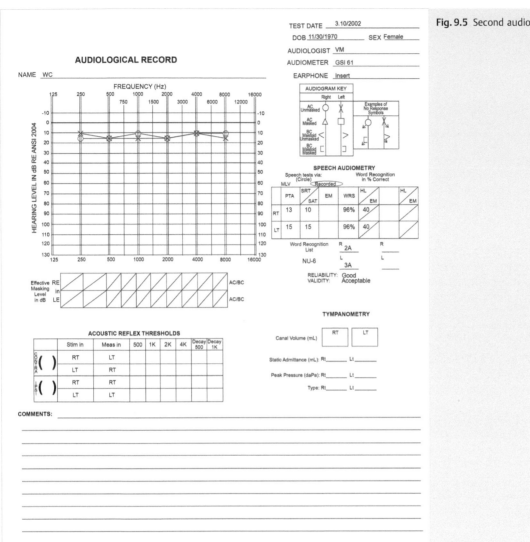

Fig. 9.5 Second audiologic re-evaluation.

- It is common practice in some states for audiologists to use audiologic results obtained within 6 months prior to a hearing aid fitting. However, the reader may consider reassessing pure-tone air conduction thresholds of patients with a history of sudden hearing loss to determine the stability of hearing sensitivity prior to the hearing aid verification process.

References

[1] Gelfand SA. Acoustic reflex threshold tenth percentiles and functional hearing impairment. J Am Acad Audiol. 1994; 5(1):10–16

[2] Martin FN. Pseudohypacusis. In: Katz J, ed. Handbook of Clinical Audiology. 5th ed. Baltimore, MD: William & Wilkins; 2002:584–596

[3] Schlauch RS, Koerner TK, Marshall L. Effective identification of functional hearing loss using behavioral threshold measures. J Speech Lang Hear Res. 2015; 58(2):453–465– [serial online]

[4] Schlauch RS, Han HJ, Yu TJ, Carney E. Pure-tone-spondee threshold relationships in functional hearing loss: a test of loudness contribution. J Speech Lang Hear Res [serial online]. 2017; 60(1):136–143

10 How Auditory Processing Deficits Can Interfere with a College Student's Success in School and Work

Jay R. Lucker

10.1 Clinical History and Description

MK is a 21-year-old female college student seen for evaluation of her auditory functioning. She reported having emotional problems (anxiety disorder) as an adolescent. Her anxiety led to her needing remedial educational services both privately and through an Individualized Education Plan (IEP) from the eighth grade through high school. Among the accommodations provided were extended time on all tests and the use of class notes given to her so she could spend her time listening and not be concerned about taking notes. These two accommodations were provided to MK because she had listening problems that the school associated with her anxiety issues. MK reported an inability to follow what teachers were saying and having problems following social conversations. Her mother confirmed these complaints. MK was evaluated twice by the school audiologist who reported MK had normal hearing. The audiologist did not investigate any additional factors other than audition even though MK consistently complained of problems tolerating certain sounds such as loud noises like sirens, fire alarms, people yelling, and noisy places like malls.

MK barely graduated high school and was enrolled at a community college, but dropped out in her first semester after midterm grades indicated she was failing all subjects. These failures occurred even though MK was provided with accommodations of a note taker in her classes and extended time for taking tests as a student with special needs. MK left college and went to work. She initially worked as a checkout at a local grocery store. The noises, failure to understand what people were saying, making errors in following through on instructions, and not responding to announcements led MK to voluntarily leave her position before she was dismissed.

MK found a second job working in a department store. Her primary responsibilities were keeping note of merchandise and follow what her supervisor told her as well as responding to questions posed by customers. Again, the noise in the work environment, confusion and lack of understanding of what her supervisors were telling her, as well as making errors in questions posed by customers, led her to quit this job. Eventually, these problems led MK to seek a comprehensive audiologic evaluation by the author.

10.2 Audiologic Testing

Results from the comprehensive audiometric evaluation revealed hearing was within normal limits at 250 to 8,000 Hz bilaterally. Speech Recognition Thresholds (SRT) and Word Recognition Scores (WRS) indicated normal ability to receive and recognize speech, respectively, bilaterally. Immittance audiometry revealed normal ear canal volume, middle ear pressure, and static compliance in each ear. Ipsilateral Acoustic Reflex Thresholds (ART) at 500 to 4,000 Hz were within normal limits bilaterally.

10.3 Questions for the Reader

1. **Based on the presenting concerns and results of the audiologic examination, what conclusions can the reader draw regarding MK's problems understanding what she hears?**
2. **Does the audiologist have sufficient information to indicate that MK's problems are not due to audiologic issues, but are more likely related to the anxiety/emotional problems reported by MK?**
3. **Does the audiologist have sufficient information to make specific recommendations for interventions for MK? If yes, what recommendations should the audiologist make?**
4. **What other tests should the audiologist perform to determine what problems are occurring with MK?**

10.4 Discussion of the Questions

1. **Based on the presenting concerns and results of the audiologic examination, what conclusions can the reader draw regarding MK's problems understanding what she hears?**

Audiologic testing reveals MK has normal hearing. The audiologic examination indicates that the presenting concerns have little to do with peripheral hearing loss.

2. **Does the audiologist have sufficient information to indicate that MK's problems are not due to audiologic issues, but are more likely related to the anxiety/emotional problems reported by MK?**

Although hearing is normal, this provides little information regarding MK's emotional state. Thus, the audiologist cannot make any conclusions regarding whether MK's problems are due to negative emotional reactions related to the reported anxiety issues. Having normal hearing, but presenting with the complaints that have been identified could contribute to negative emotional reactions that might be associated with an anxiety problem or a contributing factor to the anxiety issues reported.

3. **Does the audiologist have sufficient information to make specific recommendations for interventions for MK? If yes, what recommendations should the audiologist make?**

Based on the case history and presenting concerns, MK is having problems understanding. The audiologic test results indicate that hearing loss is not the factor contributing to the reported problems. Thus, further testing is required to determine whether MK has any other problems and the audiologist should realize this based on the audiologic test results.

4. **What other tests should the audiologist perform to determine what problems are occurring with MK?**

MK's presenting problems could be due to underlying Auditory Processing Disorders (APD), which is also labeled as Central Auditory Processing Disorder (CAPD), which needs to be evaluated.

10.5 Additional Tests

After a year of struggling to maintain her job, MK experienced an emotional breakdown. She stayed at home on medication and received psychotherapy because of increased anxiety and negative emotional reactions. Her parents questioned whether MK might have APD. Thus, MK scheduled a comprehensive auditory processing assessment.

A comprehensive auditory processing battery was completed (▶ Table 10.1). All test materials were delivered using commercially available recordings via a CD player connected to an audiometer and the material delivered via insert earphones. The following section presents the results of the test battery.

10.5.1 Auditory Hypersensitivity

Auditory hypersensitivity for loud sounds was assessed using warbled tones and narrowband noise at 250, 500, 750, 1,000, 1,500, 2,000, 3,000, 4,000, 6,000, and 8,000 Hz. Warbled tones were used to measure loudness judgment to frequency-specific stimuli, while narrowband noise provides information of tolerance to a more broadband signal rather than frequency-specific sounds. MK was instructed to raise her hand respective to the ear in which she heard the sounds. Her responses to the louder sounds were based on her behavioral responses when the sounds were presented. Intolerance was judged based on consistent negative behavioral reactions to the sounds as the intensity level was increased from 50 dB HL in 10 dB steps until two negative behavioral reactions were observed. Negative behavioral reactions could be flinching, jumping, a facial expression of surprise, grimacing, closing the eyes suddenly, and spreading the lips, etc. Results revealed tolerance thresholds of 65 to 70 dB HL,[3] which is considerably lower than normal (90 dB HL). These reduced tolerance levels were found at all frequencies for warbled tones and narrowband noise.

Table 10.1 Auditory processing test findings for MK

Test	Evaluation	Normal finding	Results
WRS (W-22) (quiet)	Right ear	88–100%	100%
	Left ear	88–100%	100%
WRS in noise (SNR + 5 dB)	Right ear		88%
	Left ear		92%
Quiet/noise difference (normal 17% or less)	Right ear	0–17%	12%
	Left ear	0–17%	8%
Auditory hypersensitivity warbled tone		Tolerance at least 90 dB HL	65–70 dB HL
Auditory hypersensitivity NB noise		Tolerance at least 90 dB HL	70 dB HL
SCAN-3A			
Auditory Figure-Ground: 0 dB		7/16th percentile or greater	9/37th percentile
Auditory Figure-Ground: + 8 dB		7/16th percentile or greater	9/37th percentile
Time Compressed Sentences		7/16th percentile or greater	8/25th percentile
Pitch Pattern Sequence	Right ear	3 tones: 75–100%	100%
	Left ear	3 tones: 75–100%	85%
Phonemic Synthesis test	Quantitative	23–25 correct	25 correct
	Qualitative	22–25 correct	25 correct
Filtered Words		7/16th percentile or greater	8/25th percentile
Competing Words: Free Recall		7/16th percentile or greater	5/5th percentile[a]
Competing Words: Directed Recall		7/16th percentile or greater	3/1st percentile[a]
Competing Sentences		7/16th percentile or greater	8/25th percentile
SSW test			
RNC	Condition	1 error	0
RC	Condition	2 errors	5[a]
LC	Condition	4 errors	8[a]
LNC	Condition	1 error	0
Ear Effect LH	RB	Difference of –3	4[a]
Reversals	RB	0 or 1	4[a]
Type A	RB	Up to 3	1
Order effect HL	RB	Difference of 3	2

Abbreviations: HL, high/low; LC, left competing; LH, low/high; LNC, left noncompeting; NB, narrowband; RB, response bias; RC, right competing; RNC, right noncompeting; SNR, signal-to-noise ratio; SSW, Staggered Spondaic Word; WRS, Word Recognition Scores.
[a]A finding outside the normal range.

10.5.2 Speech Understanding in Noise

Word recognition in noise was assessed with monosyllabic words from the Central Institute for the Deaf (CID) W-22 words lists at 40 dB SL for each ear with speech babble noise mixed with the words at 35 dB HL to create a signal-to-noise ratio (SNR) of + 5 dB. MK was instructed to repeat each word that was heard with 25 words presented per ear. Results indicated scores of 88% for the right ear and 92% for the left ear for quiet/noise difference of 12 and 8%, respectively. These results are within age level normative difference of 0 to 17% for adults based on the Buffalo Model norms.[1]

Speech understanding in noise was also measured via the Auditory Figure-Ground (AFG) subtests from the SCAN-3A Test for Auditory Processing Disorders in Adolescents and Adults – Third Edition.[2] This test has choices for SNR of 0, + 8, and + 12 dB; however, only the 0 and + 8 dB conditions were evaluated. Results were normal for the 0 and + 8 dB measures with scaled scores of 9 (37th percentile) for both. Scaled scores between 7 (16th percentile) and 13 (84th percentile) are normal.

10.5.3 Auditory Temporal Processing

Auditory temporal processing was assessed via the Time Compressed Sentence (TCS) subtest from the SCAN-3A.[3] This measure presents sentences at 60% time compression instructing MK to repeat each sentence that is heard. Key words in the sentences must be repeated correctly. MK's results were normal with a scaled score on the TCS of 8 (25th percentile).

The Pitch Patterns Perception Test developed by Musiek[4] was administered. The test requires the listener to hear a pattern of high- and low-frequency tones and the listener hums the pattern. The listener then repeats the pattern such as "high-low-high" for three tones when the first tone is a high frequency, the second tone is low frequency, and the third tone is once again high in frequency. Other patterns for the three tones were included in the test sequence. The score for normal performance is ≥ 75% for each ear.[4] MK scored 100% for the right ear and 85% for the left ear.

10.5.4 Auditory Phonological Processing

Phonological processing was assessed via the Phonemic Synthesis Test (PST).[1] The normal score for adults is correctly repeating 23 of 25 test items for a **quantitative** score and 22 of 25 for a **qualitative** score. The quantitative score relates to the number of items correctly identified when the words are divided by phoneme. For example, "cat" would be /k/-/ae/-/t/. The qualitative score is used when the response is correct. There are, however, situations when the patient repeats the word, but there is a delay (e.g., not repeating the word until the next item is presented). There can be a quick response where the patient starts to provide an answer before all phonemes are presented. Another example is "quiet rehearsal" where the patient first whispers the word, practicing what word to say, and then provides the final response. MK obtained a score of 25 for both quantitative and qualitative measures.

The Filtered Words subtest of the SCAN-3A was administered to measure auditory phonological processing.[2] This test presents words that are distorted through electronic filtering of the higher frequency sounds. The patient is instructed to repeat the words heard. MK scored in the normal range with a scaled score of 8 (25th percentile).

10.5.5 Auditory Integration (Dichotic Listening Tests)

Dichotic listening was assessed via the Competing Words (Free Recall and Directed Recall) from the SCAN-3A as well as the Staggered Spondaic Word (SSW) tests.[2,5] The Competing Words test presents different, unrelated words to each ear simultaneously. Thus, the right ear might hear "are" while the left ear hears "cat" simultaneously. The patient is instructed to repeat both words, if possible, and guess at the words for which the patient is not sure. Free Recall allows the patient to repeat the words in any order (i.e., right ear item first or left ear item first). Directed Recall measure requires the patient to repeat the right ear item for the initial list, while the second list requires the patient to repeat the left ear items first. For Free Recall, the patient obtains a correct response for each item correctly repeated regardless of the order in which the words are repeated. For Directed Recall, the patient's response is correct only if repeated in the correct order.

The SSW test also presents two words, one to each ear. However, the stimuli are spondee, compound words. Additionally, one syllable of the word is presented alone, while the other syllable is presented simultaneously to the opposite ear. For example, for the test item "airplane—wet paint," the word "air" is presented alone to the right ear (i.e., right noncompeting [RNC]), followed by "plane" again presented to the right ear (i.e., right competing [RC]) simultaneously presented with "wet" in the left ear (i.e., left competing [LC]). Then, the final word "paint" is presented alone to the left ear (i.e., left noncompeting [LNC]). The **odd items** of this 40-item test are presented with the first word starting in the right ear, while the **even items** are presented with the first word starting in the left ear. The patient is given a score of 1 for each word correctly repeated regardless of the order in which it is spoken. However, incorrectly repeating the correct order is scored qualitatively as a reversal. Normative data are available for the number of items correctly repeated for RNC, RC, LNC, and LC. Normative data are also available to assess qualitative responses such as **reversals**, **delayed responses** (not responding as soon as the test item is completely presented, but waiting and repeating the test item when the next test item is ready to be presented), and **quick responses** (starting a response before hearing all words, etc.).

Results from the Competing Words tests indicated deficits in both conditions with Free Recall having a scaled score below normal (5 [5th percentile]) and Directed Recall also having a scaled score below normal (3 [2nd percentile]). Additionally, ear difference on the SCAN-3A was abnormal for five measures, indicating significantly better performance for the right ear compared with the left.

On the SSW test, MK's scores for RC and LC were abnormal (five and eight errors, respectively). MK's **Ear Effect Score** was abnormal (low/high [LH] of four), indicating MK performed significantly better when the right ear started the sequence of words (L) compared with the left ear starting the sequence (H). The **Standard Integration Ratio (SIR)** measure from the SSW[5,6] was normal (0.68). The SIR measures the standard deviation difference between the RC and LC findings with a normal score if the SIR is below 1 SD (a score of 1.00). Thus, the integration problem may be more related to dichotic listening and coordination by the brain in processing between the two ears than to specific language-based integration problems related to familiarity with the words used. The reversals on the SSW were very abnormal (eight reversals), whereas the normal score is a maximum of one reversal for adults. Although these findings were all outside the normal range, normal results were found for the type A pattern, comparison of the two greatest error values for the eight "cardinal numbers," the eight error values for the RNC, RC, LC, and LNC for both Right Ear First (REF) and Left Ear First (LEF) presentations. Additionally, normal findings were obtained for the Order Effect, which is a measure of whether more errors were made on the first spondee word compared to the second spondee presented regardless of which ear heard the first word.

Auditory Separation was assessed via the Competing Sentences measure of the SCAN-3A.[2] Competing Sentences present different, unrelated sentences to each ear simultaneously instructing the patient to repeat only one sentence from the directed ear with the first list of 10 sentences repeating only the right ear item and the second list repeating only the left ear item. Results were normal (scaled score of 8 [25th percentile]). As such, only measures of dichotic listening, in which MK had to repeat the items from both ears, were abnormal.

10.6 Outcome

Results of the audiologic evaluation indicated normal hearing. Results, however, for the auditory processing testing revealed significant deficits related to auditory hypersensitivity to loud sounds, auditory integration problems associated with dichotic listening, and organization/sequencing problems related to the reversals found on the SSW. Thus, the complaints and problems MK has in listening and understanding are not related to hearing loss, but rather related to these auditory processing problems, which had gone undiagnosed.

Very often, adults report having "hearing" and "listening" problems. Typically, audiologists focus on peripheral auditory functioning to identify or rule out hearing loss. In the present case, MK had normal hearing, but MK was failing in college and at work and she could not understand why. MK scheduled an appointment with an audiologist after her first semester in college because she thought she had a hearing loss. The audiologist found her hearing to be normal, which agreed to results from the previous audiologic evaluations. After having difficulty maintaining employment, MK scheduled an appointment with another audiologist who found normal hearing. Neither audiologist recommended MK consider auditory processing testing.

Findings from the auditory processing assessment found MK's intolerance to sounds are related to loud sounds (i.e., hypersensitivity). MK confirmed that this intolerance is not related to specific sounds, but rather the intensity level. Since loud speech, especially with reverberation, and background noise can often reach beyond 90 dB sound pressure level (SPL) and since MK cannot tolerate sounds at 70 dB HL (which would be 90 dB SPL for speech and complex noises), it is not surprising that MK has problems understanding speech in the presence of loud noise and reverberant speech. Thus, MK requires intervention regarding her hypersensitivity to loud sounds.

It was found that the auditory hypersensitivity reported with MK led to increased negative emotional reactions that needed to be addressed.[4] The usual method to address hypersensitivity is to use earplugs to attenuate the loud and unexpected sounds. Earplugs, however, would also reduce the lecturers' voices as well as interactions between business associates and customers at work. Thus, MK might be able to wear earplugs when she is walking in the street or traveling on buses or train, but in college and at work, MK cannot use earplugs. Additionally, MK could not use earplugs in social situations. Thus, MK needs to learn to overcome her negative emotional reactions to loud sounds.

Research[3,7,8,9,10] has reported two approaches to reduce negative emotional reactions in patients with hypersensitivity. One approach is the use of a **sound therapy**, a listening program that has been found to improve auditory processing abilities[3,7,10] as well as reduce the negative emotional reactions to sounds.[3] The other approach is called **systematic desensitization**,[8,9] typically completed with a behavioral psychologist, which can lead to success in dealing with previously intolerable sounds. As for listening therapy, one program is *The Listening Program* or TLP (www.advancedbrain.com). Research has demonstrated significant improvement in auditory processing abilities following the use of TLP training.[7,10]

Auditory lexical integration, another deficit area identified, relates to one's inability to splice together pieces of auditory information, making sense of the material. This is identified by the two ears integrating verbal messages and is assessed via dichotic listening tests. Dichotic listening can be improved through programs such as *CAPDOTS* (www.capdots.com). For the lexical or linguistic component of integrative processing, a computer program such as *Fast ForWord* (www.scilearn.com) can be used. For MK, dichotic listening testing revealed the problem to be integration by the brain between the two auditory centers. Thus, CAPDOTS was the program recommended.

As for the reversal problem reported via the SSW test, learning how to use graphic organizers has been found to be helpful. The reversal problems on the SSW test relate to one's ability to organize linguistic information.[1] These organizers can be used to organize ideas for written assignments. Thus, should MK elect to re-enroll in college, she could use graphic organizers to complete class projects. Additionally, the organizers can teach MK how to organize tasks and job activities at work.

As for re-enrolling in college, MK's greatest concern was not "getting" what her instructors were presenting in class. MK could not understand their lectures and had significant difficulties following questions and answers posed between students and instructors as well as class discussions. Thus, MK should have an accommodation of recording class lectures and discussions. Many universities are using recording programs such as *Tegrity* (www.tegrity.com) in which instructor lectures and class discussions are synchronized with the Power Point presentations. Thus, MK would only need to identify where she became lost or misunderstood information in a class based on what slides were projected and MK could review the lecture and discussions related only to those slides.

Additional accommodations in college would include the continued use of a note taker, availability for tutoring, especially one-on-one tutoring, and having a quiet work environment to complete her coursework, class assignments, and complete examinations. The auditory processing problems found, especially with integration and organization, require extra time for the brain to put together the pieces of information and organize them for MK to respond. Thus, MK needs extended time for assignments and for examinations and quizzes.

With regard to work, when interacting with her supervisors, MK could ask for written outlines or notes related to any conferences and meetings they plan and for MK to have this written material to review in advance of the conference or meeting. MK could ask supervisors to outline key factors in messages they verbally present so MK understands the important pieces. MK could take these written outlines to her workstation and develop an organized way to complete the tasks required.

If followed through, these accommodations and treatments should allow MK to find and hold a job for as long as MK is willing to work. These recommendations should also lead to improved educational outcomes in college and lead MK to pursue her goal to obtain a bachelor's degree. The treatments recommended should lead to reduction in hypersensitive hearing and negative emotional reactions to annoying sounds as well as improve MK's comprehension and integration of auditory-verbal information. The organization strategies should lead to faster completion of work as well as better completed assignments.

MK followed through and is presently completing the TLP listening therapy and FastForward training. As for the organization strategies, MK reported she is waiting to hear from another college to which MK applied as a student with special needs. MK is hoping to be accepted and be provided tutoring services to assist her in organizing her work and written assignments as well as be provided with accommodations such as recording class lectures. MK agreed to return for a re-evaluation of her auditory processing abilities during MK's winter break from college. She is presently not working, but hopes to go to college when it begins in the fall (2 months from the completion of the auditory processing testing) and work part-time with greater success in school and on her job.

10.7 Key Points

- It is critical that audiologists look beyond the outer, middle, and inner ear when evaluating patients. Audiologists must learn to be sensitive to hearing/listening problems, which may be due to APD when hearing thresholds, middle ear functioning, word recognition in quiet (and in noise), and otoacoustic emissions are normal.

- Audiologists should remember that auditory processing problems could affect adults as well as children; thus, it is not merely a "childhood" and "adolescent" problem.
- When adult patients report "listening" problems and are found to have normal hearing, audiologists should complete evaluations of auditory processing or refer these patients to competent, knowledgeable audiologists for comprehensive auditory processing assessments.
- There are accommodations and treatments for auditory processing disorders for adults as well as children. The well-established treatment options for children can be applied to adults as long as the patient knows that the activities were developed for children, but the listening tasks challenge their listening abilities and thus can improve their auditory processing skills.

References

[1] Katz J. APD Evaluation to Therapy: The Buffalo Model. Available at: http://www.audiologyonline.com/articles/apd-evaluation-to-therapy-buffalo-945. Accessed July 28, 2017

[2] Keith RW. SCAN-3:A Tests for Auditory Processing Disorders in Adolescents and Adults. New York, NY: Pearson; 2008

[3] Lucker JR. Auditory hypersensitivity in children with autism spectrum disorder. Focus Autism Other Dev Disabl. 2013; 28(3):184–191

[4] Musiek F. Pitch Pattern Sequence Test. St. Louis, MO: Auditec, Inc

[5] Katz J. INT and the challenge in identifying it. SSW Reports. 2015; 37(2):1–2

[6] Katz J, Medwetsky L. Standard Integration Ratio (SIR). SSW Reports. 2015; 37(2):2–6

[7] Lucker JR, Doman A. Auditory hypersensitivity and autism spectrum disorder: an emotional response. Autism Science Digest. 2012; 4:103–108

[8] Gomes E, Rotta NT, Pedroso FS, Sleifer P, Danesi MC. Auditory hypersensitivity in children and teenagers with autistic spectrum disorder. Arquivos do Neuro-Psiquiatria. 2004;62(3). Available at: http://www.scielo.br/scielo.php?pid=S0004282X2004000500011&script=sci_arttext Google Scholar. Accessed July 28, 2017

[9] Koegel RL, Openden D, Koegel LK. A systematic desensitization paradigm to treat hypersensitivity to auditory stimuli in children with autism in family contexts. Res Practice Patients Severe Disabl. 2004; 29:122–134

[10] Vargas S, Lucker JR. A quantitative summary of The Listening Program (TLP) efficacy studies: what areas were found to improve by TLP intervention? Occup Ther Int. 2016; 23(2):206–217

Suggested Readings

[1] Geffner D, Ross-Swain D. Auditory Processing Disorders: Assessment, Management, and Treatment. 2nd ed. San Diego, CA: Plural Publishing; 2012

[2] Musiek FA, Chermak G. Handbook of Central Auditory Processing Disorders, Vol. 1. Auditory Neuroscience and Diagnosis. San Diego, CA: Plural Publishing; 2013

[3] Chermak G, Musiek FA. Handbook of Central Auditory Processing Disorders, Vol. 2. Comprehensive Intervention. 2nd ed. San Diego, CA: Plural Publishing; 2013

11 Hearing versus Auditory Processing Disorders: Are Hearing Aids Enough?

Jay R. Lucker

11.1 Clinical History and Description

TJ is a 47-year-old male who worked as a financial consultant. At 40 years, TJ began noticing problems understanding soft speech and when communicating in noisy places. Upon encouragement from his wife, TJ scheduled an appointment to see an otolaryngologist. At the examination, the physician could not find any disease process to explain his hearing problems and referred him to an audiologist whose audiometric examination revealed hearing to be within normal limits between 250 and 4,000 Hz, followed by a mild sensorineural hearing loss at 8,000 Hz. In addition, Speech Recognition Thresholds (SRT) indicated normal ability to receive speech and Word Recognition Scores (WRS) indicated normal ability to recognize speech. Finally, immittance audiometry and ipsilateral Acoustic Reflex Thresholds (ART) at 500 to 4,000 Hz indicated normal middle ear function.

Incredibly, with normal hearing through 4,000 Hz and only a mild hearing loss through 8,000 Hz, the audiologist recommended hearing aids. TJ agreed to try the hearing aids for a 30-day trial. Predictably, before the end of the second week, TJ returned the hearing aids because he found sounds and speech to be louder, but still could not understand what people said to him and he was still experiencing significant problems understanding speech in background noise. In fact, he reported that background noise was more annoying aided than unaided.

Eventually, TJ made an appointment to see a second audiologist. The audiologic test findings were the same as before and the second audiologist once again recommended a trial with hearing aids containing noise reduction. Once again, TJ tried these hearing aids for 2 weeks and returned the aids with similar reports as the first trial.

A year later, TJ reported that his problems understanding speech continued. He scheduled an appointment to see another otolaryngologist and audiologist. Again, his results were normal and the results from the audiometric examination was the same as before. The otolaryngologist referred TJ to an otologist who recommended an Auditory Brainstem Response (ABR) examination and magnetic resonance imaging (MRI). Both procedures were normal. The otologist recommended TJ make an appointment with a speech-language pathologist (SLP) for language testing. Outcomes from the SLP evaluation indicated normal, age-appropriate findings on all language and cognitive-linguistic tests administered. The SLP recommended TJ make an appointment with an audiologist specializing in Auditory Processing Disorder (APD).

A year after the evaluation with the SLP, TJ reported his hearing and understanding of conversations became worse. As a result, he withdrew from many social situations so he would not have to struggle understanding what people were saying. Eventually, TJ made an appointment for a comprehensive audiologic and APD assessment. While taking a case history, TJ disclosed having problems understanding speech since high school. At that time, he did not report the problem and worked with friends to better understand his schoolwork and did not see an audiologist or SLP. It was not until TJ was an adult and work demands increased that he began to identify still having significant problems understanding what people were saying, especially in noise.

11.2 Questions to the Reader

1. **Based on the presenting concerns and results of the audiologic examinations, what conclusion can the reader draw regarding TJ's problems understanding speech?**
2. **Does the reader have sufficient information to indicate what is causing TJ to have these problems understanding what he hears?**
3. **Does the reader have sufficient information to make specific recommendations for interventions for TJ? If yes, what recommendations would the reader make?**
4. **What other tests would the reader perform to determine what problems TJ might have?**

11.3 Discussion of the Questions

1. **Based on the presenting concerns and results of the audiologic examinations, what conclusion can the reader draw regarding TJ's problems understanding speech?**

Audiologic testing reveals TJ has normal hearing through 4,000 Hz and only a mild sensorineural hearing loss to 8,000 Hz. It is felt that this mild decrease in hearing in the high frequencies is not sufficient to account for the complaints presented by TJ. There must be some other cause to TJ's complaints. Additionally, TJ reported having problems understanding teachers in high school and this would suggest that this is not a current problem, but may have been present since childhood and was never recognized.

2. **Does the reader have sufficient information to indicate what is causing TJ to have these problems understanding what he hears?**

The reader does not have sufficient information to determine what may be causing TJ's complaints. The results of the audiometric examination, ABR, and MRI were normal. Thus, the reader can assume that TJ's problems are not associated with peripheral hearing loss or specific central auditory pathology.

3. **Does the reader have sufficient information to make specific recommendations for interventions for TJ? If yes, what recommendations would the reader make?**

The reader does not have sufficient information to provide recommendations to help TJ resolve his problems understanding speech in quiet and background noise. The only recommendation would be for further testing to investigate other factors such as auditory processing abilities.

4. **What other tests would the reader perform to determine what problems TJ might have?**

TJ's case history, along with his normal hearing and neurologic findings, suggests TJ's problems could be related to an underlying APD. Thus, TJ should undergo a comprehensive auditory processing assessment.

11.4 Additional Tests

A comprehensive auditory processing battery was once again completed (▶ Table 11.1). All test materials were delivered using commercially available recordings via a CD player connected to an audiometer and delivered via insert earphones. The following presents the results of the test battery.

11.4.1 Speech Understanding in Noise

Word recognition in noise was measured using the Central Institute for the Deaf (CID) W-22 monosyllabic words at 50 dB

HL for each ear with speech babble noise mixed with the words at 45 dB HL to create a signal-to-noise ratio (SNR) of + 5 dB. TJ was instructed to repeat each word he heard with 25 words presented per ear. Results indicated WRS decreasing from 100% in quiet to 80 and 76% in noise for the right and left ears, respectively. The quiet/noise difference was 20 and 24% for the right and left ears, respectively. These results are outside the normal limits within age level normative difference of 0 to 17% for adults based on the Buffalo Model norms.[1]

Speech understanding in noise (SIN) was also measured via the Auditory Figure-Ground (AFG) subtest from the SCAN-3A Tests of Auditory Processing Disorders for Adolescents and Adults - Third Edition.[2] This test has choices for SNR of 0, + 8, and + 12 dB; however, only the 0 and + 8 dB conditions were evaluated. Results were below normal (scaled score of 4 [2nd percentile]) for the 0 and + 8 dB (scaled score of 6 [9th percentile]) measures. Scaled scores greater than 6 (9th percentile) are within the normal range, while scores of ≤ 6 are below the normal range. The findings from these tests were abnormal for TJ, indicating he has significant deficits understanding speech in noise.

Table 11.1 Auditory processing test findings for TJ

Test	Evaluation	Normal finding	Results
WRS (W-22) (quiet)	Right ear	88–100%	100%
	Left ear	88–100%	100%
WRS in noise (SNR: + 5 dB)	Right ear		80%
	Left ear		76%
Quiet/noise difference (norm 17% or less)	Right ear	0–17%	20%*
	Left ear	0–17%	24%*
SCAN-3A			
Auditory Figure-Ground: 0 dB		7/16th percentile or greater	4/2nd percentile*
Auditory Figure-Ground: + 8 dB		7/16th percentile or greater	6/9th percentile*
Filtered Words		7/16th percentile or greater	6/9th percentile*
Competing Words: Free Recall		7/16th percentile or greater	6/9th percentile*
Competing Words: Directed Recall		7/16th percentile or greater	4/2nd percentile*
Competing Sentences		7/16th percentile or greater	10/50th percentile
Time Compressed Sentences		7/16th percentile or greater	11/63rd percentile
Pitch Pattern Sequence	Right ear	3-tones 75–100%	100%
	Left ear	3-tones 75–100%	100%
Phonemic Synthesis Test	Quantitative	23 to 25 correct	25 correct
	Qualitative	22 to 25 correct	25 correct
SSW test			
RNC	Condition	1 error	0
RC	Condition	2 errors	1
LC	Condition	4 errors	8*
LNC	Condition	1 error	0
Ear Effect LH	RB	Difference of –3	5*
Order Effect HL	RB	Difference of 3	2
Reversals	RB	0 or 1	0
Type A	RB	Up to 3	2

Abbreviations: HL, high/low; LC, left competing; LH, low/high; LNC, left noncompeting; RB, response bias; RC, right competing; RNC, right noncompeting; SNR, signal-to-noise ratio; SSW, Staggered Spondaic Word; WRS, Word Recognition Scores. * indicates a deficit problem found

11.4.2 Auditory Integration (Dichotic Listening)

Dichotic listening was assessed via the Competing Words (Free Recall and Directed Recall) from the SCAN-3:A[2] and the Staggered Spondaic Word (SSW) tests. The Competing Words test presents different, unrelated words to each ear simultaneously. Thus, the right ear might hear "are" while the left ear hears "cat" simultaneously. The patient is instructed to repeat both words, if possible, and guess at words even if the patient is not sure. Free Recall allows the patient to repeat the words in any order (i.e., right ear item first or left ear item first). Directed Recall measure requires the patient to repeat the right ear item for the initial list, while the second list requires the patient to repeat the left ear items first. For Free Recall, the patient obtains a correct response for each item correctly repeated regardless of the order in which the words are repeated. For Directed Recall, the patient's response is correct only if repeated in the correct order. Performance on both measures was below normal: scaled score of 6 [9th percentile] for the Free Recall task and scaled score of 4 [2nd percentile] for the Directed Recall task.

Another measure of dichotic listening was assessed via the Competing Sentences measure of the SCAN-3:A.[2] The Competing Sentences test presents different unrelated sentences to each ear simultaneously and the patient is instructed to repeat only one sentence from the directed ear with the first list of 10 sentences repeating only the right ear item and the second list repeating only the left ear item. TJ's performance was normal (scaled score of 10 [50th percentile]), likely because this task of auditory separation is more a measure of attention than integration in which the listener focuses on one ear while ignoring the other. Additionally, the competition is clearly separated from the primary message. Thus, the brain does not have to determine what it has to focus on since the patient is instructed to repeat only the sentence in the specified ear. TJ identified no problems with attention and focusing. His problems were when the noise was mixed with the primary speech message such as in the AFG and word recognition in noise tasks.

In addition, the SSW test was administered. This test also presents two words, one to each ear; however, the stimuli are spondee, compound words. Additionally, one syllable of each word is presented alone while the other syllable is presented simultaneously to the opposite ear. For example, for the test item "airplane—wet paint," the word "air" is presented alone to the right ear (i.e., right noncompeting [RNC]), followed by "plane" again presented to the right ear (i.e., right competing [RC]) and simultaneously presented with "wet" in the left ear (i.e., left competing [LC]). Then the final word "paint" is presented alone to the left ear (i.e., left noncompeting [LNC]). The **odd items** of this 40-item test are presented with the first word starting in the right ear, while the **even items** are presented with the first word starting in the left ear. The patient is provided a score of "1" for each word correctly repeated regardless of the order in which it is spoken. Incorrectly repeating the correct order, however, is scored *qualitatively* as a **reversal**. Normative data are available for the number of items correctly repeated for the RNC, RC, LNC, and LC conditions. Normative data are also available to assess qualitative responses such as **reversals**, **delayed responses** (not responding as soon as the

test item is completely presented, but waiting and repeating the test item when the next test item is ready to be presented), and **quick responses** (starting a response before hearing all words, etc.). Significant integration deficits were noted for TJ for the LC with eight errors. All other conditions were normal. For response biases, the Ear Effect score was abnormal (low/high [LH] of five), while all other results were normal. Ear Effect relates to the different conditions in which the words start in the right ear (Right Ear First [REF]) or in the left ear (Left Ear First [LEF]). The LH finding indicates that fewer errors were made for the REF than the LEF condition, indicating that TJ's integration was better when the information coming into the ear and being processed by the brain follows the sequence of right ear, followed by left ear rather than the opposite sequence. Findings from these dichotic listening measures indicated that TJ has auditory lexical integration problems related to integrating auditory-verbal messages to form the meaningful whole for comprehension.[3]

11.4.3 Auditory Phonological Processing

Phonological processing was assessed via the Phonemic Synthesis Test (PST).[1] The normal score for adults is correctly repeating 23 of 25 test items for a **quantitative** score and 22 of 25 for a **qualitative** score. The quantitative score relates to the number of items correctly identified when the words are divided into phonemes. For example, "cat" would be /k/-/ae/-/t/. The qualitative score is implemented when the response is correct. There are, however, situations when the patient repeats the word correctly, but there is a *delay* (e.g., not repeating the word until the next item is presented). There can be a *quick response* where the patient starts to provide an answer before all phonemes are presented. Another example is *quiet rehearsal* where the patient first whispers the word, practicing what word to say, and then provides the final response. TJ obtained a score of 25 for the quantitative and qualitative measures.

The Filtered Words subtest of the SCAN-3A was administered to measure auditory phonological processing.[2] This test presents words that are distorted through electronic filtering of the higher frequency sounds. The patient is instructed to repeat the words heard. TJ performed below normal (scaled score of 6 [9th percentile]), indicating problems processing the words he heard when they were electronically distorted by filtering. This result is related to lexical integration and not phonological processing.

11.4.4 Auditory Temporal Processing

Auditory temporal processing was assessed via the Time Compressed Sentence (TCS) subtest from the SCAN-3A and the Pitch Pattern Sequence test.[2,4] This TCS presents sentences using 60% time compression and TJ was instructed to repeat each sentence. Key words in the sentences must be repeated correctly. TJ's results were normal with a scaled score of 11 (63rd percentile).

The Pitch Patterns Sequence Test developed by Musiek was also administered.[4] This test requires the listener to hear a pattern of high- and low-frequency tones and the listener hums the pattern. The listener then repeats the pattern such as "high-low-high" for three tones when the first tone is a high frequency, the second tone is low frequency, and the third tone is once again high in frequency. Other patterns for the three tones were included in the test sequence. The score for normal performance is ≥ 75% for each ear[4] and TJ scored 100% for each ear.

11.5 Outcome

Results of the auditory processing test battery indicated problems for TJ when he hears words that are distorted by either clarity of their production (Filtered Words) or the presence of noise (SIN test). Additionally, problems with auditory lexical integration[3] were found (Competing Words Free Recall and Directed Recall[2] and the SSW test[1]). Thus, TJ integrates part of the verbal message, but cannot integrate all the information to form the meaningful whole. These factors likely contribute to TJ's problems following verbal messages, especially in noise. Additionally, these problems likely existed since childhood and contributed to TJ's problems of understanding speech in class.

For recommendations, hearing aids are not appropriate in this case because hearing aids do not improve the brain's ability for TJ to process what he hears. There are, however, materials available that could improve TJ's listening and auditory processing abilities. Some of these materials were developed for young children, but TJ could be helped by the listening and auditory processing tasks that are part of these materials.

Dichotic listening programs, such as CAPDOTS (www.capdots.com) and the Dichotic Onset Training (DOT),[1] can improve dichotic integrated listening. Working with an SLP helped improve SIN in tasks related to comprehension of verbal messages with increasing levels and meaningfulness of competing messages. The competition would start with noise well below the speaking level (i.e., Signal-to-Noise Ratio [SNR]) and then the noise is increased to create a 0 dB SNR. The competition would involve meaningless noise at the beginning and progress to meaningful speech competition with meaningful speech mixed in the same earphones during the listening tasks.

TJ worked on the DOT program and SIN training with an SLP for 1 year. At the end of the year, TJ returned to repeat his auditory processing assessment. Results of the repeated auditory processing testing revealed normal findings on all measures. WRS in noise indicated an SNR of + 5 dB and revealed a quiet/noise difference of 8 and 12% for the right and left ears, respectively. The SSW test revealed normal findings for all conditions, including only two errors for the LC condition. The Ear Effect was no longer significant (LH of one). The SCAN-3A results were normal for all measures with scaled scores of 9 (37th percentile) or better.

This case can serve to inform audiologists to look beyond the audiometric results when evaluating patients reporting problems hearing in noise, but have normal or near-normal hearing. Not all hearing problems are related to peripheral hearing loss and not all hearing problems can be helped with hearing aids.

In some cases, hearing aids are needed along with auditory training, but auditory training is typically not recommended by audiologists. In some cases, hearing aids are not the best solution. Audiologists need to investigate APD in adults and not merely think that APD is a "childhood" disorder. Most measures of auditory processing have normative values for adults and some tests provide normative data for adults older than 50 years.

TJ's case indicates that auditory processing training can be helpful for adults. TJ was very pleased when he returned for retesting because he was now better able to participate in social situations.

Adults with APD can be helped. It is important to recognize there may be APD issues present when an adult patient is scheduled for an audiologic examination. It is important for the audiologist to question the patient about auditory processing issues and complete testing of APD such as measuring SIN and dichotic listening should be conducted.

11.6 Key Points

- Adults reporting problems understanding speech may have APD.
- Hearing aids may not be appropriate to help adults with essentially normal hearing who have problems processing speech in quiet and noise.
- APD testing can be completed in adults.
- Findings from APD testing in adults can help adults better understand why they may be having problems understanding speech in quiet and noise.
- Materials are available to improve auditory processing abilities in adults.

References

[1] Katz J. APD Evaluation to Therapy: The Buffalo Model. Available at: http://www.audiologyonline.com/articles/apd-evaluation-to-therapy-buffalo-945. Accessed July 28, 2017

[2] Keith RW. SCAN-3:A Tests for Auditory Processing Disorders in Adolescents and Adults. New York, NY: Pearson; 2008

[3] Hawkins J, Lucker JR. Looking at auditory processing from a multisystem perspective. Topics in Central Auditory Processing. 2017; 2(1):4–12

[4] Musiek F. Pitch Pattern Sequence Test. St. Louis, MO: Auditec, Inc

Suggested Readings

[1] Geffner D, Ross-Swain D. Auditory Processing Disorders: Assessment, Management, and Treatment. 2nd ed. San Diego, CA: Plural Publishing; 2012

[2] Musiek FA, Chermak G. Handbook of Central Auditory Processing Disorders, Vol. 1. Auditory Neuroscience and Diagnosis. San Diego, CA: Plural Publishing; 2013

[3] Chermak G, Musiek FA. Handbook of Central Auditory Processing Disorders, Vol. 2. Comprehensive Intervention. 2nd ed. San Diego, CA: Plural Publishing; 2013

12 An Unusual Case of Fluctuating Hearing Loss

Judy Peterein

12.1 Clinical History and Description

A 31-year-old female was initially seen at the audiology clinic for roaring and ringing tinnitus, fluctuating hearing loss, and dizzy spells.

FH is now a 41-year-old female who was initially seen for comprehensive audiologic evaluation at the age of 31 years. FH reported roaring tinnitus in the left ear and ringing tinnitus in the right ear. The tinnitus varied daily. In addition, FH reported episodes of spinning vertigo lasting from approximately 30 minutes up to 1 to 2 days. FH also reported hearing loss. Hearing loss and tinnitus increased prior to an episode of vertigo. Symptoms improve near the middle of her menstrual cycle. Balance symptoms increased around the time of her period. Symptoms had been present for 1 year prior to her initial appointment at this clinic. FH had been previously followed at another clinic.

Medical history also included migraine headaches with visual aura as well as anxiety and hyperhidrosis (excessive sweating). FH was taking pentoxifylline, triamterene/hydrochlorothiazide (HCTZ), diazepam, and Paxil at the time of initial consultation with the otolaryngologist.

12.2 Audiological Evaluation

Initial audiologic test results are shown in ▶ Fig. 12.1. Pure-tone thresholds in the right ear revealed a moderate Sensorineural Hearing Loss (SNHL) from 250 to 1,000 Hz rising to a mild loss at 1,500 Hz, further rising to normal hearing at 2,000 and 3,000 Hz, and then sloping to a mild to moderate SNHL from 4,000 to 8,000 Hz. Pure-tone thresholds in the left ear revealed

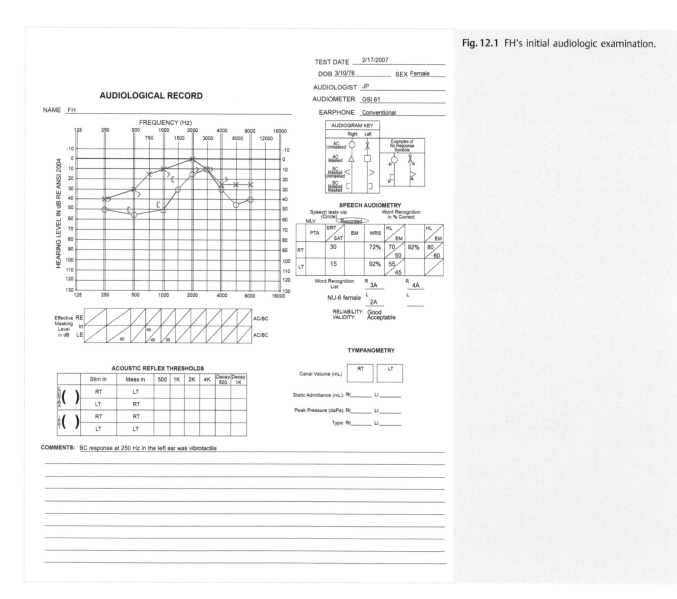

Fig. 12.1 FH's initial audiologic examination.

a mild SNHL at 250 and 500 Hz rising to normal hearing from 750 to 3,000 Hz and then sloping to a slight SNHL from 4,000 to 8,000 Hz. Speech Recognition Thresholds (SRT) revealed a mild loss in the ability to receive speech in the right ear and normal ability to receive speech in the left ear. Word Recognition Scores (WRS) revealed normal ability to recognize speech in each ear.

12.2.1 Additional Audiologic Evaluations

FH returned for follow-up audiologic testing every 6 to 12 months with more frequent testing as needed. Several follow-up comprehensive audiometric examinations were selected for review for this case report.

▶ Fig. 12.2 reports the audiologic test results 6 months later. Pure-tone thresholds in the right ear revealed significantly poorer hearing at 3,000 to 4,000 and 8,000 Hz with slightly poorer hearing noted at 2,000 and 6,000 Hz. Pure-tone results for the left ear revealed significantly poorer hearing from 250 to 8,000 Hz. SRT revealed a mild loss in the right ear and moderate loss in the left ear in the ability to receive speech. WRS

testing revealed normal ability to recognize speech in the right ear and slight difficulty in the ability to recognize speech in the left ear.

The next follow-up audiologic examination obtained 6 months later is reported in ▶ Fig. 12.3. Pure-tone thresholds in the right ear revealed significantly improved hearing at 250 to 1,000 Hz and 3,000 to 8,000 Hz. Pure-tone thresholds for the left ear revealed no significant change in hearing with the exception of a 15-dB improvement at 1,500 Hz. SRT revealed normal ability to recognize speech in the right ear with a mild loss in the left ear. WRS revealed normal ability to recognize speech in the right ear and slight difficulty in the ability to recognize speech in the left ear.

Four additional audiologic examinations are highlighted prior to the discussion of the case. ▶ Fig. 12.4 includes test results obtained 3 months after the results reported in ▶ Fig. 12.3. Pure-tone thresholds for the right ear revealed significantly poorer hearing at 1,000 and 3,000 to 8,000 Hz. Pure-tone thresholds for the left ear were relatively unchanged. SRT revealed a mild loss in the ability to receive speech, bilaterally. WRS did not significantly change in either ear.

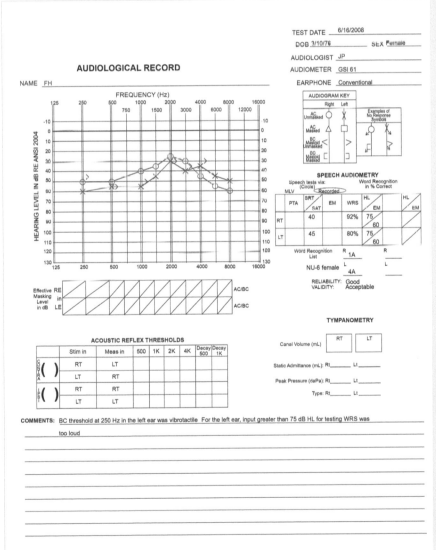

Fig. 12.2 Follow-up audiologic examination 6 months later.

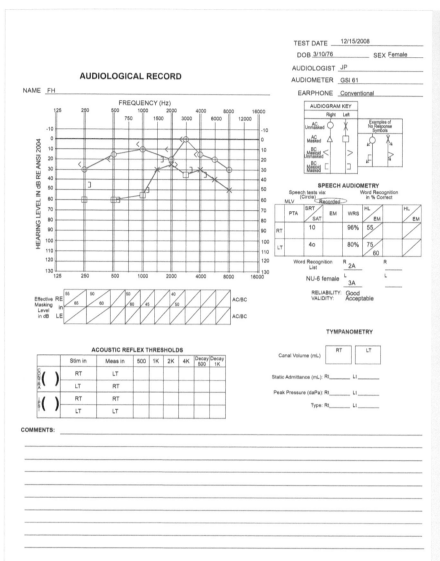

Fig. 12.3 Follow-up audiologic examination 6 months later during first pregnancy (31-week gestation).

The next audiologic examination reported in ▶ Fig. 12.5 was obtained 20 months later. Pure-tone air conduction thresholds were relatively unchanged. The right WRS was also not significantly different; however, the left WRS was significantly poorer at 58% as compared to 84% as compared to the test results in ▶ Fig. 12.4.

▶ Fig. 12.6 reports test results obtained approximately 1 year later. Pure-tone thresholds for the right ear revealed significantly improved thresholds from 250 to 8,000 Hz. Pure-tone thresholds for the left ear were not significantly different. SRT revealed normal ability to receive speech in the right ear and moderately severe loss in the left ear. WRS revealed normal ability to recognize speech in the right ear and poor ability to recognize speech in the left ear.

The final audiologic examination reported in ▶ Fig. 12.7 was obtained approximately 4 months later. Pure-tone thresholds obtained for the right ear were significantly poorer from 250 to 1,500 Hz as well as at 6,000 and 8,000 Hz. The right WRS decreased from 96 to 84%. Pure-tone thresholds for the left ear were not significantly different. The left WRS improved from 56 to 72%.

12.3 Questions to the Reader

1. **What are some potential underlying causes of the fluctuation in FH's hearing loss?**
2. **What medical treatments might be indicated based on the patient's symptoms and hearing loss fluctuation?**
3. **What audiologic recommendations could be made for FH?**

12.4 Discussion of the Questions

1. **What are some potential underlying causes of the fluctuation in FH's hearing loss?**

Several underlying causes could be considered in the case of FH. Hearing loss fluctuation could be secondary to Meniere's disease or endolymphatic hydrops. Autoimmune disease can also present with fluctuating SNHL; however, progression of hearing loss rather than intermittent improvement in hearing is the typical pattern in the case of autoimmune inner ear disease.[1] In

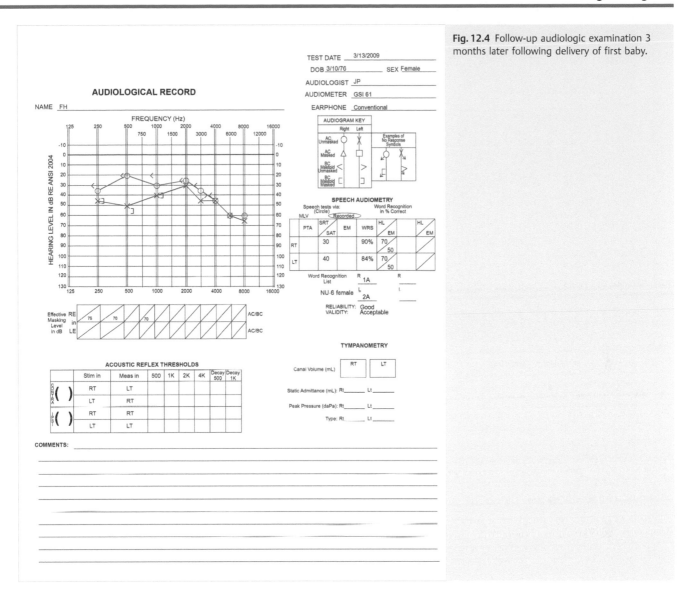

Fig. 12.4 Follow-up audiologic examination 3 months later following delivery of first baby.

addition, hormonal changes may cause hearing loss fluctuation.[2,3,4]

2. What medical treatments might be indicated based on the patient's symptoms and hearing loss fluctuation?

Meniere's disease or endolymphatic hydrops can be treated in several ways. Dietary change including salt restriction as well as salt and caffeine restriction is often the initial treatment recommendation. Diuretics can also be added to reduce fluid retention with HCTZ/triamterene, the most commonly used diuretic. Additional medications that can be prescribed include allergy medications, vestibular suppressants such as diazepam and meclizine, as well as immunosuppressants such as prednisone. Betahistine is also prescribed. Intratympanic injections using either steroids such as dexamethasone and methylprednisolone or gentamicin are often used to treat endolymphatic hydrops. The most common surgical procedure for Meniere's disease is endolymphatic sac surgery. Surgical procedures such as labyrinthectomy or vestibular nerve section are less commonly used.[5]

Less likely in the case of FH, treatment for autoimmune inner ear disease includes the use of oral corticosteroids in varying doses and varying durations. Intratympanic steroid injections are also often administered. The use of methotrexate has not been shown to be as effective as the use of steroids. The use of immunosuppressants has also been explored.[1]

If hormonal changes are associated with hearing loss fluctuation, treatment is less well documented. Progression of hearing loss during pregnancy has been documented, but improvement of hearing loss during pregnancy is less well documented. In the case of improved hearing loss during pregnancy, possible treatment following delivery might include use of oral contraceptives. In addition, treatment with gonadotropin-releasing hormone analogs such as leuprolide and nafarelin has been suggested.[6]

3. What audiologic recommendations could be made for FH?

Bilateral amplification is the recommendation in most cases of SNHL such as with FH. Following otologic consultation, hearing aids can be considered. Digital hearing aids with an adequate

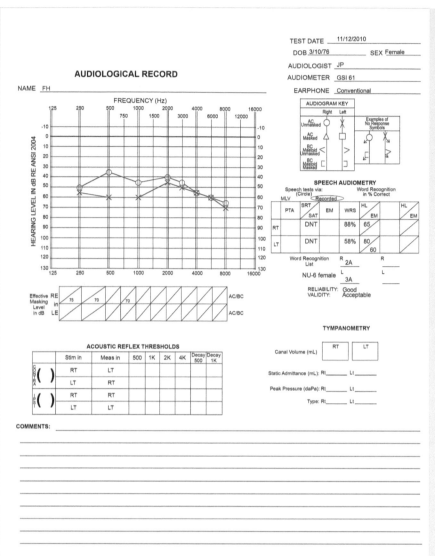

Fig. 12.5 Follow-up audiologic examination 20 months later.

number of bands to allow adjustment based on hearing loss configuration would be preferred. Capability to provide more than one hearing aid program would enable FH to choose differing amounts of amplification based on changes in hearing loss. Additional hearing-assistive devices such as FM systems and/or Bluetooth streaming devices are also recommended to improve the signal-to-noise ratio (SNR) in noisy listening environments and to provide better hearing on the telephone, television, etc. Scheduled audiologic follow-up every 6 to 12 months or more often if needed is recommended to allow for adjustment in hearing aid programming.

12.4.1 Final Diagnosis and Recommended Treatment

Initial ear, nose, and throat (ENT) diagnosis consisted of vestibular migraine; however, due to the low-frequency SNHL component and ongoing tinnitus in the left ear, Meniere's disease was also suggested. The underlying pathophysiology of both vestibular migraine and Meniere's disease is uncertain, making clinical differentiation of the two conditions difficult.

There is significant overlap in both the presentation and diagnostic criteria of the two conditions. Migraine may be a common etiology between vestibular migraine and Meniere's disease. This has not yet been proven. One possible differentiating factor between vestibular migraine and Meniere's disease is the presence of low- to mid-frequency SNHL in the case of definite Meniere's disease.[7] Medical treatment for FH included change in diet to investigate foods that triggered symptoms. FH noted that caffeine was associated with onset of symptoms. Increasing her Paxil dose was recommended to control the migraine component prophylactically. It was recommended that FH continue taking Dyazide. FH was also referred to a migraine specialist in the neurology department. Following the neurology consultation, medications included Imitrex, Paxil, and Topamax. FH also underwent a temporal bone CT scan to evaluate for possible enlarged vestibular aqueduct. CT results were negative for enlarged vestibular aqueduct. An MRI was also completed early in the diagnostic process and was negative for cerebellopontine angle lesions.

Of note is the significant improvement in hearing sensitivity in the right ear as demonstrated in ▶ Fig. 12.3 and ▶ Fig. 12.6.

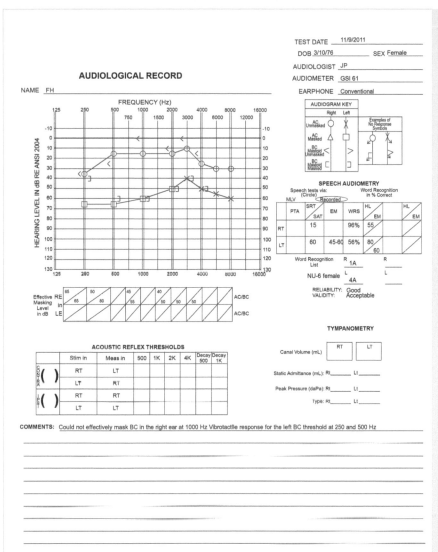

AUDIOLOGICAL RECORD

NAME FH

TEST DATE 11/9/2011

DOB 3/10/76 SEX Female

AUDIOLOGIST JP

AUDIOMETER GSI 61

EARPHONE Conventional

Fig. 12.6 Follow-up audiologic examination 1 year later during second pregnancy (24-week gestation).

COMMENTS: Could not effectively mask BC in the right ear at 1000 Hz Vibrotactile response for the left BC threshold at 250 and 500 Hz

On both test dates, FH was in the third trimester of pregnancy. Following delivery of both babies, hearing in the right ear worsened after approximately 1 week. This suggests hormonal changes significantly altered hearing sensitivity in at least the right ear. Changes in hearing associated with changes in hormone levels including estrogen in women have been supported by several studies.[2,3,4] In an attempt to treat FH's SNHL, FH was referred to the obstetrics and gynecology department. Attempts to treat her hearing loss hormonally were not successful.

Audiologic recommendations included the use of bilateral hearing aids as well as hearing-assistive devices including Bluetooth streaming for cell phone calls, television, etc. Use of amplification by FH will be discussed later.

12.5 Outcome

As previously indicated, hormonal treatment for FH's hearing loss was not successful. FH continues medical treatment for both vestibular migraine and Meniere's disease. FH is followed by an ENT physician and a neurologist. Her hearing loss remains relatively stable at this time in both ears. Her current medications include alprazolam, nortriptyline, and Paxil. FH also recently started magnesium and B2 supplement. FH is not currently experiencing vertigo, but continues to experience headaches approximately once a month.

Audiologic management includes audiologic testing every 6 to 12 months with additional testing as needed. FH started with a hearing aid in her right ear, which was her poorer hearing ear at that time. FH was successfully fitted with a conventional digital Behind-The-Ear (BTE) hearing aid and custom acrylic earmold. During her initial pregnancy, FH did not wear the hearing aid due to improved hearing, as shown in ▶ Fig. 12.3. Approximately 18 months after receiving her right hearing aid, FH was fitted with a hearing aid for her left ear. A similar conventional digital BTE hearing aid from the same manufacturer and custom acrylic earmold was chosen for the left ear. FH wore bilateral hearing aids and returned for reprograming as needed secondary to hearing loss fluctuation. During her second pregnancy, FH discontinued use of the right hearing aid, but continued use of the left hearing aid (▶ Fig. 12.6). FH was subsequently fitted with bilateral digital Receiver-In-the-Canal (RIC) hearing aids with custom acrylic earmolds. FH noted significant improvement in hearing aid performance after receiving the upgraded digital signal processing. FH also purchased a Bluetooth streamer that

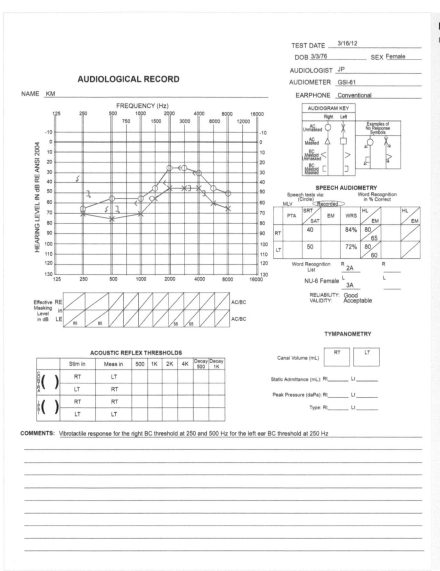

Fig. 12.7 Follow-up audiologic examination 4 months later following delivery of second baby.

allowed her to receive cell phone calls through her hearing aids. FH continues to wear this set of hearing aids successfully.

12.6 Key Points

- Vestibular migraine and Meniere's disease present with similar symptoms and should both be considered in the diagnosis of individuals with vertigo, dizziness, and imbalance. Overlap between many symptoms of vestibular migraine and Meniere's disease occurs.
- Changes in hearing including both worsening and improvement in hearing can occur secondary to hormonal changes. This case demonstrates an unusual improvement in hearing during pregnancy. The possibility of hormonal treatment for hearing loss is suggested.
- Amplification options should be offered to individuals with hearing loss regardless of underlying etiology. Available options include digital hearing aids as well as hearing-assistive devices such as Bluetooth streamers, FM (frequency modulation) devices, and personal amplifiers. Cochlear

implants are also an option in cases of severe to profound hearing loss and/or poor WRS or unsuccessful use of conventional hearing aids.

References

[1] Vambutas A, Pathak S. AAO: autoimmune and autoinflammatory (disease) in otology—what is new in immune-mediated hearing loss. Laryngoscope Investig Otolaryngol. 2016; 1(5):110–115

[2] Al-Mana D, Ceranic B, Djahanbakhch O, Luxon LM. Hormones and the auditory system: a review of physiology and pathophysiology. Neuroscience. 2008; 153(4):881–900

[3] Miller M, Gould W. Fluctuating sensorineural hearing impairment associated with the menstrual cycle. J Aud Res. 1967; 7(4):373–385

[4] Souaid JP, Rappaport JM. Fluctuating sensorineural hearing loss associated with the menstrual cycle. J Otolaryngol. 2001; 30(4):246–250

[5] Clyde JW, Oberman BS, Isildak H. Current management practices in Ménière's disease. Otol Neurotol. 2017; 38(6):e159–e167

[6] Stevens MN, Hullar TE. Improvement in sensorineural hearing loss during pregnancy. Ann Otol Rhinol Laryngol. 2014; 123(9):614–618

[7] Liu YF, Xu H. The intimate relationship between vestibular migraine and Meniere disease: a review of pathogenesis and presentation. Behav Neurol.; 2016:3182735

13 Hidden Hearing Loss

Shruti Balvalli Deshpande and Aniruddha K. Deshpande

13.1 Clinical History and Description

Individuals with similar audiograms can have vastly different speech discrimination abilities. (Central) auditory processing disorder ([C]APD) is one such condition in which, despite presenting with a normal audiometric examination, an individual might experience marked difficulties listening to speech in challenging acoustical environments. The diagnosis of (C)APD is made by an audiologist, although the assessment and differential diagnosis procedures are multidisciplinary in nature.[1]

This case demonstrates the importance of carefully studying the clinical history and conducting additional audiologic tests when deemed appropriate, for accurate audiologic diagnosis and management in cases with suspected (C)APD.

AZ, a 25-year-old female, was referred to a university audiology clinic because she reported "having a hard time understanding speech, especially in noisy listening environments." She described herself as having "a lifelong passion for music." She was a college student majoring in psychology with a minor in music. Academically, AZ described herself as being a good, attentive student and she took pride in her academic success since elementary school. As an adolescent, AZ was part of a music band. She reported purchasing a personal listening device (PLD) as a birthday present at 15 years of age and enjoyed listening to music for several hours daily. Further, AZ reported she recently noticed she was not able to tolerate very loud sounds and no longer enjoyed attending musical concerts. AZ described experiencing intermittent "buzzing" in each ear, but it did not seem to affect her daily activities or sleep. On further questioning, AZ reported she did not wear hearing protection during band practice/performances or at concerts. Also, AZ described the intensity of the music that she listened through her PLD as "my roommates think it is considerably loud." No other significant medical, educational, family, or social history was reported.

13.2 Audiological Testing

▶ Fig. 13.1 reports AZ's comprehensive audiologic evaluation. Pure-tone audiometry indicated AZ's hearing sensitivity was within normal limits, bilaterally. The pure-tone average (PTA) for the left ear was 5 dB HL and that for the right ear was 10 dB HL. AZ's Speech Awareness Threshold (SAT) was 5 dB HL for each ear. Speech Recognition Threshold (SRT) was 15 dB HL for the left ear and 20 dB HL for the right ear. Word Recognition Scores (WRS) were obtained for each ear at 40 dB SL (re: SRT) using a full list of the male talker version of Northwestern University Auditory Test Number 6 (NU-6). WRS for the left and right ears were 98 and 90%, respectively. Most Comfortable Level (MCL) was 55 dB HL for each ear and AZ's Loudness Discomfort Level (LDL) was 105 dB HL for the left ear and 100 dB HL for the right ear, which does not agree with AZ's report of intolerance to loud sounds.

Tympanometry revealed normal middle ear pressure, static compliance, and ear canal volume bilaterally. Ipsilateral Acoustic Reflex Thresholds (ARTs) were 100 dB HL at 500 and 1,000 Hz and absent at 2,000 and 4,000 Hz in each ear. Contralateral ARTs were absent from 500 to 4,000 Hz in each ear. Distortion Product Otoacoustic Emissions (DPOAEs) were present, bilaterally.

Since ipsilateral ARTs were absent at 2,000 and 4,000 Hz in each ear and contralateral ARTs were absent at all frequencies despite normal hearing sensitivity, click-evoked Auditory Brainstem Response (ABR) was performed for each ear. Starting at 90 dB nHL and at a rate of 11.1/s, single-channel ABRs (Fz: noninverting electrode; Fpz: ground electrode; ipsilateral mastoid: inverting electrode) were recorded for each ear. Alternating click stimuli were presented monaurally. Wave morphology and replicability were fair at high intensities; however, wave I amplitudes appeared to be reduced even at 90 dB nHL. Slightly elevated ABRs were recorded bilaterally (wave V was present up to 40 and 50 dB nHL in the left and right ears, respectively). Since AZ's ABRs were elevated in comparison to her audiometric thresholds, she was referred to a neuro-otologist. Clinical and radiological examinations ordered by the neuro-otologist revealed no structural abnormalities/space-occupying lesions. Computed tomographic (CT) scans and magnetic resonance imaging (MRI) of the brain and spinal cord were normal.

AZ's primary complaint was difficulty hearing in noisy environments, in the presence of a normal audiometric examination. Hence, the audiologist suspected that AZ might have (C)APD. AZ was scheduled for tests to rule out (C)APD, including the SCAN-3: for Adolescents and Adults (SCAN-3:A),[2] Quick Speech-in-Noise (QuickSIN) test,[3] Masking Level Difference (MLD),[4] and Random Gap Detection Test (RGDT).[5] Additionally, AZ was also evaluated by a psychologist and speech-language pathologist. Results indicated that she was performing within the normal range on cognitive, psychoeducational, and speech-language tests.

The SCAN-3:A[2] consists of several subtests that evaluate a variety of auditory processing skills such as temporal processing, dichotic listening, and monaural low redundancy. The SCAN-3:A includes screening, diagnostic, and supplementary subtests. The audiologist administered the screening subtests of the SCAN-3:A, which included the following:

- **Gap detection:** it measures temporal processing where the patient is instructed to indicate if he or she heard one or two tones. This measure assesses a patient's ability to detect brief gaps, which are in milliseconds.
- **Auditory figure-ground 0 dB:** in this subtest, the patient is instructed to repeat words embedded in background noise presented at the same intensity as the words. This subtest assesses auditory figure-ground or auditory closure and is a measure of monaural low redundancy.
- **Competing words—free recall:** in this subtest, different monosyllabic words are presented to each ear dichotically and the patient is instructed to repeat both words in any order. AZ's scores for the gap detection and competing words

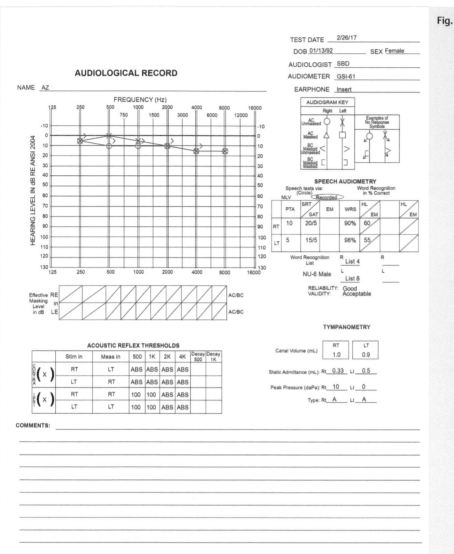

Fig. 13.1 Audiometric evaluation for AZ.

—free recall were within normal limits, but her score for the auditory figure-ground 0 dB was outside the normal range.

The **QuickSIN** test was also administered. The task of the patient on the QuickSIN[3] is to correctly identify keywords from a list of sentences in the presence of four-talker babble noise. The signal-to-noise ratio (SNR) systematically decreases in 5-dB steps from + 25 to 0 dB, making the test progressively more difficult. Based on the number of keywords correctly identified, the Signal-to-Noise Ratio Hearing Loss (SNRHL) for each ear is computed and interpreted. The test was presented at AZ's MCL for each ear (55 dB HL, bilaterally). AZ's SNRHL was 15.5 and 14.5 dB for the left and right ears, indicating severe and moderate SNRHL, respectively. These results suggest that the SNR for AZ would have to improve by approximately 15 dB in order for her performance in noise to be equal to that of a person with normal hearing.

The **MLD**[4] test assesses binaural interaction at the level of the brainstem. Individuals with typical binaural interaction as well as patients with temporal lobe lesions experience "binaural release from masking" when the phase of the signal or the noise is reversed in one ear (antiphasic condition) as opposed to when the signal and noise are in phase, binaurally (homophasic condition).[6] The binaural release from masking phenomenon is not observed in patients with lower brainstem lesions.[6] AZ experienced a release from masking of 9 dB for a 500-Hz pure tone embedded in 500-Hz narrowband noise in the antiphasic condition. She also experienced a release from masking of 8 dB for a 1,000-Hz pure-tone embedded 1,000-Hz narrowband noise in the antiphasic condition. That is, AZ's performance was within normal limits as her threshold in noise improved slightly from the homophasic to the antiphasic conditions.

The **RGDT**[5] assesses temporal processing and was presented binaurally at AZ's MCL. AZ was instructed to indicate if she heard one or two tones/clicks for octave frequencies from 500 to 4,000 Hz. The RGDT includes tones or clicks separated by interstimulus intervals (or gaps) of 0, 2, 5, 10, 15, 20, 25, 30, or 40 milliseconds. The gaps are randomly varied so that anticipatory responses can be eliminated. Results of the test indicated that AZ's RGDT threshold was 5 milliseconds and was within normal limits.

13.2.1 Diagnostic Observations

AZ's auditory profile is intriguing for several reasons:

- Her audiometric examination was "normal" and her DPOAEs were present in spite of long-term noise exposure.
- ARTs and ABRs were impacted, but were not completely absent in the presence of DPOAEs as would be expected in a "classic" case of auditory neuropathy.
- Although AZ indicated that tinnitus was present bilaterally, she was not impacted by its presence and she did not experience dizziness.
- Speech understanding tests and tests of (C)APD assessing auditory figure-ground indicated that AZ's primary complaint of difficulty listening in noisy environments was valid. However, since other auditory processes such as dichotic listening, binaural interaction, and temporal processing were within normal limits, a diagnosis of (C)APD would have been inappropriate. Note that a score of two standard deviations or more below the mean for at least one ear on at least two behavioral tests of (C)APD (assessing two different processes) is a recommended criterion for (C)APD diagnosis.[7]

While AZ's medical history did not appear to be linked with her audiologic complaints, it is worth noting that AZ had a long-standing history of exposure to music through her PLDs. An avid music lover, she was constantly exposed to loud music during band practice and at concerts. In the recent past, she also indicated difficulty tolerating loud sounds.

13.3 Questions to the Reader

1. **Is it possible to have a "hearing loss" in the presence of a "normal" audiometric examination?**
2. **What additional tests could an audiologist perform to investigate the possibility of hidden hearing loss (HHL)?**

13.4 Discussion of Questions

1. **Is it possible to have a "hearing loss" in the presence of a "normal" audiometric examination?**

Recent research has demonstrated that in some mammals (including humans), long-standing noise exposure could lead to a loss of low spontaneous rate and high threshold auditory nerve fibers (synapses) in the presence of intact hair cells in the cochlea. The low spontaneous rate and high threshold auditory nerve fibers seem to play an important role with respect to listening in the presence of background noise.[8,9,10]

Such individuals with long-standing noise exposure leading to the loss of cochlear synapses (cochlear synaptopathy) typically experience severe difficulties comprehending speech in the presence of noise and may experience tinnitus. Patients such as these have audiometric examinations that are generally "normal." Because the conventional audiometric examinations for these patients are normal and their auditory difficulties are "hidden" in nonchallenging listening environments, the condition has been termed HHL.[11]

2. **What additional tests could an audiologist perform to investigate the possibility of hidden hearing loss (HHL)?**

Exploring the possibility of HHL can be challenging. However, such an assessment not only will help with planning appropriate audiologic management, but is also an important academic/research endeavor since HHL is a relatively new phenomenon. There are only a handful of studies investigating this phenomenon in human participants.[8,9,10,11,12] Researchers are investigating the optimum test battery for identifying HHL in human participants.[12]

Some clinical measures that seem promising include extended high-frequency (EHF) audiometry, ABR, and the ratio of the summating potential (SP) to the action potential (AP) (i.e., SP/AP, measured with electrocochleography [ECochG]).[8]

13.5 Additional Testing

AZ underwent EHF audiometry and ECochG. EHF audiometry was performed for each ear using Sennheiser HDA-300 headphones. Results indicated that AZ's thresholds were 40 and 50 dB HL for the left ear and 40 and 55 dB HL for the right ear at 12,000 and 16,000 Hz, respectively. AZ's EHF thresholds indicated moderate hearing loss at 12,000 and 16,000 Hz, bilaterally.

ECochG was also performed for each ear. Using an abrasive gel, AZ's forehead and ear canals were scrubbed. A horizontal recording montage was used with the test ear (inverting), non-test ear (ground), and forehead (noninverting). Conductive gel was used to affix the gold-foil tiptrodes placed in the ear canals. The overall impedance was less than 5 kΩ with interelectrode impedances less than 2 kΩ. Each ear was individually tested. Acoustic click stimuli (100-μs clicks) were delivered in alternating polarity at 95 dB nHL at the rate of 9.1 Hz. Approximately 2,000 sweeps were averaged. A bandpass filter of 10 to 3,000 Hz was used and responses were amplified 100,000 times. An offline analysis was performed to identify SP and AP peaks (▶ Fig. 13.2 and ▶ Fig. 13.3). The SP and AP amplitudes for the waveforms were defined as the difference between peak and baseline. The SP/AP amplitude ratio was determined for each ear. The SP/AP amplitude ratio was 0.48 for the left ear and 0.53 for the right ear. These values indicated that the SP/AP amplitude ratio was abnormally large and similar to cases of Meniere's disease.[13]

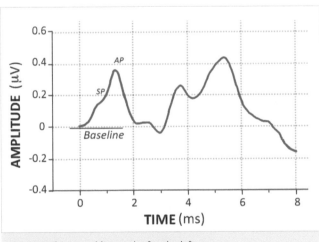

Fig. 13.2 Electrocochleography for the left ear.

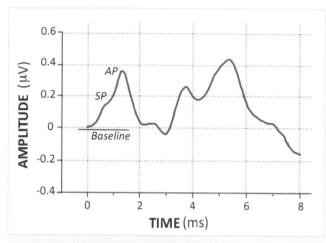

Fig. 13.3 Electrocochleography for the right ear.

13.6 Additional Questions to the Reader

1. **The development of an optimum test battery to evaluate HHL in human participants is still in its infancy. However, as described above, EHF audiometry and ECochG seem to be important clinical measures that audiologists could employ to investigate the possibility of HHL. What would be the rationale for using these measures to assess HHL?**

13.7 Discussion of the Additional Questions

1. **The development of an optimum test battery to evaluate HHL in human participants is still in its infancy. However, as described above, EHF audiometry and ECochG seem to be important clinical measures that audiologists could employ to investigate the possibility of HHL. What would be the rationale for using these measures to assess HHL?**

HHL is primarily characterized by a normal audiometric examination and difficulty understanding speech in noise. Audiologists rarely test audibility at EHF (12,000 and 16,000 Hz); however, these frequencies are crucial for speech understanding in challenging listening situations such as noise or reverberations.[14] Moreover, hearing is affected at these EHFs in cases with cochlear synaptopathy or noise-induced HHL.[8] Hence, EHF audiometry is a sensitive clinical measure of HHL.[15] It must be noted, however, that there is currently no current procedural terminology (CPT) code for EHF audiometry and therefore this procedure cannot be billed.

Animal studies indicate that cochlear synaptopathy/HHL can be objectively diagnosed by measuring the amplitude of ABR wave I, which is significantly reduced in such cases. Typically, ABR in human participants is a far-field response and variability in SNR, head shape, size, and tissue conductivity makes the ABR a less reliable measure for assessing HHL. Recall that AZ's ABRs were elevated and wave I appeared to be reduced in amplitude even at high sensation levels. Using ECochG with tiptrodes inserted deep into the ear canals, the ABR wave I (the AP) is normalized to the SP, which is generated by the cochlear hair cells.[8] In AZ's case, the SP/AP was significantly higher than the normal range.[13] While a high SP/AP generally indicates Meniere's disease, it is speculated that the pathophysiology of cochlear synaptopathy/HHL might be similar to Meniere's disease in which the mechano-electrical transduction processes of the cochlea are affected.[8] Interestingly, electron microscopic studies in Meniere's disease are characterized by deafferentation, which is very similar to the ones in microscopic studies of cochlear synaptopathy.[8]

13.8 Final Diagnosis and Recommended Treatment

AZ's audiologic profile indicates an EHF hearing loss with deficits in speech understanding in noise. Based on the history and overall results of the assessments completed by the audiologist, speech-language pathologist, psychoeducational team, as well as the neuro-otologist, it appears that AZ might have HHL.

13.8.1 Management

Upon completing the assessment protocol, AZ was counseled about the nature of her hearing loss and its impact. First and foremost, she was counseled about monitoring the volume while listening to her PLDs and encouraged to use hearing protection in noisy environments. The need for periodically assessing her hearing was also stressed. To enhance speech understanding in noisy environments such as in her classroom, AZ was encouraged to use frequency modulation (FM) systems in conjunction with preferential seating and self-advocacy. AZ also elected to participate in a series of auditory training sessions to help improve her skills of listening in challenging acoustic environments. Finally, she was provided informational counseling with respect to her tinnitus.

13.9 Outcome

A follow-up appointment 3 months later indicated that there were no changes in AZ's conventional and EHF hearing thresholds. AZ, however, reported that the management strategies and aural rehabilitation sessions significantly helped her understand the possible cause of her hearing problems, control the amount and the loudness of noise that she was exposed to, and doing significantly better with speech understanding in noisy environments. At school, AZ now uses an FM device and appropriately uses self-advocacy to excel.

13.10 Key Points

- It is important investigate beyond the conventional audiometric examination.
- A test battery incorporating subjective and objective measures often helps solve an enigmatic case.
- Audiologic assessment oftentimes needs to be followed with management and counseling—even when the initial audiometric examination appears normal, but the patient reports hearing difficulties in difficult listening environments.

13.11 Acknowledgment

The authors would like to thank Ms. Smruti Balvalli for re-creating the figures used in the case study.

References

[1] Bellis TJ. Understanding auditory processing disorders in children. American Speech-Language-Hearing Association. Available at: http//www.asha.org/public/hearing/disorders/understand-apd-hild.htm. Accessed August 22, 2017

[2] Keith RW. SCAN-3 for Adolescents and Adults: Tests for Auditory Processing Disorders. San Antonio, TX: Pearson; 2009

[3] Killion MC, Niquette PA, Gudmundsen GI, Revit LJ, Banerjee S. Development of a quick speech-in-noise test for measuring signal-to-noise ratio loss in normal-hearing and hearing-impaired listeners. J Acoust Soc Am. 2004; 116(4,) (P)(t 1):2395–2405

[4] Bilger RC, Hirsh IJ. Masking of tones by bands of noise. J Acoust Soc Am. 1956; 28(4):623–630

[5] Keith RW. Random Gap Detection Test. St. Louis, MO: Auditec; 2000:13

[6] Lynn GE, Gilroy J, Taylor PC, Leiser RP. Binaural masking level differences in neurological disorders. Arch Otolaryngol. 1981; 107(6):357–362

[7] Musiek FE, Baran JA, Bellis TJ, et al. Guidelines for the diagnosis, treatment and management of children and adults with central auditory processing disorder. American Academy of Audiology. 2010. Available at: https://www.audiology.org/publications-resources/document-library/central-auditory-processing-disorder. Accessed August 22, 2017

[8] Liberman MC, Epstein MJ, Cleveland SS, Wang H, Maison SF. Toward a differential diagnosis of hidden hearing loss in humans. PLoS One. 2016; 11(9): e0162726

[9] Guest H, Munro KJ, Prendergast G, Howe S, Plack CJ. Tinnitus with a normal audiogram: relation to noise exposure but no evidence for cochlear synaptopathy. Hear Res. 2017; 344:265–274

[10] Prendergast G, Guest H, Munro KJ, et al. Effects of noise exposure on young adults with normal audiograms I: electrophysiology. Hear Res. 2017; 344:68–81

[11] Schaette R, McAlpine D. Tinnitus with a normal audiogram: physiological evidence for hidden hearing loss and computational model. J Neurosci. 2011; 31 (38):13452–13457

[12] Bharadwaj HM, Masud S, Mehraei G, Verhulst S, Shinn-Cunningham BG. Individual differences reveal correlates of hidden hearing deficits. J Neurosci. 2015; 35(5):2161–2172

[13] Coats AC. The summating potential and Meniere's disease. I. Summating potential amplitude in Meniere and non-Meniere ears. Arch Otolaryngol. 1981; 107(4):199–208

[14] Vitela AD, Monson BB, Lotto AJ. Phoneme categorization relying solely on high-frequency energy. J Acoust Soc Am. 2015; 137(1):EL65–EL70

[15] Moore D, Hunter L, Munro K. Benefits of extended high-frequency audiometry for everyone. Hear J. 2017; 70(3):50–52

14 Auditory Dyssynchrony: A Struggle to Understand Speech in Noise

Aniruddha K. Deshpande and Shruti Balvalli Deshpande

14.1 Clinical History and Description

OP is a 25-year-old female who presented to the audiology clinic reporting difficulty hearing even moderately loud sounds. She mentioned that if speech was loud enough she understood some of the speech signal. Listening to speech in a noisy environment was especially challenging. She was not completely sure when her problem began, but indicated her hearing gradually grew worse. She experienced tinnitus intermittently, but did not consider the tinnitus to be bothersome.

OP did not report any significant medical history such as a family history of hearing loss, vertigo, ototoxicity, or noise exposure. She was a college student at a local university. She reported that it was difficult to listen to her professors or interact socially with friends and acquaintances due to her hearing loss.

14.2 Audiological Testing

▶ Fig. 14.1 reports OP's comprehensive audiologic evaluation. Pure-tone testing indicated OP had a mild to moderate severe Sensorineural Hearing Loss (SNHL) at 250 to 8,000 Hz in the left ear and a mild to severe SNHL in the right ear. There was 15-dB asymmetry, with the right ear being poorer at 500 to 8,000 Hz. Speech Recognition Thresholds (SRT) revealed a moderate severe loss in the ability to receive speech in the right ear and moderate loss in the left ear. Word Recognition Scores (WRS) were obtained at 40 dB SL (re: SRT) using the Northwestern University Auditory Test Number 6 (NU-6) list (male version) consisting of 50 phonemically balanced words. WRS for the left and right ears indicated slight difficulty in recognizing speech. Tympanometry revealed that middle ear pressure (daPa), static compliance (mL), and ear canal volume (mL) were within the normal range for each ear. Acoustic Reflex Thresholds (ARTs) were absent to ipsilateral and contralateral stimuli at 500, 1,000, 2,000, and 4,000 Hz.

14.3 Diagnosis and Recommended Treatment

Based on the results of the audiologic examination (asymmetry in hearing thresholds with the right poorer than the left ear), OP was referred to an otologist to rule out an eighth cranial nerve lesion. OP was counseled she had a hearing loss that was sufficient to interfere with communication. Since the hearing loss could not be reversed medically or surgically, being fitted with bilateral hearing aids was recommended. Upon obtaining medical clearance from her otologist, OP scheduled an appointment for her hearing aid fitting and her audiologist fitted bilateral Receiver-In-the-Canal (RIC) hearing aids (Widex Clear Fusion 440s) that were coupled to the ears via open domes.

Gain targets were verified using Real Ear Measures (REM). OP was counseled on the use and maintenance of her new hearing aids and was instructed to follow up after 2 weeks.

OP scheduled an appointment with her audiologist a week later reporting the hearing aids were not working well. She was frustrated and exclaimed: "Understanding speech in the presence of noise is a struggle for me!" Electroacoustic analysis of the hearing aids revealed the hearing aids were performing within manufacturer's specification.

The audiologist repeated the audiologic test battery to ensure reliability of responses. Results did not indicate any change with respect to the hearing status since the initial audiologic evaluation. Since OP was struggling to understand speech in noise, however, the Quick Speech-in-Noise (QuickSIN)[1] test was performed. QuickSIN is a prerecorded test assessing speech understanding in the presence of four-talker babble noise. The listener is instructed to identify keywords embedded within sentences as the signal-to-noise ratio (SNR) progressively decreases in 5 dB steps from + 25 to 0 dB, making the target speech progressively more difficult to identify. The Signal-to-Noise Ratio Hearing Loss (SNRHL) loss is then calculated, which helps provide information on how the patient is performing in noise relative to the performance of a person with normal hearing. The QuickSIN was presented at OP's most comfortable level (MCL; 95 dB HL in the left ear and 100 dB HL in the right ear). Three sentence lists were administered for each ear and the average SNRHL for each ear was 15.5 dB, indicating that OP had severe SNRHL bilaterally. In this case, the SNRHL indicates that OP would require technology to improve SNR by 15.5 dB to hear as well as a person with normal hearing in noise. That is, in order for OP to hear as well as a person with normal hearing in noise, some method of treatment would be required that could improve the SNR by 15.5 dB. This goal clearly cannot be achieved by hearing aids alone. The hearing aids would need to be supplemented with an assistive listening device such as a remote microphone or a frequency modulated (FM) system.

14.4 Questions to the Reader

1. **Based on the case history, audiologic examination, and patient feedback, what additional testing would the reader perform?**

14.5 Discussion of the Questions

1. **Based on the case history, audiologic examination, and patient feedback, what additional testing would the reader perform?**

OP's comprehensive audiometric examination clearly indicated bilateral asymmetric SNHL, which might benefit from bilateral hearing aids. OP was a young motivated college student, but during her hearing aid trial she became extremely frustrated

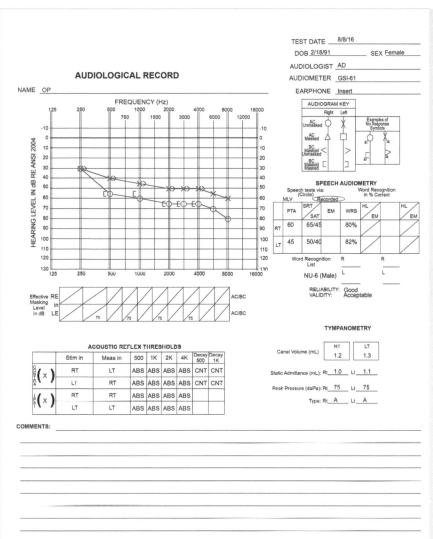

Fig. 14.1 Initial comprehensive audiologic evaluation.

with her hearing aids' performance in noisy situations. A reevaluation 7 days into her hearing aid trial did not indicate any significant change in her hearing or the function of her hearing aids. The QuickSIN, however, indicated that OP's complaints about her frustration of listening to speech in noise were valid. Extreme difficulty with understanding speech in noise could be a cardinal symptom of audiologic disorders such as, but not limited to, space occupying lesions, auditory dyssynchrony/auditory neuropathy/auditory neuropathy spectrum disorder, cochlear synaptopathy, central auditory processing disorder, or central presbycusis. Site-of-lesion assessments including a minimum of Otoacoustic Emissions (OAE) and Auditory Brainstem Response (ABR) are warranted in the above-mentioned audiologic disorders.

14.6 Additional Testing

As part of the additional site of lesion assessment, OP underwent Transient Evoked Otoacoustic Emissions (TEOAE) presented bilaterally and an ABR. The results from TEOAE are provided in ▶ Table 14.1 for the right and left ears.

Table 14.1 TEOAE results (OAE amplitude, noise amplitude, SNR, and confidence levels at five frequencies) of OP for the right and left ears

Right ear				
Frequency	OAE	Noise	Confidence	SNR
1,000	0.4	−6.3	82.4	6.7
1,414	9.9	−3.6	95.7	13.5
2,000	2.4	−9.8	94.2	12.1
2,828	11.0	−9.0	99.0	20.0
4,000	7.7	−9.5	98.1	17.2
Left ear				
1,000	7.2	−11.1	98.6	18.4
1,414	12.1	−9.0	99.2	21.1
2,000	17.5	−10.3	99.8	27.8
2,828	10.8	−9.4	99.0	20.2
4,000	15.5	−10.2	99.7	25.7

Abbreviations: SNR, signal-to-noise ratio; TOAE, transient evoked otoacoustic emission.

Since TEOAEs were present despite the moderate and moderately severe SNHL in the left and right ears, respectively, the audiologist investigated if presentation of white noise contralateral to the ear in which OAEs were being recorded led to any changes in the OAE amplitudes. Typically, such a presentation of noise would lead to suppression of OAE amplitude. For OP, contralateral efferent suppression of OAEs was absent, bilaterally.

Additionally, click-evoked ABR was completed at 100 dB nHL at a rate of 9.1/s in each ear using condensation, rarefaction, and alternate stimulus polarities. Wave morphology was poor and waves I, III, and V could not be detected in either ear. Cochlear microphonics (CMs), however, were present and were inverted on reversal of stimulus polarity from condensation to rarefaction.

14.7 Additional Questions to the Reader

1. **Based on the results of the additional objective audiologic tests, what is the probable diagnosis of OP's hearing loss?**

14.7.1 Discussion of the Additional Questions

1. **Based on the results of the additional objective audiologic tests, what is the probable diagnosis of OP's hearing loss?**

OP's bilaterally present TEOAEs, absent contralateral efferent suppression of OAEs, absent waveforms on the ABR, and the presence of robust CMs indicate a classic profile of bilateral auditory neuropathy (AN) or auditory dyssynchrony (AD). In AN/AD, while the outer hair cells (OHCs) seem to be functioning well, different levels of dyssynchrony may exist with respect to signal processing at the level of the inner hair cells (IHCs), synapses between the IHCs and the auditory neurons, and/or at the level of the auditory nerve fibers (ANFs).[2,3,4] Thus, TEOAEs and CMs, which are primarily a product of the active processes of the OHCs, are present. The waveforms of the ABR and the contralateral efferent suppression of OAEs, which are mediated by the auditory neural synapses and the ANFs, however, are absent or disordered.

The poor wave morphology and absent ABR waveforms are indicative of a compromised afferent pathway. The CM, however, is present due to intact active processes of the OHCs. It is important to distinguish the CM from wave I of the ABR. Thus, it is vital to collect ABR waveforms in both single-polarity modes (condensation and rarefaction). The CM peak will invert with reversal of stimulus polarity, while a "true" wave I peak will not.

Suppression of OAEs via noise presented to the contralateral ear is an excellent clinical method for investigating the integrity of the efferent pathway.[5] In cases of unilateral AN/AD, noise presented to the unaffected ear will travel to the brainstem via a normal afferent pathway, but will fail to suppress OAEs in the affected ear due to a compromised efferent pathway. In OP's case, it is difficult to confirm that the lack of suppression of OAEs is due to a faulty efferent pathway, as both afferent pathways are affected as well (indicated by absent ABR waveforms).

Patients with AN/AD will also typically demonstrate absent ARTs and have extreme difficulty with understanding speech, especially in the presence of noise.

14.8 Diagnosis and Recommended Treatment

Based on the audiologic profile, OP's diagnosis is consistent with AN/AD. She was referred to a neurologist for a comprehensive otoneurological assessment, results of which were within normal limits.

The audiologist reprogrammed her hearing aids by adding three programs to assist in improving performance in noise:
- A program for listening to speech in noise that operates by activating directional microphones.
- A program for adaptive noise reduction that operates on the principle of gain reduction in those channels of the digital signal processor that detect noise.
- A telecoil program to access electromagnetic signals in places equipped with a loop system such as auditoriums and classrooms.

Additionally, OP was recommended a personal FM system to assist with listening in classrooms and/or in noisy environments. After trying two FM systems (Phonak Roger and Widex SCOLA), OP chose the SCOLA system because she preferred its sound quality. The SCOLA Talk FM transmitter was combined with the SCOLA Flex FM receiver paired to one of her hearing aids as a slide-on audio shoe. The QuickSIN was re-administered at OP's MCL for sound field (90 dB HL) via two loudspeakers placed at 45- and 315-degree azimuths. Three-sentence lists were administered and the average SNR loss was 5.5 dB, indicating a mild SNR loss. Thus, there was a +10 dB improvement in SNR after implementing the suggested modifications.

Finally, OP was counseled concerning the nature of her hearing loss and encouraged to communicate about her hearing loss and accompanying difficulties with communication partners who might be unaware (e.g., a new professor) so they can create strategies to improve the effectiveness of communication. OP also chose to attend aural rehabilitation (AR) sessions to maximize her potential for effective communication. She was also provided information on cochlear implantation (CI) as another possible option.

14.9 Outcome

Six months later, a comprehensive audiologic re-evaluation indicated that OP's hearing status had not changed significantly (▶ Fig. 14.2). She reported benefit with her hearing aids, the FM system, and the AR sessions. The audiologist re-administered the QuickSIN to quantify OP's reported benefit with the FM system. The QuickSIN was administered at OP's MCL for sound field (95 dB HL) via two loudspeakers placed at 45- and 315-degree azimuths. Three-sentence lists were administered and the average SNR loss was 6 dB, indicating a mild SNRHL loss. Thus, the improvement in SNR was maintained over a 6-month period. Finally, OP reported she considered the CI, but did not want to pursue it as she was satisfied with the hearing aid–FM combination.

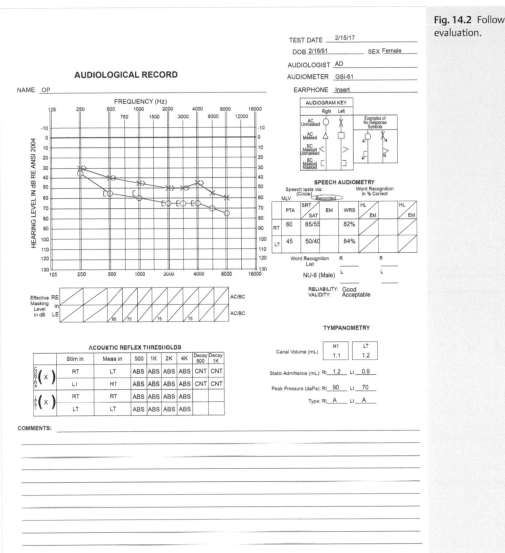

Fig. 14.2 Follow-up comprehensive audiologic evaluation.

14.10 Key Points

- Careful re-evaluation of a patient's reports even after hearing aids have been fitted is crucial in order to arrive at an accurate diagnosis.
- Subjective and objective hearing tests provide invaluable information about the possible site of lesion.
- The role of assistive listening devices, AR, and counseling for the management of individuals with hearing loss and AN/AD cannot be overstated.

References

[1] Niquette P, Gudmundsen G, Killion M. QuickSIN Speech-in-Noise Test. Version 1.3. Elk Grove Village, IL: Etymotic Research; 2001

[2] Berlin CI. Auditory neuropathy: using OAEs and ABRs from screening to management. Semin Hear. 1999; 20(4):307–314

[3] Berlin CI, Bordelon J, St John P, et al. Reversing click polarity may uncover auditory neuropathy in infants. Ear Hear. 1998; 19(1):37–47

[4] Hood LJ. Auditory neuropathy: what is it and what can we do about it? Hear J. 1998; 51(8):10–18

[5] Abdala C, Sininger YS, Starr A. Distortion product otoacoustic emission suppression in subjects with auditory neuropathy. Ear Hear. 2000; 21(6):542–553

15 Auditory Processing Disorder Therapy for Mitochondrial Myopathy

Jack Katz and Lainey Lake

15.1 Clinical History and Description

BL, a 40-year-old female, was diagnosed with mitochondrial myopathy (MM), a degenerative neurological disorder that causes damage to the mitochondria in the body. This disorder affects approximately 1 in 5,000 people.[1] At 47 years of age, BL was referred by her MM specialist and a speech-language pathologist (SLP) for an Auditory Processing Disorder (APD) evaluation. As a child, BL had some difficulties with reading and attention, but overall, performed well in school. At 20 years of age, BL began noticing some difficulties reading, understanding speech, particularly in background noise, and had poor handwriting skills. Over time, she developed significant problems with speech, short-term memory, reading, and writing.

Mitochondria are the energy sources in almost every body cell. The diagnosis of MM suggests that her certain mitochondria lost their energy, for example, decreasing to 30% of normal function.[2] Typically, MM is diagnosed by a physician taking the patient's medical history, and then proceeding with physical and neurological examinations. Some of the hallmark symptoms of MM are muscle weakness, exercise intolerance, hearing impairment, ataxia, seizures, learning disabilities, heart defects, diabetes, and stunted growth. A combination of three or more of these symptoms strongly points to mitochondrial disease, especially when the symptoms involve more than one organ system.[3] This is typically diagnosed/noted in childhood; however, it appeared in BL when she was 20 years old. This can cause organs to shut down and increase the patient's need for more sleep each day. The disorder is progressive and there is no cure.

Her sister completed the case history because BL was unable to write. BL dictated her responses and said the reason for the appointment was "because no one knows how to treat me" and the SLP suspected APD. The SLP told BL: "In his 30 years of practice, I'm the worst case he has seen in the ability to focus on one thing, and I had extremely sound-sensitive ears." Her sister indicated that BL had hearing, speech-language, social, and emotional problems. When BL arrived for the APD evaluation, she could hardly speak. It sounded like a machine gun of single unrelated speech sounds.

BL's condition had gradually worsened until she was diagnosed with MM after losing her ability to read. At that time, she also had increased difficulties in word finding, which was extremely frustrating for her. She added: "I get very angry quickly and snap at people I don't even know, just out of frustration. No more reading, spelling, or math." Before the onset of MM, BL had graduated from college, was effective in business, and was very athletic.

15.2 Audiologic Testing

BL's initial audiologic examination performed by her audiologist revealed normal hearing bilaterally as shown in ▶ Fig. 15.1.

15.3 Questions to the Reader

1. **What audiometric indications would suggest that the problem was not peripheral hearing loss, but more likely a central processing problem?**
2. **How could MM impact the function of the brain?**
3. **Do you believe her anxiety and tension exacerbated her clinical difficulties?**

15.4 Discussion of Questions

1. **What audiometric indications would suggest that the problem was not peripheral hearing loss, but more likely a central processing problem?**

Normal pure-tone thresholds, Speech Recognition Thresholds (SRT), and Word Recognition Scores (WRS) would indicate that the peripheral auditory system was normal, but the auditory-related symptoms suggested that the problems were higher in the auditory system.

2. **How could MM impact the function of the brain?**

MM is a group of neuromuscular diseases caused by damage to the mitochondria. Mitochondria are small, energy-producing structures that serve as the cells' "power plants." Nerve cells in the brain and muscles require a great deal of energy and thus appear to be particularly impaired when mitochondrial dysfunction occurs.[3]

3. **Do you believe her anxiety and tension exacerbated her clinical difficulties?**

Anxiety and tension can adversely affect the brain's capacity and interfere with executive function. This exacerbates one's difficulties. If BL's mitochondria or "power cells" are already impaired, adding complexities or worry will further reduce their capacity.

15.5 Additional Testing

BL and her sister completed the Buffalo Model Questionnaire (BMQ)[4,5,6] which provides insight into a patient's processing difficulties. The Buffalo Model is a conceptualization of auditory processing (AP) based on years of experience with patients with central auditory nervous system (CANS) lesions.[7,8] The Buffalo Model includes tests and test signs that are sensitive to CANS related regions.[8] This enabled the authors to categorize these signs and later relate them to specific academic and communicative disabilities.[9,10] BMQ (and the newer revision BMQ-R) enables adult patients or parents and teachers of children to indicate common characteristics, of the individual, that are associated with the four categories of the Buffalo Model. The Buffalo Model includes therapeutic techniques for each category that are successful in remediating auditory difficulties.[11]

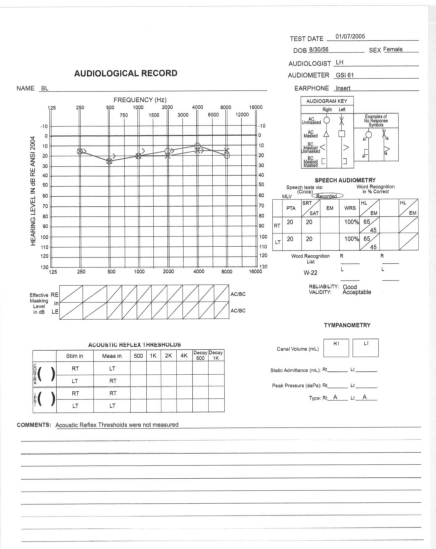

Fig. 15.1 Results of the audiometric evaluation of BL.

By using the three Buffalo Model tests (discussed later) and multidimensional scoring, we had 40 indicators that could provide multiple signs of each APD category.[11,12] The categories are Decoding (DEC), Tolerance-Fading Memory (TFM), Integration (INT), and Organization (ORG).[11] DEC determines if the person can quickly and accurately process speech. TFM involves difficulty understanding speech in background noise as well as short-term auditory memory. INT involves the ability to combine information from various parts of the brain, especially the interaction between the two hemispheres. ORG involves the ability to maintain proper sequence of auditory information and organization.

▶ Table 15.1 shows the number of BL's affirmative responses to 21 of the 32 questions related to APD categories. These results are especially severe for an adult patient. The responses to the questionnaire suggested that BL had three categories of APD. They are DEC, TFM, and INT. TFM appears a little more severe than the other two. This may be because of BL's anxiety and emotional issues that may exacerbate the TFM signs. TFM is associated with the anterior temporal and/or frontal functions when investigated in patients with brain lesion.[9]

Table 15.1 BMQ results for BL compared to the norms and number of questions for each category

Category	DEC	TFM	INT	ORG	Total
BL	5	9	4	0	18
Norms	0	2	0	1	3
No. of items	9	14	6	3	32

Abbreviations: BMQ, Buffalo Model Questionnaire; DEC, decoding; INT, Integration; ORG, organization; TFM, Tolerance-Fading Memory.
Note: Auditory Processing Disorder (APD) categories scored from the BMQ. APD ≥ 2 categories.

Clinically, BL appeared to be slow and inefficient in processing speech (DEC). In addition, BL had speech-in-noise, memory, and distraction problems (TFM). She also seemed to have difficulty transferring information from one hemisphere to the other (INT).

The AP battery included the Staggered Spondaic Word (SSW), Phonemic Synthesis (PS), and the Speech-in-Noise tests. The SSW is a widely used test of central auditory function.[13] This complex listening task not only provides a measure of dichotic listening but also contributes to the assessment of all four APD categories.[11,14] PS is a sound-by-sound presentation of words and the patient is instructed to combine the sounds and indicate the word that it forms. This requires important skills primarily associated with the auditory cortex.[15,16,17,18] The W-22 is a conventional word recognition test that is combined with speech spectrum noise to evaluate, understanding speech in the presence of background noise.

15.6 Final Diagnosis and Recommended Treatment

On the AP evaluation, BL's SSW score was 18 standard deviations (SDs) below normal, the PS score was 16 SDs below normal, and her Speech-in-Noise score was only mildly affected (right ear = 76%, the norm for which is 82%; left ear = 80%, the norm for which is 81%). She was diagnosed with DEC and TFM deficits. Initially, BL was not diagnosed with INT, because the most important sign (type A) was likely masked by her numerous DEC and TFM errors. However, using the two new additional measures (Standard Integration Ratio and Two-By-Three), INT would also be significant. Therapy addresses the simplest and the most basic skills first (e.g., DEC and TFM) and then the more complex category (INT), if needed.

15.7 Therapy

The Buffalo Model therapy procedure has been used effectively for decades.[18,19,20,21,22] AP training involves 14 sessions, one time per week, lasting 50 minutes each. One of the DEC training procedures is the Phonemic Training Program (PTP), which refines the patient's knowledge of what each phoneme sounds like and associates it with the phonic symbol. PS training is a recorded program that enables the patient to combine phonemes into words and reinforces the PTP training.[23] Words-In-Noise Training (WINT) was also administered. This speech in noise training increases the patient's ability to pull speech out, in the presence of background noise, by decreasing the signal-to-noise ratio (SNR) gradually over time.[11] Short-Term Auditory

Memory Training (STAM), which is part of TFM therapy, increases memory span for digits, words, and/or working memory using rote memory tasks. Finally, a dichotic listening INT task, Dichotic Offset Training (DOT), was used. This auditory therapy begins with presentation of four letters of the alphabet, two to each ear (similar to the SSW test using letters of the alphabet).[11] The competing words are separated by 500 ms. As the person improves, this separation gradually decreases to 0 ms. DOT helps to train the patient how to listen effectively to different stimuli in each ear. After each group of 14 sessions, BL was retested using the Central Test Battery to evaluate her progress.

15.8 Outcome

With auditory training, BL's AP skills began to improve, and within 4 years of therapy her SSW score improved to 5 SDs below normal. Her PS is essentially within normal limits. At one point, BL's physician told her that, when she started AP therapy, her vital signs and other functions improved. After 2 years of therapy, he informed BL that she would have to continue this therapy, for the remainder of her life, because of her regression when she had long vacations between therapy sessions. BL has now been in therapy for 12 years and will soon be 60 years old. Her audiometric pure-tone averages have remained essentially unchanged from 2005 to 2015 (▶ Fig. 15.2).

▶ Fig. 15.3 shows the results of BL's total SSW scores from 2005 to 2017, which show initial benefit from therapy and despite some fluctuations, her performance (2008–2009) has remained essentially unchanged over the past 7 years despite her degenerative condition. BL's number of errors decreased from 37 in 2005 to approximately 14 in 2017. ▶ Fig. 15.4 indicates her percentage correct on speech-in-noise testing over the years and ▶ Fig. 15.5 shows the PS testing results in total number correct. In recent years, therapy was directed to dichotic listening and auditory working memory, instead of DEC, because of her improved basic skills. This enabled BL to succeed with these more challenging tasks. We have noticed in the past few years that both Speech-in-Noise test and PS need to be addressed again due to the gradual decrease in these scores. Overall, after the 4 years of improvement her scores

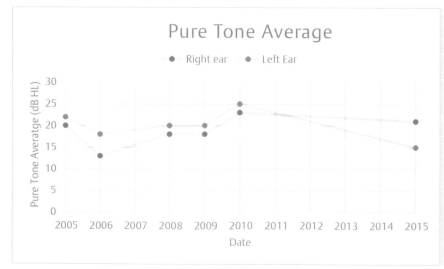

Fig. 15.2 Pure-tone average (dB HL) for the right and left ears from 2005 to 2017.

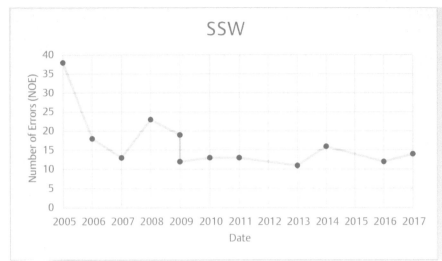

Fig. 15.3 Total number of error scores for the Staggered Spondaic Word (SSW) from 2005 to 2017. In 2009, the SSW was administered twice.

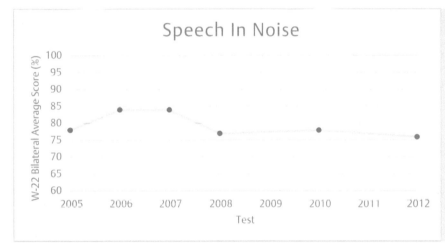

Fig. 15.4 Word Recognition Scores in noise from 2005 to 2012.

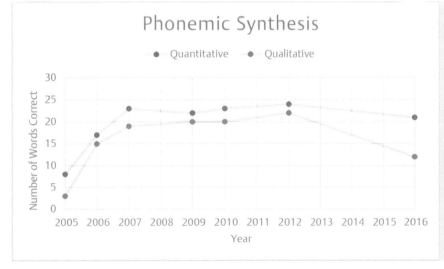

Fig. 15.5 Quantitative and qualitative number of words correct on the Phonemic Synthesis Test from 2005 to 2016.

fluctuated, but have essentially plateaued. Despite a decade of expected neurological "decline," APD therapy seems to have helped BL improve and then maintain her important auditory functions.

As noted earlier, recently, especially with longer vacation periods, BL has had some difficulties holding onto skills without further therapy. Generally, BL quickly regained what she lost when she returned to therapy although in the last few years it has taken longer to recover. The therapy has enabled BL to take part in her social life even in the presence of background noise. After 40 years of MM and 12 years of therapy, at the age of 60 years, BL's processing scores suggest she is generally maintaining her initial improvement despite the degenerative influences.

These impressive results with BL, and others we see with neurological impairment, encourage us to suggest to the reader not to deny therapy because of the presence of a serious diagnosis. We recommend providing therapy at a level to suit the person's status and to make the tasks more difficult as the person progresses.

15.9 Key Points

- APD can arise as part of a neurological or disease process such as degenerative disorders.
- Patients with degenerative diseases can benefit from Auditory Processing Therapy.
- Auditory Processing Therapy may help maintain the brain's ability to process or at least slow down the degenerative nature.

References

[1] Gorman GS, Schaefer AM, Ng Y, et al. Prevalence of nuclear and mitochondrial DNA mutations related to adult mitochondrial disease. Ann Neurol. 2015; 77 (5):753–759

[2] Muscular Dystrophy Associated Inc. Mitochondrial Myopathies. Available at: https://www.mda.org/disease/mitochondrial-myopathies/diagnosis. Accessed October 16, 2017

[3] BrainFacts.org. Neurological Diseases & Disorders A-Z from NINDS. Mitochondrial Myopathies. 2017. Available at: http://www.brainfacts.org/diseases-disorders/diseases-a-to-z-from-ninds/mitochondrial-myopathies/. Accessed October 16, 2017

[4] Katz J. The Buffalo Model Questionnaire (BMQ). SSW Reports. 2004; 26:5–6

[5] Katz J. The Buffalo Model Questionnaire: follow-up. SSW Reports.. 2006; 28: 1–3

[6] Pavlick M, Zalewski T, Gonzalez J, Duncan M. (C)APD screening instrument for the Buffalo model diagnostic test battery. J Edu Audiol Assoc. 2010; 16:4–13

[7] Katz J. The SSW test: an interim report. J Speech Hear Disord. 1968; 33(2): 132–146

[8] Katz J, Pack G. New developments in differential diagnosis using the SSW test. In: Sullivan, ed. Central Auditory Processing Disorders. Lincoln, NE: University of Nebraska Press; 1975:85–107

[9] Katz J. Classification of auditory processing disorders. In: Katz J, Stecker N, Henderson D. eds. Central Auditory Processing: A Transdisciplinary View. Chicago, IL: Mosby Yearbook; 1992:81–92

[10] Gallun FJ, Diedesch AC, Kubli LR, et al. Performance on tests of central auditory processing by individuals exposed to high-intensity blasts. J Rehabil Res Dev. 2012; 49(7):1005–1025

[11] Katz J. Therapy for Auditory Processing Disorders: Simple Effective Procedures. Pittsburgh, PA: Educational Audiology Association; 2009

[12] Katz J. APD evaluation to therapy: The Buffalo model. AudiologyOnline. 2007. Available at: http://www.audiologyonline.com/articles/apd-evaluation-to-therapy-buffalo-945

[13] Emanuel DC, Ficca KN, Korczak P. Survey of the diagnosis and management of auditory processing disorder. Am J Audiol. 2011; 20(1):48–60

[14] Jutras B, Loubert M, Dupuis JL, Marcoux C, Dumont V, Baril M. Applicability of central auditory processing disorder models. Am J Audiol. 2007; 16(2):100–106

[15] Katz J, Smith P. The Staggered Spondaic Word Test. A ten minute look at the central nervous system through the ears. Ann N Y Acad Sci. 1991; 620:233–252

[16] Luria A. Higher Cortical Functions in Man. New York, NY: Basic Books; 1966

[17] Luria A. Traumatic Aphasia: Its Syndromes, Psychology, and Treatment. The Hague: Mouton and Co.; 1970

[18] Katz J, Medol E. The use of phonemic synthesis in speech therapy. Menorah Med J. 1972; 3:10–13

[19] Katz J, Harmon C. Phonemic synthesis: diagnostic and training program. In: Keith R, ed. Central Auditory and Language Disorders in Children. San Diego, CA: College-Hill Press; 1981:145–157

[20] Katz J, King J. CAP approach for people with cochlear implants. Contact.. 2001; 14(4):39–42

[21] Kaul K, Lucker J. Auditory processing training with children diagnosed with auditory processing disorder: therapy based on the Buffalo model. J Educ Ped Habil Audiol. 2016; 22:1–10

[22] Reeves C, Lucker J. Analysis of changes in auditory processing after therapy. Topics Central Aud Process. 2017; 2(3):6–9

[23] Katz J. Phonemic training and phonemic synthesis programs. In: Geffner D, Ross-Swain D, eds. Auditory Processing Disorders: Management and Treatment. San Diego, CA: Plural Publishing Co; 2007:255–265

Suggested Readings

[1] Davis C. Mitochondrial Disease. Medicine Net. 2011. Available at: http://www.medicinenet.com/mitochondrial_disease/article.htm. Accessed July 10, 2017

[2] Katz J. Therapy for Auditory Processing Disorders: Simple Effective Procedures. Pittsburgh, PA: Educational Audiology Association

[3] Pfeffer G, Chinnery PF. Diagnosis and treatment of mitochondrial myopathies. Ann Med. 2013; 45(1):4–16

16 Asymmetric Hearing Loss: Evaluation, Diagnosis, and Treatment

Cathryn Collopy, Adam Voss, and Michael Valente

16.1 Clinical History and Description

EG is a 66-year-old male patient seen for an initial audiologic evaluation. EG reported gradual hearing loss that deteriorated slowly over the past 2 years. He reported the hearing in his right ear is better than his left ear. EG also reported constant tinnitus, slight aural fullness in the left ear, and increased difficulty hearing in background noise. In addition, EG reported that he finds himself asking for repetitions more often than in the past. EG denied otalgia or dizziness and reported a long history of unprotected noise exposure from working in factories for many years and using rifles held on the right shoulder.

16.2 Audiologic Testing

A comprehensive audiologic evaluation was performed. Otoscopic examination revealed clear external ear canals bilaterally. Pure-tone thresholds (▶ Fig. 16.1) in the right ear indicated hearing was normal at 250 to 500 Hz and then sloping from a mild sensorineural hearing loss (SNHL) at 1,000 to 2,000 Hz to a moderately severe SNHL at 4,000 to 8,000 Hz. Pure-tone thresholds in the left ear indicated hearing was normal at 250 to 500 Hz and then sloping from a mild SNHL at 1,000 Hz to a severe SNHL at 4,000 to 8,000 Hz. Speech Recognition Thresholds indicated a slight loss in the ability to receive speech in the right ear and a mild loss in the ability to receive speech in the left ear. Word Recognition Scores revealed normal ability to recognize speech in the right ear and slight difficulty in the ability to recognize speech in the left ear. Immittance revealed normal middle ear pressure (daPa), ear canal volume (mL), and static admittance (mL) in each ear. Ipsilateral acoustic reflex thresholds (ARTs) were normal at 500 to 2,000 Hz and absent at 4,000 Hz in the right ear. Ipsilateral ARTs were normal at 500 Hz, elevated at 1,000 and 2,000 Hz, and absent at 4,000 Hz in the left ear. Contralateral ARTs were normal at 500 Hz and absent at all other frequencies probe left and within normal limits at 500 and 1,000 Hz and absent at all other frequencies probe right. Reflex decay was normal in the right ear and could not be tested in the left ear. Elevated ARTs correlate with a cochlear loss, while absent ARTs indicate a severe cochlear loss or the presence of a retrocochlear pathology.[1]

16.3 Questions to the Reader

1. **In the audiologic examination of EG, what "red flag(s)" are present? Based on these results, what disorder might be suspected?**
2. **What recommendation(s) should be made for EG?**
3. **How should EG be counseled at this time?**

16.4 Discussion of Questions

1. **In the audiologic examination of EG, what "red flag(s)" are present? Based on these results, what disorder might be suspected?**

The "red flags" present are asymmetric hearing loss, left-sided tinnitus, and left-sided aural fullness. Also, the tinnitus and aural fullness are on the ear with poorer hearing, illustrating an asymmetry of auditory symptoms.[2] These results suggest possible retrocochlear pathology. Studies report incidence rates of retrocochlear pathology when asymmetric hearing loss is present to be between 2 and 8%, depending on the definition of asymmetric hearing loss.[3] When a retrocochlear pathology is suspected, a physician referral is mandated in order to determine if hearing aid use is contraindicated.[4]

2. **What recommendation(s) should be made for EG?**

Due to possible left-sided retrocochlear pathology, EG should be referred to an otologist for further examination. The otologist may order an Auditory Brainstem Response (ABR) and/or a Magnetic Resonance Imaging (MRI).

3. **How should EG be counseled at this time?**

The audiologist should counsel EG on the results of the audiologic examination. Possibility of pathology past the cochlea should be discussed. EG should be counseled to schedule an appointment with an otologist for further medical examination. Amplification should be discussed, noting that medical clearance must be provided. Hearing protection in noise should also be recommended.

16.5 Diagnosis and Recommended Treatment

EG was referred to Otology due to his asymmetry in hearing thresholds, unilateral tinnitus, and aural fullness on the same side as the poorer hearing ear. After the initial otologic evaluation, no obvious reasons for the asymmetry were reported, except the possibility of asymmetry strictly due to noise exposure (recall EG was a right-handed rifle shooter). In many clinics, EG may not have even been referred to Otology due to the assumption that noise exposure was the sole cause of the asymmetry in hearing and symptoms. Audiologists practicing under best practice guidelines[5] should learn to "assume the worst" until proven otherwise; in other words, refer to Otology for further evaluation when asymmetric symptoms are present, even if there appears to be a cause. This may lead to some "overreferrals," but may be a better strategy than not referring at all. The otologist ordered an ABR to determine neural function and an

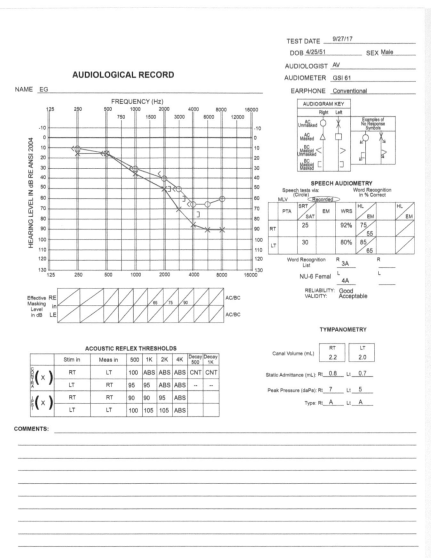

Fig. 16.1 Initial audiologic examination.

MRI of the internal auditory canal region to rule out any retrocochlear pathology. ABR testing was completed utilizing rarefaction polarity click stimuli presented at 11.1 and 71.3 clicks per second. A presentation level of 90 dBnHL was utilized and technical recording quality was excellent. In each ear, absolute and interpeak latency for waves I to V were normal. ABR test results did not suggest auditory nerve or auditory brainstem dysfunction. EG underwent an MRI with and without contrast. Results indicated normal internal auditory canals bilaterally (i.e., clear of retrocochlear pathology). EG was scheduled for a follow-up visit with Otology to review and discuss the results of the ABR and MRI. At that visit, EG was cleared to pursue amplification (i.e., hearing aids and hearing assistive technology).

16.6 Hearing Aid Evaluation

After receiving medical clearance from the otologist, EG returned for a hearing aid evaluation (HAE). At the appointment, unaided QuickSIN[6] assessment was performed binaurally in the sound field with the signal presented at 40 dB HL from a loudspeaker located at 0-degree azimuth and multi-talker

babble presented from 180-degree azimuth. The signal is a female talker reciting lists of sentences. The patient is instructed to repeat what he hears and is encouraged to guess. Each list has six sentences, one sentence at each Signal-to-Noise Ratio (SNR) of 25, 20, 15, 10, 5, and 0 dB. These SNRs encompass the range of normal to severely impaired performance in noise. Each sentence has five keywords that are scored as correct or incorrect.[6] An unaided Signal-to-Noise Ratio Hearling Loss (SNRHL) of 14 dB was measured (moderate loss). An SNRHL of 14 dB suggests that hearing aids alone could not provide sufficient amplification to improve EG's primary complaint of difficulty in hearing speech in noise. Devices such as the remote microphone should be considered to assist hearing aids for better performance in background noise or challenging listening environments. Loudness Discomfort Levels (LDLs)[7] were evaluated using TDH-50 earphones. EG was provided a printed sheet with Contour Loudness categories and instructed to make loudness judgments (1–7) as the presentation level increased[7]:

7. Uncomfortably loud

6. Loud, but okay

5. Comfortable, but slightly loud

4. Comfortable
3. Comfortable, but slightly soft
2. Soft
1. Very soft

This procedure was repeated until the category "loud, but okay" (number 6) was measured. A series of ascending pulsed warble-tone stimuli were used at 500, 1,000, 2,000, and 4,000 Hz.[7] EG's LDLs were found to be within the normal range at all frequencies tested. These results are used in order to determine if the Real Ear Saturation Response (RESR) using a loud sweep signal is below the LDL. For a successful hearing aid fit, it is important that hearing aids never exceed what EG perceived as "too loud." The unaided Client Oriented Scale of Improvement (COSI)[8] was collected (▶ Fig. 16.2). EG reported he would like to improve hearing when (1) watching television, (2) at a restaurant with his wife, and (3) hearing his grandchildren. After discussing the differences between levels of hearing aid technology including the number of channels and bands, sophistication of the hearing aid's automatic program, and flexibility in the direct streaming iPhone applications, EG elected to pursue bilateral ReSound LiNX 3D 9 62 RIC (receiver in canal) hearing aids and a ReSound wireless remote Multi Mic. EG understood that his hearing aids would be under warranty with the manufacturer for 3 years, which would include all services at the clinic, manufacturer repairs to the hearing aids, and a one-time loss and damage policy for each device. At the end of 3 years, EG acknowledged that he would have the choice of extending the warranty for another year or to let the warranty expire. Should EG choose to not extend the warranty, he understood that the clinic adopts an unbundled approach and would expect fees for hearing aid maintenance, replacement of receivers, and any reprogramming. He also understood that there would be a fee attached to any repair completed by the manufacturer. Bilateral silicone impressions were taken without incident. The patient was scheduled for a Hearing Aid Fitting (HAF) in 2 weeks. After the HAE, the audiologist completed the manufacturer hearing aid and earmold order forms which were sent with the impressions to ReSound for processing. One and a half weeks following the order, EG's hearing aids arrived at the clinic. All characteristics including hearing aid model, color, receiver wire length, and power were correct. The earmold features, such as the vent size, bore length, color, and material, were ensured to be as ordered. Verification testing was completed using the ANSI S3.22–2009 test with each hearing aid in test mode on a FONIX 8000 Hearing Aid Test System from Frye Electronics. Testing met manufacturer specifications for each aid. Verification of the directional microphone performance was completed on a FONIX 8000 and indicated the directional microphones were operating properly.

National Acoustic Laboratories
A division of Australian Hearing

NAL
CLIENT ORIENTED SCALE OF IMPROVEMENT

Name : E.G. Category. New X Return
Audiologist : Audiologist
Date : 1. Needs Established HAE
2. Outcome Assessed HAA

Degree of Change

Final Ability (with hearing aid)
Person can hear
10% 25% 50% 75% 95%

SPECIFIC NEEDS

Indicate Order of Significance

Specific need	Worse	No Difference	Slightly Better	Better	Much Better	CATEGORY	Hardly Ever	Occasionally	Half the Time	Most of Time	Almost Always
1 Hearing my wife better in noisy restaurants				X						X	
2 Hearing my grandchildren better than I currently do				X						X	
3 Hearing and understanding my TV, and the volume be lower					X						X

Categories
1. Conversation with 1 or 2 in quiet
2. Conversation with 1 or 2 in noise
3. Conversation with group in quiet
4. Conversation with group in noise
5. Television/Radio @ normal volume
6. Familiar speaker on phone
7. Unfamiliar speaker on phone
8. Hearing phone ring from another room
9. Hear front door bell or knock
10. Hear traffic
11. Increased social contact
12. Feel embarrassed or stupid
13. Feeling left out
14. Feeling upset or angry
15. Church or meeting
16. Other

Fig. 16.2 Unaided and aided COSI.

16.7 Hearing Aid Fitting

The hearing aids were connected to the manufacturer's fitting software within the NOAH fitting module. Real-Ear Measurements (REM) were performed on the FONIX 8000 to establish appropriate prescriptive real-ear insertion gain (corrected for 17 channel summation and binaural summation [3–5 dB]). REM for nonlinear hearing aids were performed with input levels of 50, 65, and 80 dB SPL (sound pressure level) that provided appropriate gain and a smooth frequency response. Aided loudness judgments was performed with a composite speech signal provided by the FONIX 8000 and EG reported 50 dB SPL as "soft," 65 dB SPL as "comfortable," and 80 dB SPL as "loud, but okay." An RESR90 was performed at 90 dB SPL and the patient did not report loudness discomfort. Maximum output of the hearing aids was programmed so that each frequency did not exceed the unaided LDLs[7] at each frequency. The following programs were activated in EG's hearing aid settings: All-Around, Restaurant, Party, and T-coil. The hearing aids were paired to EG's iPhone for direct streaming of cellphone calls to his hearing aids as well as for utilizing the Smart 3D app. He was counseled on how to wirelessly stream signals from the remote Multi Mic and in which situations it may be helpful. In addition, he was shown how to deactivate his hearing aid microphones and just receive input from the Multi Mic in noisy environments (accessed in the iPhone app). Next, EG was counseled on all the special features of the Smart 3D app (i.e., reducing background noise and "narrowing the beam" of speech input in the Restaurant and Party programs) and when to switch his hearing aids from program to program. He was also counseled on potential use of the telecoil (T-coil) within the hearing aids that can be activated for use in environments with looping capability. EG was then counseled on the use and maintenance of the hearing aids and earmolds. Warranty information was reviewed and questions were answered. The hearing aid contract was reviewed and signed. EG scheduled a follow-up visit in 2 weeks.

16.8 Hearing Aid Assessment and Outcome

Two weeks after the HAF, EG returned for a hearing aid assessment. EG reported doing well with the hearing aids in most listening situations, but was still having difficulty hearing and understanding speech in noisy places. EG reported that he prefers using the iPhone app to adjust volume and settings. EG reported hearing well when using his cellphone through direct streaming. EG reported he had not utilized the Multi Mic much. EG was counseled on the importance of using the remote Multi Mic when he finds his hearing aids are not providing adequate benefit in noise. He was counseled to use the microphone to correct for background noise, reverberation, and distance. Next, his hearing aids were connected to the fitting software, and the Restaurant and Party programs were modified and the frequency response was adjusted to provide more high-frequency emphasis and the noise reduction was programmed to be stronger. He was re-counseled on utilizing the features in the Smart 3D app where he can adjust the noise reduction and "beam focus" of the speech signal. EG then completed the aided COSI[8] (▶ Fig. 16.2). Results of the aided COSI[8] revealed that with

hearing aids, EG is hearing better or much better in his listening environments as compared to performance without hearing aids. Aided QuickSIN[6] testing was performed and EG demonstrated significant improvement when compared to unaided performance. His aided SNRHL was 6 dB (mild SNR loss) as compared to 14 dB (moderate SNR loss) at the HAE. Although improved from unaided, a 6 dB SNRHL is still not within the normal range and since EG was still having difficulty hearing in background noise, this is further proof of how remote microphone technology could help him in noise. EG was encouraged to utilize the Multi Mic in noisy listening environments. Lastly, a 2cc coupler measurement (electroacoustic analysis) was performed on the FONIX 8000 at user settings and will be used as a baseline measurement for future tests. EG returned 2 weeks later and reported he has been hearing significantly better and using the Multi Mic has been a significant help. EG is scheduled for a hearing aid check (HAC) in 6 months and will return sooner if needed. At the 6 month HAC, EG's hearing aids will be cleaned and evaluated. Electroacoustic analysis will be performed again and the results will be compared to the baseline measurement. EG's hearing needs will be assessed and any programming adjustments will be made in the software, if required. EG will be provided with any supplies (wax guards, sanitizer spray, etc.), as needed.

16.9 Key Points

- When a patient presents with asymmetrical SNHL, unilateral tinnitus, and aural fullness, a referral to Otology is necessary to rule out any retrocochlear disorder.
- It is important to acknowledge the time and expense required by the patient, audiologist, and otologist to resolve a possible retrocochlear disorder (i.e., audiologic evaluation, otology visit, ABR, MRI, follow-up, etc.). As a result, it may be expected that an otologist may adopt a "watch and wait" medical treatment plan, especially for elderly patients, and recommend reevaluation of hearing in 6 months or a year to determine if further testing is warranted.
- ABR assesses auditory nerve and brainstem function/dysfunction. The MRI is an objective, structural imaging test. Often, otologists will order MRI immediately in cases of asymmetrical symptoms and forego the ABR since if an ABR is abnormal, an MRI will likely be ordered.
- Hearing aids and assistive technology are important treatment options for significantly improving hearing and the quality of life for patients with hearing loss.

References

[1] Silman S, Gelfand SA. The relationship between magnitude of hearing loss and acoustic reflex threshold levels. J Speech Hear Disord. 1981; 46(3):312–316

[2] Acoustic Neuroma. Consens Statement. 1991; 9(4):1–24

[3] Kesser BW. Clinical thresholds for when to test for retrocochlear lesions: con. Arch Otolaryngol Head Neck Surg. 2010; 136(7):727–729

[4] Food and Drugs Administration. Code of Federal Regulations, Title 21: Food and drugs, Subchapter H, Part 801, Subpart H §801.421. Fed Regist. 1977; 42: 9286–9296

[5] Valente M, Abrams H, Benson D, et al. Guidelines for the audiologic management of adult hearing impairment. Task Force. Available at: https://audiol-

ogy-web.s3.amazonaws.com/migrated/haguidelines.
pdf_53994876e92e42.70908344.pdf. 2006

[6] Killion MC, Niquette PA, Gudmundsen GI, Revit LJ, Banerjee S. Development of a quick speech-in-noise test for measuring signal-to-noise ratio loss in normal-hearing and hearing-impaired listeners. J Acoust Soc Am. 2004; 116(4 Pt 1):2395–2405

[7] Formby C, Payne J, Yang X, Wu D, Parton JM. Repeated measurement of absolute and relative judgements of loudness: clinical relevance for prescriptive fitting of aided target gains for soft, comfortable, and loud, but ok sound levels. Semin Hear. 2017; 38(1):2G–52

[8] Dillon H, James A, Ginis J. Client Oriented Scale of Improvement (COSI) and its relationship to several other measures of benefit and satisfaction provided by hearing aids. J Am Acad Audiol. 1997; 8(1):27–43

17 The Origins of Physiologic Modulation of a Low-Noise Microphone in a Human Ear Canal

Hannah R. Burrick, Deepa Suneel, Richard A. Chole, Craig A. Buchman, Spencer B. Smith, Choongheon Lee, Ken E. Hancock, Glenis R. Long, Sumitrajit Dhar, Amanda J. Ortmann, Bryan K. Ward, and Jeffery T. Lichtenhan

17.1 Introduction

Clinicians often encounter patients with vague or intermittent auditory symptoms or difficult to interpret auditory measurements. New diagnostic tests may help expand our understanding of these irregularities. Idiosyncratic signals such as those found here may lead to new clinical tests and perhaps a better understanding of auditory physiology.

17.2 Clinical History and Description

A 23-year-old female volunteered to be a participant in a research study in the Department of Otolaryngology, Head & Neck Surgery, at Washington University School of Medicine in St. Louis. All procedures were approved by the Institutional Review Board of Washington University in St. Louis. The participant was asymptomatic. She passed a hearing screening at 20 dB HL from 250 to 8,000 Hz and denied specific otologic symptoms including tinnitus, otalgia, aural fullness, dizziness, or vertigo. She denied any current medications, a family history of hearing loss, or a personal history of otitis media, head or neck surgery, head trauma or skull fracture, chemotherapy, or radiation therapy. No spontaneous otoacoustic emissions (OAEs), in the traditional sense, were detectable above an average noise floor of –20 dB SPL (sound pressure level). Traditionally, spontaneous OAEs are steady state, ongoing sounds. The measures found in our participant were transient.

17.3 Clinical Testing

17.3.1 Audiologic Testing

Measurements were made from the participant seated in a sound-treated room using the Eaton Peabody Laboratories Cochlear Function Test Suite used with an ER-10C Distortion Product Otoacoustic Emissions (DPOAEs) probe system. In situ calibration was completed before each series of measurements. DPOAE amplitudes were within normal limits; however, there were modulations of the noise floor, or "spikes" large enough to disrupt DPOAE measurements (▶ Fig. 17.1a).

After observing the spikes, the authors stopped delivering tones to the ear making DPOAE measurements and completed ear canal measurements in the absence of any external sound. Modulations of the noise floor continued demonstrating that external stimuli used to elicit DPOAEs were not causing these spikes. The measurements discussed below are from one 20 Hz spectral bin (typically centered at 2,840 Hz) from a low-noise microphone without any external sounds such as those used for DPOAE measurements. The authors, however, found that the spike is broadband in that all spectral bins up to 20,000 Hz would "spike" simultaneously (data not shown).

The participant was instructed not to swallow in order for the measures to be accurate because swallowing caused a modulation of the noise floor during the measurements similar to the modulations the authors were documenting. The participant was instructed to report if a swallow occurred while measurements were being made and those runs were eliminated from the analysis.

Patulous Eustachian Tube Dysfunction: Ruled Out

It is well known that patients with Patulous Eustachian Tube Dysfunction (PETD) can alter ear canal admittance measurements with breathing manipulations such as ipsilateral nasal breathing.[1] The participant completed a series of voluntarily forced breathing manipulations over 60 seconds, and no change in spikes were observed that coincided with nasal breathing (▶ Fig. 17.1b–e). The authors completed the same breathing manipulations on a standard clinical admittance meter and did not find changes indicative of PETD (data not shown), thereby ruling out PETD as an origin of the participant's physiologic modulation of the low-noise ear canal microphone.

Saccade-Induced Tympanic Membrane Movements: Ruled Out

Saccadic eye movements trigger tympanic membrane movements opposite the eye movement, followed by an oscillation, and have been detected by an in-ear microphone.[2] Voluntary saccades also reduce in amplitude when the eyes are closed.[3] The participant shifted gaze multiple times during 60-second measurement runs, with her eyes both open and closed (▶ Fig. 17.1f,g). The number of spikes was unchanged compared to other runs and the amplitude of the spike was not affected by eyes-closed saccades. The authors ruled out saccade-induced tympanic-membrane movements as an origin of physiologic modulation of the low-noise microphone in this participant's ear canal.

Postural-Induced Intracranial Pressure Changes: Ruled Out

Voluntary alterations of intracranial pressure can be performed with postural changes.[4] The authors made measurements with the participant sitting upright at 90 degrees (▶ Fig. 17.1h), lying supine at 0 degrees (▶ Fig. 17.1i), and reclined back in a chair at 30 degrees (▶ Fig. 17.1j), which has been the baseline posture. In each of these postural conditions, the spikes remained, with no changes in amplitude or frequency of occurrence. The authors concluded that intracranial pressure changes due to changes in posture did not have an influence on this participant's spikes.

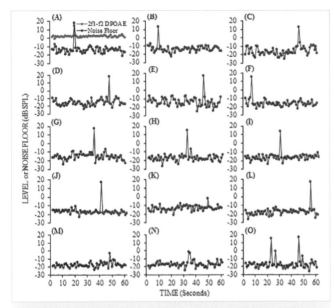

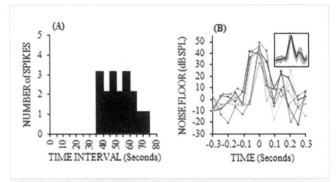

Fig. 17.2 (a) The frequency of occurrence and (b) time course of physiologic modulation of a low-noise microphone in the ear canal, or "spike." Noise floor measurements were recorded four times, each for a duration of 5 minutes. The time between spikes was quantified. (a) The maximal time intervals between spikes ranged from 35 to 75 seconds. The authors lowered the duration of the recording buffer to the smallest value available, which was 50 ms. This gave the authors 1,280 samples per minute. The spikes measured during these recordings are expressed in panel B relative to the maximum sound pressure level (SPL) of the noise floor modulation. The mean (black) ± 1 standard deviation (gray) is presented in the panel inset. A second, smaller spike may perhaps be seen with shorter recording buffer duration. The faster sampling resolution effectively lessened the duration of non-spiking measurements in the mean spike and yielded a more accurate measure of just how intense our participant's physiologic modulation of the low-noise microphone can be: 42.35 (± 5.58) dB SPL.

Fig. 17.1 (a) Noise floor of a low-noise microphone in the ear canal as a function of measurement time. Measures of distortion product otoacoustic emission (DPOAE) amplitude at $2f_1$–f_2 DPOAE (red) and noise floor (black) show that biological modulation of the noise floor, or a "spike," can be large enough to disrupt DPOAE amplitude measurements (155.1). (Within this figure legend, the authors list the run number after the panel identifier for record keeping purposes.) The participant performed forced inspiration and expiration through (b) right nostril (123.1), (c) left nostril (124.1), (d) both nostrils (126.1), (e) and held her breath (137.1). (f) Gaze shifts with eyes open (116.1) (g) and eyes closed (114.1) did not increase the number of spikes. Changing posture from 90-degree (h) upright position (178.1), (i) supine position (148.1), (j) and 30-degree reclining back (174.1) did not alter spikes. (k) A spike could be recorded in the left ear, but to a smaller extent (143.1). Changing blood pressure did change the spike: (o) After the typical course of a measurement (110.1), the participant applied pressure to the (p) right neck to occlude the jugular vein (171.1) (q) and left neck (175.1). The amplitude of physiological modulation of a low-noise microphone noise floor was clearly reduced by applying the pressure to the neck over the jugular vein. (h) Increasing heart rate with 50 jumping jacks increased the spike rate (177.1).

Contraction of Mouth Musculature: Ruled Out

The authors considered involuntary jaw musculature contraction as an origin of the spikes. A measurement was made with the participant's jaw slightly open. The authors hypothesized that opening the jaw would increase the area over which a contraction would occur and reduce the SPL of the spike. With the participant's mouth open, the spike remained at 20 dB SPL, the baseline amplitude of the modulation (data not shown).

17.3.2 Otologic Examination

With a Toynbee stethoscope (Toynbee tube[5]) positioned over the participant's ear canals, the otologist (RAC) reported that he could hear a faint "click" from both ear canals, with the right ear more audible than the left. RAC's auditory function was normal when tested in a double walled acoustic booth. His

pure-tone average was 8.3 dB HL in the right ear and 10 dB HL in the left ear and the Speech Reception Threshold (SRT) was 10 dB HL bilaterally.

Myoclonus or Tremor: Ruled Out

Myoclonus or tremor of the stapedius, tensor tympani, tensor veli palatini, or levator veli palatini muscles was considered. Palatal tremor and tympanic membrane movements were not observed. The frequencies of these otologic tremors are significantly greater than what the authors observed.[6,7] While rates of otologic myoclonus and tremors have some variation across patients, they all occur at a much higher rate than the interspike interval of 35 to 75 seconds measured from the participant (▶ Fig. 17.2). Middle ear myoclonus is typically audible to patients because they report hearing periodic clicking sounds. These clicking sounds can coincide with tympanic membrane movements that are visible with a binocular microscopy examination of the ear. It is unknown if there are milder forms that go unnoticed by the person and not visible to the otologist. Our participant could not hear her spikes and no tympanic membrane movements were observed.

Paragangliomas (Glomus Tumors): Ruled Out

Paragangliomas (glomus tympanicum or glomus jugulare) are benign, highly vascular tumors of the temporal bone. Pulsatile sounds from these tumors become audible to patients because of the blood flow near the ear or when they contact the tympanic membrane, round window, or the ossicular chain. These vascular sounds of the tumor are transmitted to the inner ear.

The sounds are usually audible and are coincident with the pulse. The participant's spikes were not audible to her and were not coincident with her pulse. On binocular microscopy, the participant had normal appearing tympanic membranes and aerated middle ears, ruling out a glomus tympanicum tumor and a glomus jugulare tumor invading the middle ear.

17.4 Questions to the Reader

1. **How did the authors know the modulations are not from an equipment malfunction?**
2. **Clinicians and scientists often ask the authors if the spikes were audible to the participant.**
3. **What is the relationship between eardrum excursions and audibility?**

17.5 Discussion of Questions

1. **How did the authors know the modulations are not from an equipment malfunction?**

The authors completed similar measurements on over 100 other study participants in whom the authors did not see physiologic modulation of the OAE probe microphone. Additionally, when making measurements on the participant of this case study, the authors completed some measurement runs with the DPOAE probe system hanging outside of her ear canal resting on her body. The noise floor measures were stable without significant modulations, meaning that the modulations are unique to this participant and her ear canal.

2. **Clinicians and scientists often ask the authors if the spikes were audible to the participant.**

The spikes were inaudible to the participant. The authors lowered the duration of the recording buffer to the smallest value available, which was 50 ms. This gave the authors 1,280 samples per minute. This allowed the authors to exclude more non-spiking moments of time in the sample. The authors found that the spike could be as intense as 50 dB SPL when the authors did not include non-spiking moments of time (▶ Fig. 17.2b). Nevertheless, the spikes were not audible to the participant.

3. **What is the relationship between eardrum excursions and audibility?**

The participant could not hear her spikes. Patients with superior canal dehiscence syndrome sometimes have audible pulsations that can be measurable with immittance, and these patients often have pulsatile tinnitus. Patients with patulous eustachian tube can have observable ear drum movements and be asymptomatic.[8] There must likely be a threshold at which eardrum pulsations become audible, but this is unknown.

17.6 Description of the Disorder and Recommended Treatment

While the authors do not yet know what is causing the modulations of the low-noise microphone, the authors found a few manipulations that altered the physiologic modulation in amplitude, frequency of occurrence, or both.

17.6.1 Switching the OAE Probe from the Right to Left Ear

All measurements discussed thus far were made in the participant's right ear canal. On switching the probe into the left ear, the modulation was present, but had decreased amplitude (▶ Fig. 17.1k). This finding is consistent with the louder audible click heard by the otologist when listening with a Toynbee tube in the participant's right ear canal. The otologist was unaware that lower amplitude spikes had been measured in the participant's left ear canal. These results show the amplitude of the physiologic modulation of the low-noise microphone is ear dependent in our participant.

17.6.2 Applying Light Pressure to the Neck

The participant used her hands to lightly apply pressure to her left or right neck in the area of the jugular veins throughout the duration of a measurement run. Neck pressure altered the amplitude of the spikes (▶ Fig. 17.1l-n), regardless of the side compressed. The modulation was notable even with an increased variability in the measurement noise floor during the recordings, suggesting that the blood flow, and perhaps a jugular vein, may play a role in spike generation. However, the authors do not suspect vascular anomalies. Dehiscences in the bony covering of the carotid artery or the jugular venous system can cause a swishing or pulsing sound in the ear. These sounds are clearly different than those observed in this participant in that they are pulsatile and coincident with the pulse.

17.6.3 Alterations with Activity

Measurements were made immediately after increased physical activity. The participant performed 50 jumping jacks prior to a measurement. This increased the frequency of occurrence of the modulations, with two large amplitude and two smaller amplitude modulations over 60 seconds (▶ Fig. 17.1o). This activity not only increased the frequency of the typically seen modulations, but also added smaller modulations immediately after the typically seen modulations, which the authors had not observed previously. A finding consistent with this observation is that a greater frequency of spiking was often found at the beginning of a test session, or right after a break, as the participant started to relax (data not shown).

17.7 Outcome

While it is too soon to make a clear statement about what is causing the modulations of the biological noise floor, the authors can hypothesize. The auditory system can be thought of as a bank of filters. The middle ear, for example, is a bandpass filter that is associated with the frequency range over which a mammal can hear. While the authors measured the spike at only one frequency bin, all frequency bins up to 20,000 Hz were affected, suggesting that middle ear filtering influences our measures of the spikes. There are many other "acoustic filters" within, and around, the head and neck, not only within ear. It is possible that one of these filters is being rung by the participant's physiologic noise, causing the spiking that was measured.

The consistency of the spiking is notable, occurring over the days, weeks, and months of performing the various manipulations for this case study. While the participant may remain asymptomatic regarding this consistent anomaly for the remainder of her life, there is a chance later she will develop audiologic symptoms. A patient or research participant with unexplained audiologic symptoms should be monitored. As audiologists and individuals involved with hearing health it is our duty to study abnormalities to achieve best practice.

17.8 Key Points

- At the time of the modulations, the normal DPOAE measurements were altered in both amplitude and signal-to-noise ratio (SNR). If clinical DPOAE measurements were taken at the point of occurrence of this modulation, the audiologist could incorrectly conclude absent or abnormal DPOAEs based on the minimal SNR. For example, when making DPOAE frequency sweeps in the clinic, randomly spaced amplitude measures with poor SNR may perhaps be related to physiologic modulation of the DPOAE probe microphone.
- Aberrant middle ear muscle reflexes measurements can happen from time to time and disappear when measurements are repeated. It may be possible that any patient may perhaps have similar "spiking" as our participant.

- Anomalous findings occur in the lab and clinic. This report is a demonstration of troubleshooting following such an anomalous finding. The authors believe they have addressed many possible causes. What remains is a poorly understood biologic phenomenon that may perhaps in time tell clinicians something not known about how the auditory system works.

References

[1] Henry DF, DiBartolomeo JR. Patulous eustachian tube identification using tympanometry. J Am Acad Audiol. 1993; 4(1):53–57

[2] Gruters KG, Murphy DLK, Jenson CD, Smith DW, Shera CA, Groh JM. The eardrums move when the eyes move: a multisensory effect on the mechanics of hearing. Proc Natl Acad Sci U S A. 2018; 115(6):E1309–E1318

[3] Shaikh AG, Wong AL, Optican LM, Miura K, Solomon D, Zee DS. Sustained eye closure slows saccades. Vision Res. 2010; 50(17):1665–1675

[4] Chapman PH, Cosman ER, Arnold MA. The relationship between ventricular fluid pressure and body position in normal subjects and subjects with shunts: a telemetric study. Neurosurgery. 1990; 26(2):181–189

[5] Toynbee J. The Diseases of the Ear: Their Nature, Diagnosis and Treatment. London: John Churchill; 1860:190–191

[6] Jamieson DR, Mann C, O'Reilly B, Thomas AM. Ear clicks in palatal tremor caused by activity of the levator veli palatini. Neurology. 1996; 46(4):1168–1169

[7] Ellenstein A, Yusuf N, Hallett M. Middle ear myoclonus: two informative cases and a systematic discussion of myogenic tinnitus. Tremor Other Hyperkinet Mov (N Y). 2013; 3:3

[8] Ward BK, Ashry Y, Poe DS. Patulous eustachian tube dysfunction: patient demographics and comorbidities. Otol Neurotol. 2017; 38(9):1362–1369

18 Occupational Noise-Induced Hearing Loss in a Zumba Instructor: Identification and Management

Oscar M. Cañete and Abin Kuruvilla-Mathew

18.1 Clinical History and Description

PM (a 27-year-old female) was referred to our Audiology clinic by a friend in August 2016. PM reported no difficulties communicating in groups or in noisy listening environments. She reported, however, a history of intermittent bilateral "buzzing" after listening to music via headphones for long periods. The "buzzing" lasted only for a few minutes without any noticeable change in hearing. PM presented with excellent health and provided a negative history of otologic diseases. PM has been working as a part-time Zumba fitness instructor for the past 2 years (six classes per week, 45–50 minutes each class). Classes are taught to large groups in a space large enough to accommodate 100 participants.

18.2 Audiologic Examination

Otoscopy revealed easily identifiable tympanic membranes bilaterally. Pure-tone air conduction audiometry indicated normal hearing bilaterally with the exception of a notch of 30 dB HL at 6,000 Hz in the left ear (▸ Fig. 18.1). Word Recognition Scores (WRS) were assessed using monitored live-voice presentation of disyllabic words (a 25-word list). A score of 100% was obtained in each ear at a presentation level of 40 dB HL. Immittance audiometry indicated Type A tympanograms bilaterally with normal ear canal volume (mL), middle ear pressure (daPa), and static admittance (mL). Ipsilateral acoustic reflex thresholds (ARTs) were within normal limits for 500, 1,000, 2,000, and 4,000 Hz bilaterally. Contralateral ARTs were not measured.

18.3 Additional Testing

Due to the history of work-related noise exposure, Distortion Product Otoacoustic Emissions (DPOAEs) and Transient Otoacoustic Emissions (TOAEs) were measured to detect subtle noise-induced changes in outer hair cell function. DPOAE amplitudes in the right ear were within normal range (0 > dB SPL, Sound Pressure Level, and ≥ 7 dB SNR, Signal-to-Noise Ratio)[1] for all test frequencies except at 3,500 Hz and 6,250 Hz. The left ear revealed a similar pattern up to 4,500 Hz with the exception of frequencies between 4,750 and 6,500 Hz (seven frequencies) that were present, but at a significantly lower amplitude (< 0 dB SPL)[1] (▸ Fig. 18.2). TOAEs responses, however, were within the normal range values (> 20 dB SPL)[1] for all test frequencies in both ears (▸ Fig. 18.3). In addition, Auditory Brainstem Response (ABR) was obtained to assess cochlear nerve integrity. Click stimuli was presented at 70 dB nHL in both ears separately at 45.1/s in alternating polarity. Absolute and interpeak latencies for Waves I, III, and V were normal for each ear (▸ Fig. 18.4). All electrophysiologic measures were obtained using the Interacoustics Eclipse EP25 (v4.5) for ABRs,

Eclipse TOAE25 (v3.04.2) for transient OAEs, and Eclipse DPOAE20 (v1.03.1) for DPOAEs.

18.3.1 Second Visit

Pure-tone audiometry did not reveal any change in hearing thresholds for the audiometric frequencies in both ears between visits. DPOAEs were repeated and a similar pattern with low response amplitude across selected frequencies was observed in both ears (▸ Fig. 18.2). In addition, PM was asked to complete a questionnaire (Knowledge, Attitudes, and Behavior, KAB)[2] concerning hearing loss prevention in order to determine PM's attitude toward hearing conservation. The attitude score in an individual could range from –50 (negative attitude) to +50 (positive attitude). PM's scores on to the questionnaire indicated that PM had an average knowledge (56.3%) concerning the impact of noise on the auditory system.[2] Positive scores on benefit (e.g., believing that hearing well is important), severity (e.g., believing that a hearing loss would have negative consequences), and barriers (e.g., perceiving few negative influences to protecting hearing) suggest that PM shows a positive attitude toward hearing loss prevention. However, because PM's self-efficacy score (e.g., believing one has the knowledge and abilities to protect hearing) was negative (– 12.5), it is unlikely that PM will make lifestyle changes related to preventing hearing loss. Overall, PM reported she did not experience any hearing symptoms that warranted the need for hearing protection.

18.4 Questions to the Reader

1. **Given that PM has no reported listening difficulties, is additional testing warranted?**
2. **If yes, what further testing should be pursued to help shed light on the possible etiology?**
3. **Is it important to assess PM's attitude toward noise, hearing loss, and hearing protection?**

18.5 Discussion of Questions

1. **Given that PM has no reported listening difficulties, is additional testing warranted?**

Although PM had no self-reported complaints of hearing difficulties, a more comprehensive assessment was recommended due to the nature of her occupation and the risks associated with high-noise exposure levels. The disabling effects of hearing loss in adults due to occupational noise exposure is estimated to be approximately 16% worldwide, ranging from 7 to 21%.[3] Noise-Induced Hearing Loss (NIHL) causes permanent sensorineural hearing loss and is usually characterized by a notch in the pure-tone audiogram at 3,000, 4,000, or 6,000 Hz with recovery at 8,000 Hz.[4] Occupations or recreational activities where people are exposed to high-noise levels include

Fig. 18.1 PM's audiologic examination.

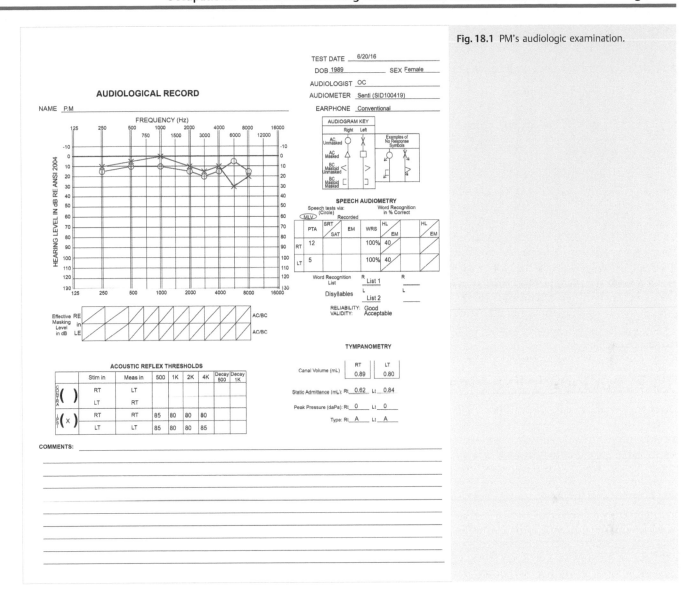

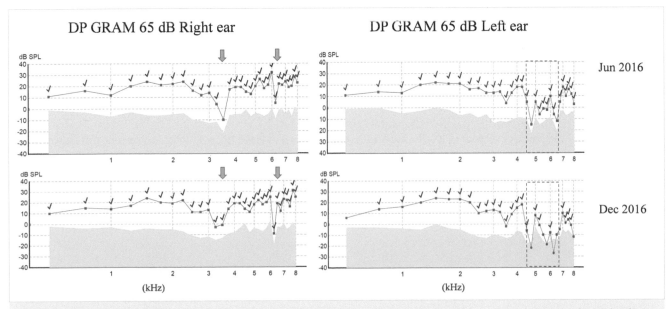

Fig. 18.2 DPOAE amplitude for right and left ears (7 dB S/N). DP-gram diagnostic protocol including 31 frequencies, $f_2/f_1 = 1.2$, $L_1/L_2 = 65/55$ dB SPL. Noise rejection level was 20 dB SPL. A probe check-fit procedure was conducted prior to each measurement to ensure that the primary levels were ±5 dB. Top panel reports results for the first visit. Bottom panel reports results for the second visit.

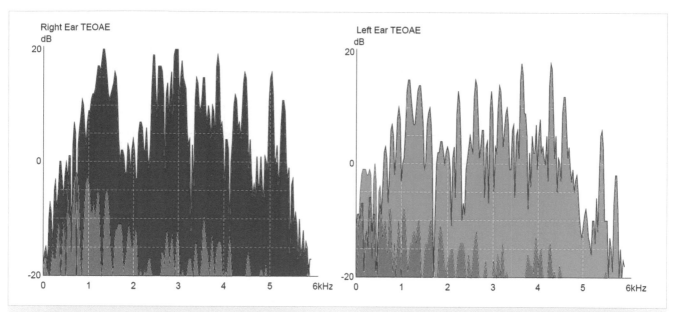

Fig. 18.3 TOAE amplitudes for right and left ears. Responses were measured at 500 to 5,500 Hz at 83 dB SPL using 1,000 replications (>90% reproducibility).

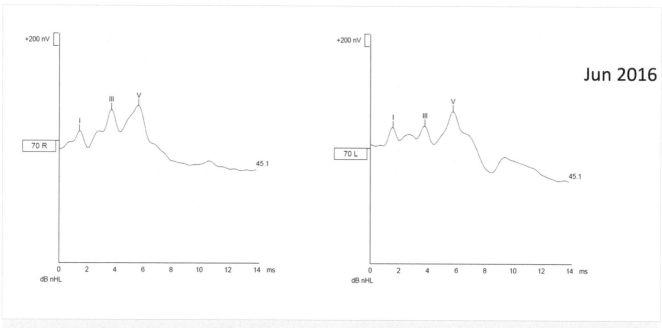

Fig. 18.4 PM's ABR waveforms obtained using 70 dB nHL click stimuli.

construction workers, musicians, miners, army personnel, concerts, and nightclubs where people in these situations are more at risk to present with NIHL.[5,6,7,8] More recently, attention has been directed to other forms of noise exposure such as fitness classes where noise levels have been reported between 83 and 96 dBA.[9,10] For instance, Zumba class levels can reach 91.2 dBA over 60 minutes, which has shown to induce hearing-thresholds shifts between pre- and postclass.[11] This is especially relevant to the instructors as they are exposed to high levels of music on a regular basis and are at a higher risk of NIHL. According to the National Institute for Occupational Safety and Health guidelines

for noise exposure, 8 hours exposure at 85 dBA in 1 day would be the limit to prevent an NIHL.[12] Unilateral or asymmetrical hearing loss is important to discern regardless of the severity because it can be a sign of a retrocochlear pathology and in such cases further investigation is required (e.g., electrophysiological testing).

2. If yes, what further testing should be pursued to help shed light on the possible etiology?

Electrophysiologic testing serves as an objective cross-check to pure-tone audiometry. OAE measurements are useful for early diagnosis and monitoring of NIHL and has been shown to identify a dysfunction before changes are seen in the pure-tone audiogram across a range of octave and interoctave frequencies.[1] PM's TOAE whole-wave response was within normal limits. DPOAE measurement allowed for a more frequency-specific (octave and interoctave) detection of cochlear dysfunction (**Fig. 50.2**). While the current audiologic testing primarily suggested hearing impairment only in PM's left ear (30 dB HL at 6,000 Hz), a bilateral hearing impairment may become present with further exposure to loud noise levels. The presence of an asymmetric NIHL has been reported previously in the literature.[13,14,15] A possible explanation to the left ear being more susceptible can be that the noise source was closer to one ear than the other (head shadow effect), along with other factors such as differences in recovery rate and weaker efferent mechanisms.[13,16] In the case of PM, however, these factors are open for speculation until all ambient exogenous and/or endogenous factors of NIHL are carefully considered.

The current test protocol and results clearly highlight the importance to record at least eight frequencies per octave when performing diagnostic DPOAEs. This allows for detailed assessment of cochlear processing of sound over a wide frequency range. This protocol is not time consuming (~ 5 minutes per ear) and allows for detection of dips (dysfunction) in the interoctave regions that may be reflective of the early stages of NIHL[1,17,18,19] as evidenced by a reduction of DPOAEs amplitudes in a range of specific frequencies.

Recent research, along with evidence from animal studies, have suggested that reduced or variable ABR Wave I amplitude across adults with normal hearing thresholds might be related to differences in noise exposure levels.[16,20] Reports indicated that Wave I amplitude is reduced in the noise-exposed animals compare to controls at suprathreshold stimulation levels (> 40 dB SPL) suggesting that ABR at suprathreshold levels are more sensitive to reflect an auditory damage than at threshold levels. Unfortunately, clinicians are not able to study these noise-induced damaging effects with ABRs recorded to only a single presentation level (e.g., 70 dB nHL for PM) and hence future evaluations should include amplitude intensity functions for ABR waves.

3. Is it important to assess PM's attitude toward noise, hearing loss, and hearing protection?

It is common for people to underestimate the effects of hearing loss on communication and quality of life.[21,22] Therefore, hearing protection approaches to avoid noise damage on the auditory system are often underutilized.[23,24] Occupational NIHL is commonly associated with activities related to construction, mining, military, and musicians. When people, however, are exposed to loud noise during fitness classes and other leisure activities, they are at risk for permanent hearing damage later in life. The risk of hearing damage also increases when working long days (e.g., summer holidays) during peak seasons.

The results from the KAB questionnaire revealed that PM did not experience any hearing symptoms and was not concerned about her hearing. It is, however, important for clinicians to relate attitudes to actual hearing status and tailor their counselling to highlight the potential dangers of exposing oneself to loud noise and try to achieve attitudinal change. It is also important to use such self-reported questionnaires in the

follow-up visits, not only to monitor changes in attitude and its relation to the hearing status, but also to ensure that frequent visits and counselling have not induced anxiety and fear.

The use of hearing protection is more closely associated to beliefs than knowledge. Prevention should consider strategies to reduce noise levels at the occupational environment and the noise levels transmitted to the person's inner ear. The use of personal earplugs could help to reduce noise exposure, but this would require some degree of training for proper insertion to obtain maximum sound attenuation. Overall, the improvement of awareness and knowledge about NIHL would be relevant in inducing changes in behavior regarding the use of hearing protection.

18.6 Final Diagnosis and Recommended Treatment

PM's assessment reveals normal hearing sensitivity bilaterally with the exception of a 30 dB HL notch at 6,000 Hz in the left ear. It is, however, possible to observe low DPOAEs amplitudes (< 0 dB SPL) in the range of 4,500 to 8,000 Hz. Also, PM's DPAOAE results revealed low amplitude responses at specific frequencies. This abnormal DPOAE finding may suggest outer hair cell dysfunction (e.g., reduced amplitude).[17] OAEs can be reduced in amplitude for a broader frequency range than an increase of threshold in the pure-tone octave frequencies which indicates an early stage of cochlear damage,[19] suggesting preclinical damage that cannot be necessarily evident in the pure-tone audiogram.[18]

There are some limitations that the reader should be aware of. First, it was not possible to obtain PM's baseline DPOAEs (i.e., previous to noise exposure) so the authors cannot rule out previous cochlear dysfunction. Second, it was not possible to measure the specific noise levels PM was exposed too during the classes. This limits the information available to determine PM's noise exposure and dose levels more accurately. Also, information about the classroom setting (e.g., loudspeaker locations) was not available at the time of testing, which could have provided more information on loudspeaker location relative to each ear and the extent of the ear asymmetry observed in PM's hearing.

As PM is exposed to occupational noise, it was recommended she use protection devices such as earplugs. It is important to remember that actual attenuation of these devices can be influenced by certain conditions, such as the quality of the material, the working environment, and proper insertion.

There are a number of reasons people do not use hearing protection during fitness classes. First, foam earplugs block and muffle the sound of the environment so participants cannot hear the instructor or the music. Second, there are only few sizes available and not all people have the same ear size. Third, hearing protectors can be uncomfortable and result in some people feeling embarrassed to use them publicly.

Most "conventional" earplugs reduce the sound more in the high than low- and mid-frequencies, thereby producing unnatural muted sound. Currently, high-fidelity earplugs (e.g., musician earplugs) are available that can reduce the sound (e.g., 9, 15, and 25 dB) equally across all frequencies, allowing for speech and music to remain clear. This implies that use of these musician earplugs can reduce the volume of the music to a safer and more comfortable level, but concurrently allow for hearing the music and the instructor still clearly.

Periodic measurements of noise levels in the fitness room could help reduce the noise level to a safer limit (lower than 85 dBA), which reduces the risk of NIHL. It is also important to determine appropriate loudspeaker location and distance from the instructors and participants to ensure safer exposure levels,[11] less strain on the voice of instructors, and reduce noise-induced symptoms or symptoms such as tinnitus.

Information and knowledge about the risk of damage due to noise exposure are relevant to promote behavioral changes; however, actions to bring about these changes can be quite challenging as benefits are not easily perceived by people (e.g., use of hearing protective devices). Using questionnaires such as the KAB may be helpful in identifying reasons as to why a person is unwilling to take action in preventing hearing loss (e.g., idea of uncomfortable ear protectors, hearing proctors not available in the fitness center, etc.). As in PM's case, since she presents with an overall positive attitude toward hearing protection, it is important henceforth to identify and intervene in areas that will facilitate a behavioral change.

18.7 Key Points

- Clinicians should consider Zumba fitness classes as equivalent to occupations associated with the risk of NIHL and identify early symptoms or signs of hearing loss.
- Regularly scheduled hearing assessment, even in presence of normal hearing sensitivity, should be considered with people exposed to high noise levels.
- The use of questionnaires/self-report measures will provide additional information concerning the level of awareness and knowledge about the risk of damage due to noise exposure in order to promote protection behavioral changes.
- DPOAEs (detailed/extended) can be a fast and objective tool to monitor hearing function in people exposed to hazardous noise levels.

References

[1] Dhar S, Hall JW. Otoacoustic Emissions: Principles, Procedures, and Protocols. San Diego, CA: Plural Publishing; 2011:230

[2] Saunders GH, Dann SM, Griest SE, Frederick MT. Development and evaluation of a questionnaire to assess knowledge, attitudes, and behaviors towards hearing loss prevention. Int J Audiol. 2014; 53(4):209–218

[3] Nelson DI, Nelson RY, Concha-Barrientos M, Fingerhut M. The global burden of occupational noise-induced hearing loss. Am J Ind Med. 2005; 48(6):446–458

[4] Mirza R, Kirchner DB, Dobie RA, Crawford J, ACOEM Task Force on Occupational Hearing Loss. Occupational noise-induced hearing loss. J Occup Environ Med. 2018; 60(9):e498–e501

[5] Feder K, Michaud D, McNamee J, Fitzpatrick E, Davies H, Leroux T. Prevalence of hazardous occupational noise exposure, hearing loss, and hearing protection usage among a representative sample of working Canadians. J Occup Environ Med. 2017; 59(1):92–113

[6] Leensen MCJ, van Duivenbooden JC, Dreschler WA. A retrospective analysis of noise-induced hearing loss in the Dutch construction industry. Int Arch Occup Environ Health. 2011; 84(5):577–590

[7] Vogel I, Brug J, Van der Ploeg CPB, Raat H. Discotheques and the risk of hearing loss among youth: risky listening behavior and its psychosocial correlates. Health Educ Res. 2010; 25(5):737–747

[8] Carter L, Williams W, Black D, Bundy A. The leisure-noise dilemma: hearing loss or hearsay? What does the literature tell us? Ear Hear. 2014; 35(5):491–505

[9] Nassar G. The human temporary threshold shift after exposure to 60 minutes' noise in an aerobics class. Br J Audiol. 2001; 35(1):99–101

[10] Torre P, III, Howell JC. Noise levels during aerobics and the potential effects on distortion product otoacoustic emissions. J Commun Disord. 2008; 41(6):501–511

[11] Gaeta LJA. Work out your body, not your ears! Audiology Today 2016; 28(6):18–27

[12] Sriwattanatamma P, Breysse P. Comparison of NIOSH noise criteria and OSHA hearing conservation criteria. Am J Ind Med. 2000; 37(4):334–338

[13] Sturman CJ, Frampton CM, Ten Cate WJF. Hearing loss asymmetry due to chronic occupational noise exposure. Otol Neurotol. 2018; 39(8):e627–e634

[14] Fernandes SV, Fernandes CM. Medicolegal significance of asymmetrical hearing loss in cases of industrial noise exposure. J Laryngol Otol. 2010; 124(10):1051–1055

[15] Hong O. Hearing loss among operating engineers in American construction industry. Int Arch Occup Environ Health. 2005; 78(7):565–574

[16] Maison SF, Liberman MC. Predicting vulnerability to acoustic injury with a noninvasive assay of olivocochlear reflex strength. J Neurosci. 2000; 20(12):4701–4707

[17] Attias J, Horovitz G, El-Hatib N, Nageris B. Detection and clinical diagnosis of noise-induced hearing loss by otoacoustic emissions. Noise Health. 2001; 3(12):19–31

[18] Job A, Raynal M, Kossowski M, et al. Otoacoustic detection of risk of early hearing loss in ears with normal audiograms: a 3-year follow-up study. Hear Res. 2009; 251(1–2):10–16

[19] Helleman HW, Jansen EJM, Dreschler WA. Otoacoustic emissions in a hearing conservation program: general applicability in longitudinal monitoring and the relation to changes in pure-tone thresholds. Int J Audiol. 2010; 49(6):410–419

[20] Konrad-Martin D, Dille MF, McMillan G, et al. Age-related changes in the auditory brainstem response. J Am Acad Audiol. 2012; 23(1):18–35, quiz 74–75

[21] Arlinger S. Negative consequences of uncorrected hearing loss–a review. Int J Audiol. 2003; 42 Suppl 2:S17–S20

[22] Chia E-M, Wang JJ, Rochtchina E, Cumming RR, Newall P, Mitchell P. Hearing impairment and health-related quality of life: the Blue Mountains Hearing Study. Ear Hear. 2007; 28(2):187–195

[23] Carter L, Black D. More to lose? Noise risk perceptions of young adults with hearing impairment. Semin Hear. 2017; 38(4):319–331

[24] Beach E, Williams W, Gilliver M. Hearing protection for clubbers is music to their ears. Health Promot J Austr. 2010; 21(3):215–221

Suggested Reading

[1] Tikka C, Verbeek JH, Kateman E, Morata TC, Dreschler WA, Ferrite S. Interventions to prevent occupational noise-induced hearing loss. Cochrane Database Syst Rev. 2017; 7(7):CD006396

[2] Stucken EZ, Hong RS. Noise-induced hearing loss: an occupational medicine perspective. Curr Opin Otolaryngol Head Neck Surg. 2014; 22(5):388–393

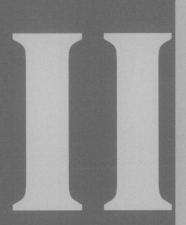

Part II

Diagnostic Examination—Auditory Function

II

19 Nonorganic Hearing Loss: A Case Study

Alicia Restrepo and Gail Whitelaw

19.1 Clinical History and Description

YP is a 45-year-old female who was referred to otolaryngology in June 2016. She reported an infection in the left ear that began following an upper respiratory infection (URI) in May 2016. She was treated with an antibiotic and referred to audiology and otolaryngology by her primary care physician (PCP). YP reported otalgia, aural fullness, and a decrease in hearing in the left ear during her appointment with otolaryngology. Her physical examination was unremarkable with the exception of reported tenderness in the left external auditory canal during otoscopy.

YP provided the otolaryngologist with the results from an audiometric examination completed at another facility (▶ Fig. 19.1). The audiometric results demonstrated a mild flat sensorineural hearing loss (SNHL) in the right ear and a flat severe mixed hearing loss in the left ear. There was significant interaural asymmetry, with the hearing in the left ear being poorer than the right ear. A Speech Recognition Threshold (SRT) was obtained at 30 dB Hearing Level (HL) in the right ear and 80 dB HL in the left ear, which were consistent with the Pure-Tone Average (PTA) bilaterally. These results indicated a mild loss in the ability to receive speech in the right ear and a severe loss in the left ear. Word Recognition Scores (WRS) were administered at 70 dB HL in the right ear and at 105 dB HL in the left ear with 80 dB HL of contralateral masking. The results indicated normal ability to recognize speech in the right ear and moderate difficulty in the left ear. Tympanometry indicated normal middle ear pressure, ear canal volume, and compliance bilaterally.

The otolaryngologist recommended either oral steroids or an Intratympanic (IT) steroid injection based on YP's reported symptoms and the previous audiometric findings, which were suggestive of a Sudden Sensorineural Hearing Loss (SSNHL). YP was counseled that steroids might not improve her hearing

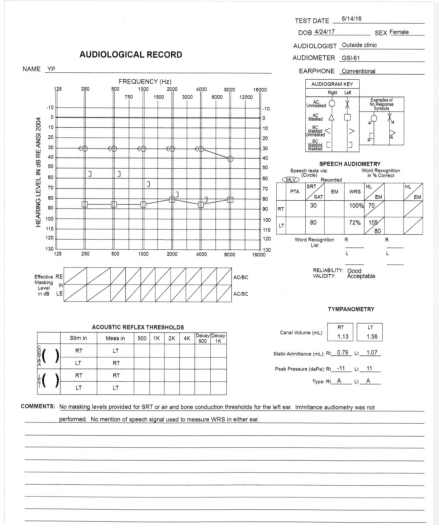

Fig. 19.1 Initial audiologic examination from an outside clinic.

since a month had passed since she initially noted a decrease in her hearing in the left ear. Patients who follow up with a physician less than a week after noticing an SSNHL have greater chances in regaining hearing compared to patients who wait more than 1 week.[1] YP elected to undergo the IT injection. The procedure was performed and YP was scheduled for a follow-up comprehensive audiologic evaluation 2 weeks later to determine the impact that the IT injection had on her hearing.

19.2 Audiological Testing

A follow-up audiologic evaluation was performed in June 2016 (▶ Fig. 19.2). The audiologist noted poor reliability during pure-tone testing because YP demonstrated difficulty responding consistently throughout the evaluation. An ascending approach was utilized for the threshold measure rather than the conventional descending approach.

The initial audiogram (▶ Fig. 19.2) demonstrated a slight to mild flat SNHL in the right ear and a flat moderately severe SNHL in the left ear. An SRT was measured at 35 dB HL in the right ear and 75 dB HL in the left ear, which was in agreement with the PTA of 33 dB HL in the right ear and 68 dB HL in the left ear. YP was reinstructed due to poor reliability, and air conduc-

tion thresholds and SRT were repeated for the left ear (▶ Fig. 19.3). An improvement was noted in air conduction thresholds after reinstruction; however, the SRT (40 dB HL) and PTA (51 dB HL) were no longer in agreement. The SRT and PTA should not differ by more than 8 dB HL[2] in most cases. A positive pure-tone Stenger was obtained at 250 to 8,000 Hz, which is suggestive of a nonorganic hearing loss.

Bone conduction testing was performed with the bone conductor placed on the right mastoid and thresholds were consistent with air conduction thresholds for the right ear. The bone conductor was transferred to the left mastoid and unmasked BC thresholds were measured. Interestingly, there was a significant threshold shift (i.e., the left ear BC thresholds were significantly poorer than the right ear BC thresholds [▶ Fig. 19.2]). Interaural attenuation for BC is considered to be 0 dB HL because both cochleas are located within the temporal bone of the skull, allowing vibration through the bone oscillator to stimulate both cochleas simultaneously.[3] A significant difference in unmasked interaural BC thresholds should not occur in a case of "true" asymmetry. Average interaural attenuation of a signal transmitted through BC is 5 to 10 dB.[4] YP's unmasked BC thresholds on the left ear should have been consistent with the unmasked BC thresholds on the right ear within 5 to 10 dB.

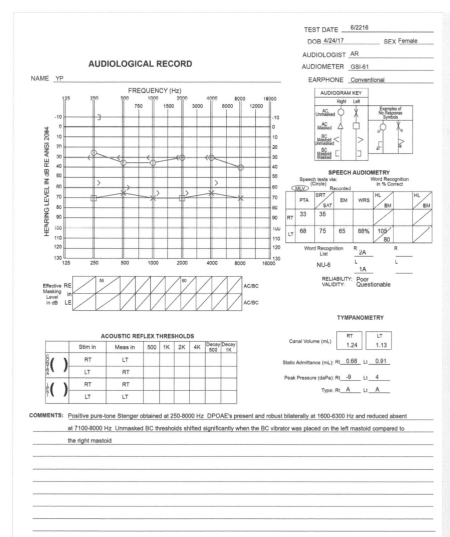

Fig. 19.2 Follow-up audiometric examination.

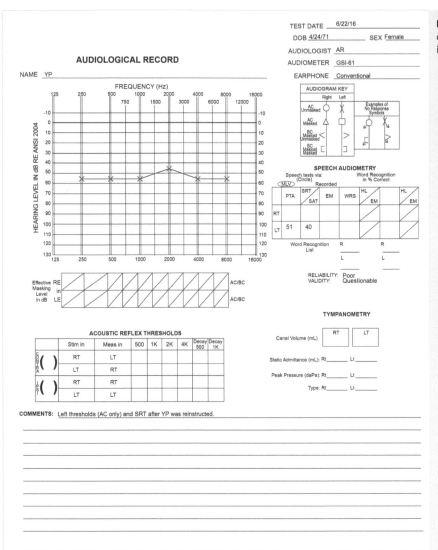

Fig. 19.3 Repeat of measuring AC (air conduction) thresholds in the left ear due to initial unreliable thresholds.

WRS were performed using Monitored Live Voice (MLV) of a half-list of NU-6 (Northwestern University Auditory Test No.6) word list using a female talker. The presentation level was 105 dB HL, with 85 dB HL of contralateral effective masking. The results were suggestive of slight difficulty in recognizing speech in the left ear. The audiologist elected to discontinue testing due to inconsistent responses and WRS was not measured in the right ear. YP was scheduled to follow-up with the otolaryngologist who was notified of the test findings.

Tympanometry indicated normal middle ear pressure, ear canal volume, and compliance bilaterally. Distortion Product Otoacoustic Emissions (DPOAEs) were present and robust at 1,600 to 6,300 Hz and reduced or absent at 7,100 to 8,000 Hz. This is suggestive of normal or near-normal hearing bilaterally.

19.3 Questions to the Reader

1. **Explain the Stenger phenomenon and how it is useful in identifying patients with nonorganic hearing loss.**
2. **Compare the results of the DPOAEs and the audiogram in the left ear. Were these results expected?**

3. **Explain why this patient was misdiagnosed with an SSNHL and the ramifications of this misdiagnosis.**
4. **Why is it recommended for an audiologist to use an ascending approach rather than the standard descending approach with patients who are suspected of malingering?**

19.4 Discussion of Questions

1. **Explain the Stenger phenomenon and how it is useful in identifying patients with nonorganic hearing loss.**

The Stenger phenomenon occurs when a pure-tone of the same frequency or spondee words is presented at different presentation levels bilaterally. Although the stimulus is presented bilaterally, the patient should only perceive the stimulus having the higher presentation level. An audiologist may utilize the Stenger to help identify patients who are suspected of exaggerating hearing loss (i.e., malingering) by presenting a pure tone at 10 dB HL above the measured threshold of the better ear and simultaneously presenting a pure tone at the same frequency at

10 dB HL below the measured threshold in the poorer ear. A patient with a "true" asymmetry will respond to this stimulus because he or she is unable to hear the stimulus presented to the poorer ear; however, the stimulus presented to the better ear is audible. A patient who is malingering will not respond to the stimulus because he or she is unaware of the tone being presented to the better ear and is attempting to feign a hearing loss in the poorer ear. The Stenger may also be used with spondee words.[3]

2. Compare the results of the DPOAEs and the audiogram in the left ear. Were these results expected?

DPOAEs in the left ear were present and robust at 1,600 to 6,300 Hz and reduced or absent at 7,100 to 8,000 Hz. This finding is suggestive of overall normal or near-normal hearing. DPOAEs are an objective, quick measure with high sensitivity and specificity in relation to audiometric thresholds. DPOAEs are a valuable test for audiologists to utilize for patients with suspected nonorganic hearing losses. It is important to note, however, that patients with a "true" SSNHL may continue to have measurable DPOAEs. DPOAEs present in patients with SSNHL have a higher chance of recovering hearing sensitivity than patients having absent DPOAEs following SSNHL.[5,6]

3. Explain why this patient was misdiagnosed with an SSNHL and the ramifications of this misdiagnosis.

YP was incorrectly diagnosed with an SSNHL because the previous audiologist did not utilize a comprehensive approach to ensure accurate test results. It is useful to employ the Stenger for any newly diagnosed asymmetric hearing loss. The Stenger is easy to perform and does not take a significant amount of time. It would have been useful for this audiologist to utilize DPOAEs, if possible, because DPOAEs provide insight into cochlear integrity. Every audiologist must pay close attention and document the reliability of the results patients provide during the audiometric evaluation. Every audiologic examination must include the audiologist's perception of the patient's reliability and validity.

The misdiagnosis of YP's audiometric results led to an unnecessary medical procedure that has the potential to cause unfavorable side effects such as pain at the injection site, sensation of burning, increase in the loudness of tinnitus, and temporary dizziness.[7] In addition to an unnecessary medical procedure being performed based on inaccurate audiologic results, the procedure was an unnecessary expense, adding to increased health care costs.

4. Why is it recommended for an audiologist to use an ascending approach rather than the standard descending approach with patients who are suspected of malingering?

An ascending approach, or beginning the threshold search below a patient's threshold, is recommended for patients who are suspected of malingering. If the audiologist chooses to utilize the descending approach, he or she will present a suprathreshold pure-tone, allowing the patient to establish a reference level.[3] This allows the patient to respond at a false level with greater consistency.

19.5 Description of Disorder and Recommended Treatment

Nonorganic hearing loss can be divided into two distinct categories: those who are feigning hearing loss intentionally (i.e., malingering) and those who are doing so unintentionally (i.e., conversion deafness). Conversion deafness is rare and is more commonly seen in pediatric patients than adult patients and is thought to be related to psychological factors.[8]

One common reason a patient may intentionally feign hearing loss is for financial compensation, whether it be through Veterans Affairs, Workers' Compensation, or due to a personal injury such as an automobile accident. Another reason may be to avoid certain responsibilities at work or school. A patient may present with conversion deafness for psychological reasons, such as seeking attention or because he or she is performing poorly at work or school. For example, he or she has poor grades or is unable to perform the duties expected at work.[3] Unfortunately, YP's motivation is unknown.

19.6 Outcome

YP was scheduled to follow up with otolaryngology the day after her comprehensive audiologic evaluation and the otolaryngologist was notified of the findings. YP cancelled the follow-up appointment via telephone and did not reschedule. The reason for this is unknown; however, the authors speculate that it is because the patient became aware that the audiologist suspected she was malingering.

19.7 Key Points

- A comprehensive audiologic evaluation will often help determine the course of treatment that the otolaryngologist chooses for a patient. It is essential to evaluate every patient carefully to ensure that an inaccurate evaluation does not lead to inappropriate medical treatment
- It is essential to utilize multiple diagnostic tools whenever possible, especially with instances of SSNHL in order to rule out a nonorganic hearing loss.
- The Stenger and DPOAEs are important tools for audiologists to consider when assessing the hearing of patients suspected of nonorganic hearing loss.

References

[1] Kuhn M, Heman-Ackah SE, Shaikh JA, Roehm PC. Sudden sensorineural hearing loss: a review of diagnosis, treatment, and prognosis. Trends Amplif. 2011; 15(3):91–105

[2] Roeser R, Clark J. Clinical masking. In: Roeser R, Valente M, Hosford-Dunn H, eds. Audiology Diagnosis. 2nd ed. New York, NY: Thieme Medical Publishers; 2007:261–287

[3] Shoup A, Roeser R. Audiologic evaluation of special populations. In: Roeser R, Valente M, Hosford-Dunn H, ed. Audiology: Diagnosis. 2nd ed. New York, NY: Thieme Medical Publishers; 2007:314–334

[4] Stenfelt S. Transcranial attenuation of bone-conducted sound when stimulation is at the mastoid and at the bone conduction hearing aid position. Otol Neurotol. 2012; 33(2):105–114

[5] Nemati S, Naghavi S, Kazemnejad E, Banan R. Otoacoustic emissions in sudden sensorineural hearing loss: changes of measures with treatment. Iran J Otorhinolaryngol. 2011; 23(1):37–44

[6] Ishida IM, Sugiura M, Teranishi M, Katayama N, Nakashima T. Otoacoustic emissions, ear fullness and tinnitus in the recovery course of sudden deafness. Auris Nasus Larynx. 2008; 35(1):41–46

[7] Liu Y, Chi F, Yang T, Liu T. Assessment of complications due to intratympanic injections. Word J Otorhinolaryngol-Head Neck Surg. 2016; 2:13–16

[8] Wang YP, Wang MC, Lin HC, Lee KS. Conversion deafness presenting as sudden hearing loss. J Chin Med Assoc. 2006; 69(6):289–293

Suggested Readings

[1] Austen S, Lynch C. Non-organic hearing loss redefined: understanding, categorizing and managing non-organic behaviour. Int J Audiol. 2004; 43(8):449–457

[2] Kinstler DB, Phelan JG, Lavender RW. The Stenger and Speech Stenger tests in functional hearing loss. Audiology. 1972; 11(3):187–193

[3] Lin J, Staecker H. Nonorganic hearing loss. Semin Neurol. 2006; 26(3):321–330

Part III

Diagnostic Examination—Vestibular Function

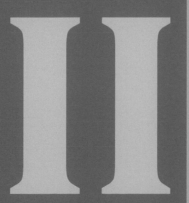

20 Central Vestibular Dysfunction: A Case of Wernicke's Encephalopathy

Amy K. Winston and Patricia McCarthy

20.1 Clinical History and Description

JD, a 52-year-old female, was referred by her neurologist for videonystagmography (VNG) to investigate the etiology of the patient's persistent dizziness and ataxia.

JD reported persistent movement in her visual field, dizziness, and severe postural unsteadiness. Symptom onset followed an acute episode in which the patient demonstrated altered mental status with confusion and memory loss. This incident occurred one evening when JD was at a restaurant with her husband. During the meal, JD excused herself to go to the restroom; her husband became alarmed when she failed to return. Ultimately, JD was found naked in the restroom, deliriously searching for her bed, which she believed to be nearby. JD was then taken by ambulance to a local emergency room (ER). When queried later, she denied any memory of the event in the restaurant.

While in the hospital after this incident, JD began complaining of dizziness and blurred vision. She also reported onset of decreased sensation in both feet, stating that her toes were "numb and tingly." She was observed to be ataxic and was identified as a High Fall Risk. In addition, nurses documented episodes of tremors of her extremities and tongue as well as intermittent word-finding difficulties, stuttering, and halting speech.

When seen for VNG testing, JD's gait was wide (i.e., feet wide apart) and characterized by short, cautious, and shuffling strides. She reported several falls since getting out of the hospital; these falls were in all directions—to the side, front, and back. She had resorted to using a walker for stability because of daily "near falls" and a resultant intense fear of falling. JD confirmed experiencing persistent dizziness and unsteadiness. When describing her dizziness, she denied any perception of rotation, either of herself or of her environment, but she complained of unclear vision, noting that her eyes and head did not seem to move together. She identified specific head movements —including looking up, turning the head left or right, and bending forward—that increased the intensity of her dizziness and made her more likely to fall. JD was not nauseated and had not vomited, and she reported no perceptible change in hearing since dizziness onset. As was observed during her hospital stay, JD demonstrated word-finding difficulties and halting speech, but when asked about her speech, she denied having any problem. Her answers to intake questions were somewhat rambling and unfocused. Overall, JD's disposition ranged from pleasant to tearful to confused during her appointment. At times, she became quite upset about her condition, and she repeatedly asked when her dizziness would go away and when she would be "back to normal."

JD's medical history was otherwise significant for chronic alcohol abuse, major depressive disorder, and obesity. Her surgical history was significant only for gastric bypass surgery, which was performed approximately 3 years ago.

20.2 Vestibular Testing

20.2.1 Videonystagmography

VNG test results were abnormal. Significant findings were noted as follows.

Spontaneous Nystagmus Testing

An 11 deg/s down-beating spontaneous nystagmus was measured with fixation (i.e., with the presentation of a visual target; ▶ Fig. 20.1a; ▶ Fig. 20.2); this nystagmus enhanced to 16 deg/s without fixation (▶ Fig. 20.1b).

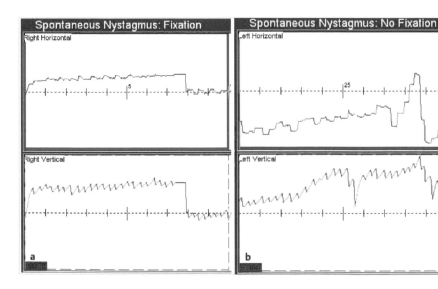

Fig. 20.1 Down-beating spontaneous nystagmus present **(a)** with fixation and **(b)** without fixation.

Gaze Testing

An 8 to 10 deg/s down-beating nystagmus was recorded in all gaze conditions (right, left, up, and down) with fixation; nystagmus velocity was stable or increased (8–14 deg/s) without fixation. The documented gaze nystagmus was noted to be essentially consistent with the identified spontaneous nystagmus. Eye movements were conjugate in all gaze conditions.

Horizontal Random Saccade Testing

Tracings (▶ Fig. 20.3) were noted to be extremely disorganized; results revealed reduced response velocity and prolonged latency measures.

Smooth Pursuit Testing

Horizontal visual pursuit test tracings were characterized by intrusions from the down-beating spontaneous nystagmus. Overall measures for gain and symmetry were within normal limits at all test frequencies.

Optokinetic Testing

JD had symmetrical responses with reduced gain at both the 20 and 40 deg/s target velocities (▶ Fig. 20.4).

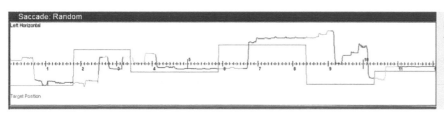

Fig. 20.2 Visual pursuit tracings with intrusions from down-beating spontaneous nystagmus.

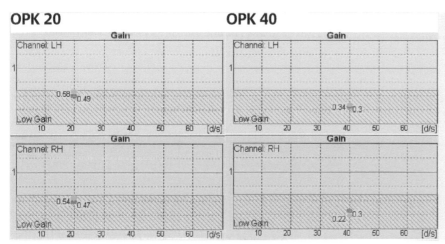

Fig. 20.3 Optokinetic test findings revealing symmetrical results with reduced gain at both target velocities.

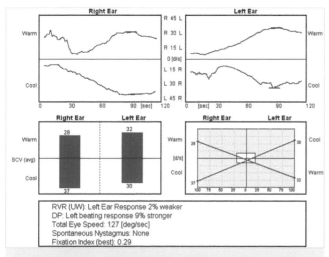

Fig. 20.4 Bithermal caloric summary. Note the robust caloric response and normal fixation suppression results.

Positional Testing

Positional testing revealed a 15 to 19 deg/s down-beating nystagmus in all positions with fixation that enhanced to a 21 to 26 deg/s down-beating nystagmus without fixation.

Bithermal Caloric Testing

Bithermal caloric responses were robust and symmetrical, with no significant caloric weakness or directional preponderance. JD was able to adequately suppress this caloric-induced horizontal nystagmus. Note that, as expected, the spontaneous down-beating nystagmus was recorded in all tracings.

VNG findings of down-beating spontaneous nystagmus and abnormal results on random saccade and optokinetic testing strongly suggest a central etiology for JD's dizziness and ataxia.

20.3 Questions to the Reader

1. **Is JD experiencing vertigo?**
2. **What information can you glean from observation of JD's gait?**
3. **Why is down-beating spontaneous nystagmus typically considered a strong sign of central vestibular dysfunction?**

20.4 Discussion of Questions

1. Is JD experiencing vertigo?

Vertigo is a term that involves the false perception of movement of oneself or of one's surrounding environment when no movement is actually occurring. True vertigo may be experienced as spinning sensation or as a rocking or tilting movement. JD's description of her persistent dizziness is inconsistent with true vertigo. Vertigo results from an imbalance in vestibular neural activity, which may originate from peripheral and/or central vestibular dysfunction. The three paired semicircular canals are most sensitive to angular acceleration (head movement with increasing velocity). Unilateral dysfunction in these end organs or their neural projection will often produce a spinning sensation. Impairment of inputs from the paired otolith organs, the utricle, and saccule, which are sensitive to linear acceleration, can generate a feeling of tilting. A central vestibular lesion may or may not result in a true sensation of vertigo.

2. What information can you glean from observation of JD's gait?

The three primary inputs to balance are (1) vision, (2) the peripheral vestibular system, and (3) somatosensory cues, including sensory inputs from the skin, joints, muscles, and tendons. In a healthy system, all three inputs contribute information to the central system that is then processed, primarily by the cerebellum, to determine where the head and body are in space and to direct appropriate motor responses to keep a person upright and stable. If one or more of these inputs are impaired and/or if they are in conflict with one another, the central vestibular system must decide which input is likely most accurate and direct the motor response accordingly. In situations in which the support surface is flat and stable, somatosensory cues will typically dominate.

Assessing the patient's gait can often provide important clues as to possible site of lesion. JD was observed to use a wide gait with a shortened stride and intermittent shuffling. By shortening her stride and shuffling, JD is maximizing the somatosensory cues available to her central vestibular system. Use of a wide gait essentially widens JD's normal base of support, which lowers her center of gravity and makes her less likely to fall. JD reported unclear vision and stated that her eyes and head do not seem to move together. This would suggest that her visual inputs to balance are inaccurate. Her heavy reliance on somatosensory cues also suggests that she is either not receiving or is not able to effectively use information from her peripheral vestibular system.

3. Why is down-beating spontaneous nystagmus typically considered a strong sign of central vestibular dysfunction?

Ewald's first law states that eye and head movements occur in the plane of the semicircular canal that is being stimulated.[1] Through the vestibulo-ocular reflex (VOR), each semicircular canal directs eye movements in the same plane as its physical orientation. With this, stimulation of a horizontal canal results in a rightward or leftward horizontal eye movement; stimulation of an anterior canal results in an eye movement that is primarily upward with a leftward or rightward torsional component; and stimulation of a posterior canal triggers an eye movement that is primarily downward with a leftward or rightward torsional component. Given these relationships, generation of a pure down-beating spontaneous nystagmus of peripheral origin is essentially impossible. In contrast, abnormal eye movements that develop secondary to a central vestibular lesion may not follow Ewald's first law, because they do not reflect peripheral vestibular function or the predictable relationships that underscore the VOR. Central vestibular nystagmus may be vertical, horizontal, torsional, or oblique; it may be of fixed direction, but it can also change directions. Down-beating spontaneous nystagmus, then, is assumed to be of central origin.

20.5 Additional Testing

20.5.1 Magnetic Resonance Imaging

JD underwent FLAIR (fluid-attenuated inversion recovery) magnetic resonance imaging (MRI) testing. This evaluation method is typically used to examine areas such as the brain and spinal cord that are covered in or surrounded by cerebrospinal fluid (CSF) in order to minimize interference from the CSF, which appears bright on imaging. MRI findings revealed abnormal hyperintensities in the periventricular region of the brain. These results indicated lesions in the cerebral white matter around both ventricles. There was no evidence of intracranial hemorrhage or tumor.

20.5.2 Blood Work

An extensive panel of blood tests was completed. Results indicated an abnormally low blood level of thiamine (vitamin B1). Thiamine is a water-soluble vitamin that is typically ingested as part of a healthy diet. It can be found in many foods—including whole grains, eggs, meat, fish, legumes, and leafy, green vegetables—and is absorbed into the bloodstream in the small intestine. Thiamine helps break down sugars in the body and is a necessary component for several critical body functions, including neurotransmitter production, carbohydrate metabolism, and lipid metabolism.[2,3]

20.6 Diagnosis and Recommended Treatment

Diagnostic test findings and patient presentation were determined to be consistent with Wernicke's encephalopathy (WE). WE is a neurological disorder caused by thiamine deficiency, which results in neuronal damage and loss. Classic presentation of this disorder is characterized by three cardinal symptoms: ataxia, eye movement disorder, and mental confusion.[4,5,6] These patients will most typically present with ophthalmoplegia—a paralysis or weakness of the extraocular muscles—and/or nystagmus. Vertical nystagmus, either up beating or down beating, may be present; in rare cases, the direction of the nystagmus can change with gaze or during disease progression.[7,8] The direction of the nystagmus reflects the central structures that have been damaged. Down-beating nystagmus often reflects changes in the vestibulocerebellum (nodulus, uvula, flocculus, and paraflocculus). Patients with WE may also have other neurological signs, including tremors or peripheral neuropathy, usually involving the lower extremities.[9]

JD's constellation of symptoms—confusion, memory loss, down-beating nystagmus, ataxia, tremors, and peripheral neuropathy—includes this hallmark WE triad. The abnormally low thiamine level found in JD's bloodwork strongly supports the diagnosis, and her MRI results are also consistent with WE. Depending on the disease progression, MRI abnormalities may or may not be noted in cases of WE, but when present, lesions are most commonly found in the medial thalami and the periventricular regions of the third ventricle.[10,11]

JD's medical history includes two key factors known to predispose one to developing WE: chronic alcohol abuse and bariatric surgery. WE is most commonly associated with chronic alcohol abuse. Over time, exposure to alcohol damages the intestinal mucosa, effectively reducing the amount of thiamine that can be absorbed from the gastrointestinal system by as much as 90%.[5,6] In addition, many alcoholics develop poor diets as they begin to replace food with alcohol, further reducing their overall thiamine intake.[4,10] JD also underwent gastric bypass surgery, which as a primary concern may reduce overall thiamine intake due to resultant dietary restrictions (in content and quantity), and as a secondary concern can result in excessive vomiting, which is also known to reduce thiamine levels.[6,12]

The treatment for acute WE is intravenous administration of thiamine along with other supportive vitamins and minerals in which the patient is likely to be deficient. This treatment continues until there is no longer any evidence of clinical improvement.[4] Oral thiamine may be used in supportive care after the acute phase has passed, but poor patient compliance and impaired thiamine absorption can reduce effectiveness in some cases.[4] If treated promptly and effectively, WE-associated ataxia, confusion, and eye-movement disorders improve

relatively quickly, though residual postural instability may remain. Nystagmus and memory issues, particularly short-term memory problems, will persist in some patients following treatment.[5,6,13,14]

JD was treated with intravenous thiamine as an inpatient and was placed on an oral thiamine regimen after being discharged from the hospital. In addition, she was referred to physical therapy for vestibular therapy and fall prevention and was placed under the care of a psychotherapist to begin addressing her substance abuse. Since beginning treatment, JD's symptoms have improved, but significant residual deficits remain. Physical therapy reports indicate that JD's ataxia is less severe than at onset. She has transitioned from a walker to a quad cane for support, but she is still at high risk for falling. Regarding her mental state, JD's initial confusion has receded, but, per her neurologist, she demonstrates ongoing short-term memory issues. The persistent down-beating nystagmus remains and continues to interfere with JD's vision and sense of stability. Neurology recently initiated treatment with gabapentin in an attempt to reduce the severity of the nystagmus. Other methods of reducing the functional effects of the nystagmus, including base-down prism glasses, have been discussed with JD but have not yet been introduced. The long-term prognosis for JD is unclear, as notes in her medical record suggest she has continued to drink heavily.

20.7 Key Points

- WE is a neurological disorder caused by thiamine deficiency. Classic presentation of WE includes the triad of ataxia, an eye movement disorder, and mental confusion.
- Individuals with poor nutritional intake of thiamine or who have conditions that impair or limit absorption of thiamine are at risk for developing WE. Research indicates that patients with a history of long-term alcohol abuse and those who have undergone bariatric surgery are particularly susceptible.
- Oculomotor abnormalities in VNG testing, including down-beating spontaneous nystagmus present both with and without fixation, reduced velocity on saccade testing, and reduced gain on OPK, are all consistent with an underlying central vestibular site of lesion.
- Intravenous administration of thiamine is the primary treatment for WE. Resolution of presenting symptoms is often incomplete, with residual nystagmus and memory issues most commonly persisting post treatment. Additional interventions to address underlying contributing conditions or residual symptoms are typically necessary. Drug therapy may be considered to alleviate vertical nystagmus.

References

[1] Leigh RJ, Zee DS. The Neurology of Eye Movements. 4th ed. New York, NY: Oxford University Press; 2006

[2] Mayo Clinic Staff. Thiamine (vitamin B1). The Mayo Clinic. http://www.mayoclinic.org/drugs-supplements/thiamine/background/hrb-20060129. Updated November 1, 2013. Accessed November 3, 2016

[3] Medscape. Vitamin B1 (thiamine). http://emedicine.medscape.com/article/2088582-overview. Updated February 5, 2014. Accessed October 20, 2016

[4] Thompson AD, Guerrini I, Marshall EJ. Wernicke's encephalopathy: role of thiamine. Pract Gastroenterol. 2009; 33(6):21–30

[5] Thomson AD, Marshall EJ. The natural history and pathophysiology of Wernicke's encephalopathy and Korsakoff's psychosis. Alcohol Alcohol. 2006; 41 (2):151–158

[6] Sechi G, Serra A. Wernicke's encephalopathy: new clinical settings and recent advances in diagnosis and management. Lancet Neurol. 2007; 6(5):442–455

[7] Mejia NI, Pless M. Downbeat nystagmus in Wernicke encephalopathy. Neuro-ophthalmology. 2009; 33(4):178–179

[8] Abouaf L, Vighetto A, Magnin E, Nove-Josserand A, Mouton S, Tilikete C. Primary position upbeat nystagmus in Wernicke's encephalopathy. Eur Neurol. 2011; 65(3):160–163

[9] Medscape. Wernicke encephalopathy clinical presentation. http://emedicine. medscape.com/article/794583-clinical. Updated October 28, 2015. Accessed October 20, 2016

[10] Sullivan EV, Pfefferbaum A. Neuroimaging of the Wernicke-Korsakoff syndrome. Alcohol Alcohol. 2009; 44(2):155–165

[11] Zuccoli G, Pipitone N. Neuroimaging findings in acute Wernicke's encephalopathy: review of the literature. AJR Am J Roentgenol. 2009; 192(2):501–508

[12] Aasheim ET. Wernicke encephalopathy after bariatric surgery: a systematic review. Ann Surg. 2008; 248(5):714–720

[13] Medscape. Wernicke encephalopathy treatment & management. http://emedicine.medscape.com/article/794583-treatment. Updated October 28, 2015. Accessed November 3, 2016

[14] Paparrigopoulos T, Tzavellas E, Karaiskos D, Kouzoupis A, Liappas I. Complete recovery from undertreated Wernicke-Korsakoff syndrome following aggressive thiamine treatment. In Vivo. 2010; 24(2):231–233

Suggested Readings

[1] Sechi G, Serra A. Wernicke's encephalopathy: new clinical settings and recent advances in diagnosis and management. Lancet Neurol. 2007; 6(5):442–455

[2] Thomson AD, Marshall EJ. The natural history and pathophysiology of Wernicke's encephalopathy and Korsakoff's psychosis. Alcohol Alcohol. 2006; 41 (2):151–158

21 Hearing Disorders: Vestibular Schwannomas and Sudden Sensorineural Hearing Loss

Alison M. Brockmeyer-Lauer

21.1 Clinical History and Description

KB is a 30-year-old female who presented for an audiologic evaluation for sudden hearing loss in the right ear. She reported that the hearing in her right ear declined abruptly 2 days prior to the appointment. She also reported constant tinnitus in the right ear and slight imbalance since the decline in hearing, as well as increased sensitivity to loud sounds in the right ear. She reported right aural fullness, but denied otalgia, a history of ear infections, as well as excessive noise exposure. When sudden hearing loss is caused by a viral infection, the patient may report cold-like symptoms from an upper respiratory infection (URI),[1] but KB denied any symptoms of a URI or any other illnesses at the time of the hearing loss. Finally, she stated that her left ear had not been affected and she had not noticed any hearing issues in her left ear.

21.2 Clinical Testing

A comprehensive audiologic evaluation was performed (▶ Fig. 21.1). Pure-tone audiometry revealed hearing sensitivity within normal limits from 250 to 8,000 Hz in the left ear and normal hearing at 250 Hz, sloping to a moderately severe to severe sensorineural hearing loss from 750 to 8,000 Hz in the right ear. Speech Recognition Threshold (SRT) testing revealed normal ability to receive speech in the left ear and a moderately severe loss in the ability to receive speech in the right ear. Word Recognition Scores (WRS) were obtained using a recorded version of Northwestern University Auditory Test No. 6 (NU-6) monosyllabic word

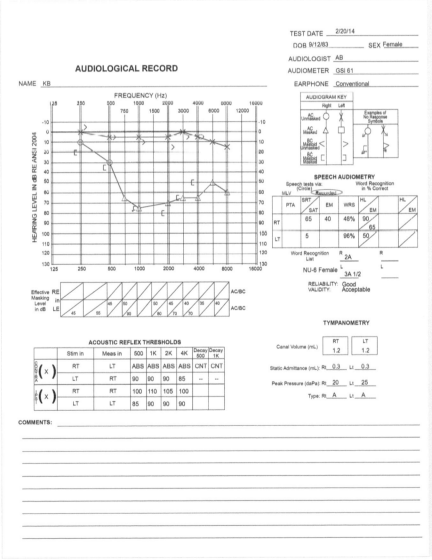

Fig. 21.1 Initial audiological examination following sudden hearing loss.

lists with a female speaker. Words were presented at most intelligible level (MIL), corresponding to a 45 dB sensation level (dB SL) relative to the SRT in the left ear and a 25 dB SL relative to the SRT in the right ear. A score of 96% was obtained in the left ear, demonstrating normal word recognition ability. A score of 48% was obtained in the right ear, demonstrating very poor word recognition ability. Immittance audiometry was performed. Tympanograms were within normal limits, bilaterally. With stimulation to the left ear, ipsilateral and contralateral Acoustic Reflex Thresholds (ART) were present within normal limits at 500 to 4,000 Hz. Ipsilateral ART with stimulation to the right ear were present within normal limits at 500 and 4,000 Hz, and present, but elevated at 1,000 and 2,000 Hz. Contralateral ART with stimulation in the right ear were absent at 500 to 4,000 Hz. Contralateral acoustic reflex decay testing was negative with stimulation to the left ear at 500 and 1,000 Hz and could not be tested with stimulation to the right ear due to absent reflex thresholds. Due to the sudden onset of unilateral hearing loss, KB followed up with an otologist. KB was prescribed oral steroids (12-day taper of prednisone) and an ABR was ordered.

21.3 Questions to the Reader

1. **Why did the otologist order an ABR? What aspects of the case history and clinical testing could be consistent with a retrocochlear lesion?**
2. **What is the incidence of vestibular schwannoma (VS) in patients with sudden sensorineural hearing loss (SSNHL)?**

21.4 Discussion of Questions

1. **Why did the otologist order an ABR? What aspects of the case history and clinical testing could be consistent with a retrocochlear lesion?**

The ABR is a test that evaluates auditory function and can detect auditory dysfunction caused by acoustic tumors, infection, metabolic disease, and degenerative disease. The ABR suggests auditory nerve or auditory brainstem dysfunction in approximately 90% of the cases with VS that are greater than 1.5 cm and 70% of the time with VS smaller than 1.5 cm.[2] Patients with VS may have variable symptoms, including hearing loss, tinnitus, and dizziness.[3]

2. **What is the incidence of vestibular schwannoma (VS) in patients with sudden sensorineural hearing loss (SSNHL)?**

Approximately 1 to 4% of patients with VS present with SSNHL.[3,4,5] SSNHL is more frequently encountered with small (< 1 cm) and medium-sized (1.1–2.9 cm) tumors rather than larger tumors (> 3 cm). Also, lateral tumors originating from or extending to the internal auditory canal (IAC) more often lead to SSNHL compared to medial tumors, which would indicate that compression of the cochlear nerve is the mechanism of the SSNHL.[3,4,5]

21.5 Additional Testing

KB returned for an ABR 2 weeks after her original audiologic evaluation and otology consultation. At the ABR appointment, KB reported she completed her oral steroids and her hearing in the right ear improved significantly and appeared to return to normal. She stated she could use the phone again with either ear and could not detect a difference in the sound when using either. KB reported that she still had occasional tinnitus in the right ear, but denied any other otologic symptoms.

Due to her reports of improved hearing in the right ear, a repeat audiologic evaluation was performed (▶ Fig. 21.2). This evaluation reported normal hearing sensitivity from 250 to 8,000 Hz bilaterally, except for a slight sensorineural hearing loss at 4,000 Hz in the right ear only. SRT testing revealed normal ability to receive speech bilaterally. WRS were obtained using a recorded version of NU-6 monosyllabic word lists with a female speaker. Words were presented at MIL, corresponding to a 45 dB SL relative to the SRT in both ears. A WRS of 100% was obtained in the left ear and 96% in the right ear, demonstrating normal word recognition ability in both ears. Immittance audiometry was performed. Tympanograms were within normal limits, bilaterally. Ipsilateral and contralateral ARTs were present within normal limits in both ears and acoustic reflex decay testing was negative at 500 and 1,000 Hz in both ears. KB was counseled that the hearing in her right ear had improved significantly.

Despite the improvement in hearing in the right ear, an ABR was still performed (▶ Fig. 21.3). ABR testing was completed utilizing rarefaction and alternating polarity click stimuli presented at 11.1 and 71.1 clicks per second. Stimulus presentation levels of 80 and 85 dBnHL were utilized in the left and right ears, respectively. Technical recording quality was good. In ▶ Fig. 21.3, waveforms for the left ear are on the left, labeled A1, and waveforms for the right ear are on the right, labeled B1. ABR results revealed normal absolute latencies for Waves I, III, and V on the left side and normal interpeak latencies for Waves I to III, III to V, and I to V on the left side. Also, a normal shift in Wave V latency was observed with increased stimulus repetition rate on the left side. ABR results on the right side revealed a normal absolute latency for Wave I, but delayed absolute latencies for Waves III and V. Interpeak latency from Waves III to V on the right side was normal, but interpeak latencies from Waves I to III and I to V were prolonged. A normal shift in Wave V latency was observed with increased stimulus repetition rate on the right side, but Wave V interaural latency difference was abnormal. ABR results suggested retrocochlear dysfunction on the right side.

Clinical correlation was recommended due to the abnormal ABR results. The otologist ordered an MRI scan, which revealed a medium-sized (2.1-cm) solitary right VS. While hearing loss is present in 95% of patients with VS, cases have been reported of VS in patients with normal hearing.[6] Unilateral tinnitus is usually still reported in these cases.[6] It is important to note that KB reported continued occasional tinnitus in the right ear even after recovery of hearing.

21.6 Additional Questions to the Reader

1. **Is recovery of hearing typical in cases of SSNHL instigated by VS?**
2. **Why was the MRI needed for clinical correlation if the ABR results indicated retrocochlear pathology?**
3. **What are the typical treatment options for VS?**

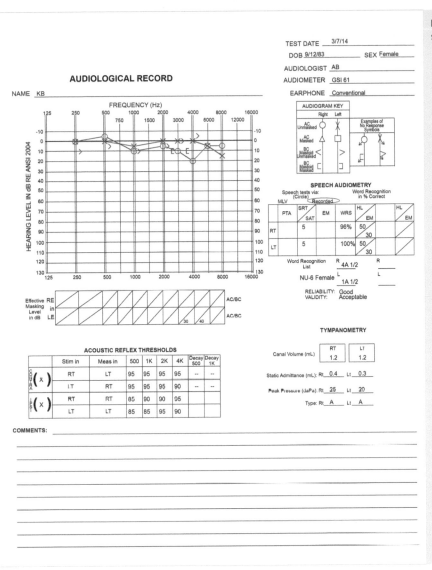

Fig. 21.2 Audiological examination following steroid treatment and hearing recovery.

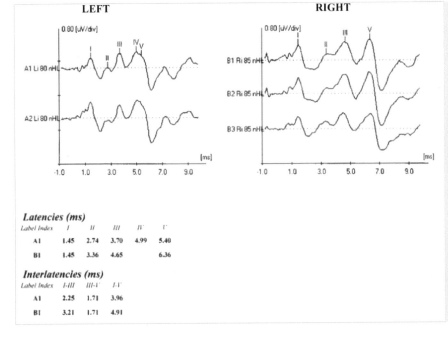

Fig. 21.3 Auditory brainstem response waveforms. Waveforms for the left ear are on the left (A1), waveforms for the right ear are on the right (B1).

Latencies (ms)

Label Index	I	II	III	IV	V
A1	1.45	2.74	3.70	4.99	5.40
B1	1.45	3.36	4.65		6.36

Interlatencies (ms)

Label Index	I-III	III-V	I-V
A1	2.25	1.71	3.96
B1	3.21	1.71	4.91

21.7 Discussion of Additional Questions

1. **Is recovery of hearing typical in cases of SSNHL instigated by VS?**

Recovery of hearing is not discussed frequently in cases of SSNHL with VS. A retrospective study, however, reviewed 295 cases of SSNHL. Of the 295 patients, 12 (4%) were found to have a VS. Of the 12 patients with VS, 4 (33%) showed good recovery with corticosteroid treatment.[4]

2. **Why was the MRI needed for clinical correlation if the ABR results indicated retrocochlear pathology?**

As discussed above, the ABR is a test that evaluates auditory function and can detect auditory nerve or auditory brainstem dysfunction caused by acoustic tumors, infections, metabolic disease, and degenerative disease. The MRI assesses anatomical structures and reports structural changes in the eighth nerve, which may lead to auditory dysfunction. Therefore, the MRI is the "gold standard" in the diagnosis of VS and is needed to diagnose a VS as the cause of the auditory dysfunction reported in the ABR. The MRI is also needed to confirm position of the tumor as well as quantify size.[2]

3. **What are the typical treatment options for VS?**

Current management of VS includes three treatment options: watchful waiting, surgical resection, and radiation therapy. The primary focus of each treatment option is preservation of facial nerve function and hearing while avoiding complications related to tumor growth or treatment. Watchful waiting, or observation, has become a common treatment approach as VS are often diagnosed at small sizes with minimal symptoms due to improved imaging strategies. Serial imaging is required with this treatment approach and loss to follow-up is a potential risk, as annual imaging is recommended. Advantages of watchful waiting include preserving a minimally symptomatic period and avoiding treatment-related complications and side effects.[7,8]

The goal of surgical resection is to remove as much of the tumor as possible without damaging the surrounding structures. Surgical resection may be recommended in cases where tumor growth is observed, vestibular symptoms are present, or there is any doubt of the diagnosis. There are three different surgical approaches: retrosigmoid, middle fossa, and translabyrinthine. Hearing preservation can be accomplished using either the retrosigmoid or middle fossa approach, and most patients maintain the immediate postoperative hearing result over long-term follow-up. When hearing preservation is desired, intraoperative ABR monitoring can be performed to provide feedback to the surgeon(s) on hearing status during surgery. ABR monitoring is reliable, but feedback to the surgeon(s) occurs in a delayed manner. The presence of Wave V at the conclusion of surgery is a predictor of hearing preservation. When no usable hearing is present in the affected ear at the time of surgery, the translabyrinthine surgical approach is preferred.[7,8]

The goal of radiation therapy is to stop tumor growth without damaging the structures surrounding the tumor. The primary indication for radiation therapy is tumor growth. This treatment option would not likely be recommended in cases with vestibular symptoms, prior radiation therapy, or if there is any doubt about the diagnosis. Hearing preservation varies with the length of time after treatment as hearing loss can be a late effect of radiation therapy.[7,8] As a result, annual audiologic evaluations are recommended for patients that undergo radiation therapy.

A period of observation is usually recommended for small tumors, while surgical resection or radiation therapy is reserved for growing or symptomatic tumors. The optimal treatment strategy for VS is based on the individual and the patient's initial hearing status, vestibular symptoms, age, medical comorbidities, and importance of hearing preservation need to be considered.[7]

21.8 Diagnosis and Recommended Treatment

KB was diagnosed with a medium-sized right solitary VS, which is a single tumor that originates in the vestibular portion of the eighth cranial nerve, just within the IAC. Different treatment options were discussed and due to the tumor's size and compression on the eighth nerve, surgical resection was recommended. The patient's hearing in the affected ear following steroid treatment was essentially normal. Therefore, hearing preservation was an important goal and the retrosigmoid surgical approach was recommended. ABR testing would be used in the operating room to provide feedback on the hearing status.

21.9 Outcome

KB underwent surgical resection of the right solitary VS using the retrosigmoid approach. Intraoperative ABR monitoring was performed. The tumor was successfully removed, but the ABR diminished upon opening of the craniotomy and was lost soon after tumor resection began. As a result, KB lost all hearing in the right ear following surgery. KB also had significant balance issues following surgery, which improved with physical therapy. KB did not pursue any amplification options following the loss of hearing in the right ear. It was recommended, however, that she consider either Contralateral Routing of Signal (CROS) amplification or the bone-anchored Baha device for single-sided deafness.

21.10 Key Points

- SSNHL can occur in patients with VS. Therefore, ruling out retrocochlear pathology is important in cases of SSNHL. It is important that the ABR and MRI still be completed even if hearing recovers.
- Steroid treatment is not necessarily contraindicated in cases of SSNHL with VS and there are several documented cases of hearing recovery following steroid treatment. The patient, however, needs to be extensively counseled on the possible effects of VS on hearing status, especially if hearing recovers.
- MRI is the "gold standard" in the diagnosis of VS, but the ABR can reveal auditory dysfunction secondary to acoustic tumors, infections, degenerative disease, and metabolic disorders.

- The management of VS is individualized and several treatment approaches may be recommended, including watchful waiting, surgical resection, and radiation therapy.

References

[1] Cadoni G, Agostino S, Scipione S, et al. Sudden sensorineural hearing loss: our experience in diagnosis, treatment, and outcome. J Otolaryngol. 2005; 34(6): 395–401

[2] Peterein JL, Neely JG. Auditory brainstem response testing in neurodiagnosis: structure versus function. J Am Acad Audiol. 2012; 23(4):269–275

[3] Jeong KH, Choi JW, Shin JE, Kim CH. Abnormal magnetic resonance imaging findings in patients with sudden sensorineural hearing loss: vestibular schwannoma as the most common cause of MRI abnormality. Medicine (Baltimore). 2016; 95(17):e3557

[4] Lee JD, Lee BD, Hwang SC. Vestibular schwannoma in patients with sudden sensorineural hearing loss. Skull Base. 2011; 21(2):75–78

[5] Lin C, Gong Q, Zuo W, Zhang R, Zhou A. The clinical characteristics and treatment for sudden sensorineural hearing loss with vestibular schwannoma. Eur Arch Otorhinolaryngol. 2015; 272(4):839–842

[6] Valente M, Peterein J, Goebel J, Neely JG. Four cases of acoustic neuromas with normal hearing. J Am Acad Audiol. 1995; 6(3):203–210

[7] Quesnel AM, McKenna MJ. Current strategies in management of intracanalicular vestibular schwannoma. Curr Opin Otolaryngol Head Neck Surg. 2011; 19(5):335–340

[8] Liu W, Ni M, Jia W, et al. How to address small- and medium-sized acoustic neuromas with hearing: a systematic review and decision analysis. World Neurosurg. 2015; 84(2):283–291.e1

22 A Classic Case of Vestibular Neuritis

Heather Monroe

22.1 Clinical History and Description

DT is a 40-year-old male who scheduled an appointment with otolaryngology citing a 5-year history of persistent dizziness and postural instability that began after a single, severe attack of vertigo. The patient described the vertiginous attack as a severe spinning sensation of unspecified direction, which lasted all day and was accompanied by nausea and vomiting. DT stated that he did not lose consciousness. Two weeks after this episode, he experienced significant postural instability. Initially he was evaluated by a physician in his hometown and underwent physical therapy, but the patient reported only minimal improvement in his symptoms. For the 5 years since the vertiginous attack, he had a constant sensation of dizziness and imbalance. In addition, he reported motion-induced visual blurring with rightward head turns, a sensation of fullness on the right side of his head, significant difficulty driving at night, and difficulty in busy visual environments such as a crowded supermarket. He denied tinnitus, aural fullness, and did not experience any changes in his hearing.

22.2 Vestibular Testing

Bithermal caloric irrigation revealed a 100% right reduced vestibular response. Otherwise, video-oculography (VOG) results were within normal limits. The video Head Impulse Test (vHIT) revealed covert saccades and reduced gain for rightward impulses in the horizontal plane (▶ Fig. 22.1). Leftward impulses and impulses in the planes of the anterior and posterior canals in both ears were within normal limits, indicating that the patient was able to maintain fixation. Cervical vestibular-evoked myogenic potential (cVEMP) responses were obtained and replicated in both ears at normal thresholds (▶ Fig. 22.2). Ocular vestibular-evoked myogenic potential (oVEMP) responses were present in the left ear and absent in the right ear (▶ Fig. 22.3). The patient refused rotational chair testing due to claustrophobia.

22.3 Questions to the Reader

1. **What is the significance of the patient's reported symptoms of motion-induced visual blurring with rightward head turns?**
2. **What information did the audiologist gain from the vestibular test results?**
3. **What additional information would have rotational chair testing provided?**
4. **Why is an accurate diagnosis and quantitative assessment of remaining function important?**

22.4 Discussion of Questions

1. **What is the significance of the patient's reported symptoms of motion-induced visual blurring with rightward head turns?**

The patient's report of his vision blurring when he moves his head to the right provided the audiologist with an important clue regarding the status of his inner ear. Motion-induced visual blurring with head movement to the right indicates failure of the vestibuloocular reflex (VOR) to maintain visual fixation during rightward head movement and suggests uncompensated unilateral peripheral dysfunction in the right ear.

2. **What information did the audiologist gain from the vestibular test results?**

The ability of clinical audiologists to evaluate the vestibular system continues to expand. With the recent additions of vHIT and VEMP to the clinical repertoire, it is now possible to provide objective data regarding the function of the VOR within the range of natural head movement for all six semicircular canal pairs and evaluate the pathway of the otolith organs and individual branches of the vestibular nerve. In this case, valuable and distinct information obtained from caloric testing, VEMPs, and vHIT contributed to the patient's diagnosis.

- **Calorics.** First introduced over 100 years ago, the caloric test is one of the oldest components of the vestibular

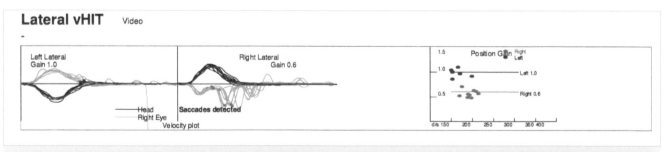

Fig. 22.1 Video head impulse test tracings for the right lateral semicircular canal revealed covert saccades, indicating DT's eyes slipped off the target and a corrective saccade during the head movement was required to return DT's eyes to the target. The gain value for the right lateral canal is 0.5 and is outside of the normal range. Tracings for the left lateral canal are consistent with normal function. The patient's eyes remain on the target throughout the head movement and the gain value is 1.0, indicating that eye movement was equal and opposite to head movement. Gain values between 0.7 and 1.0 are considered within normal limits. Reduced gain is consistent with vestibuloocular reflex dysfunction.

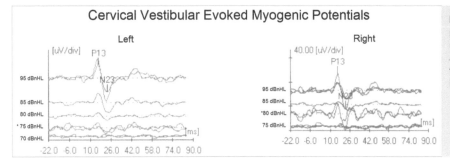

Cervical Vestibular Evoked Myogenic Potentials

Fig. 22.2 Cervical vestibular-evoked myogenic potential responses were present in both ears at normal thresholds of 75 and 80 dBnHL for the left and right ears, respectively. This suggests normal function in the pathway of the saccule and inferior branch of the vestibular nerve.

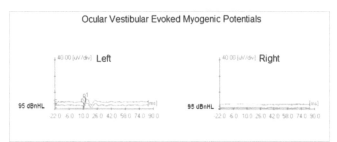

Fig. 22.3 Ocular vestibular-evoked myogenic potential responses were obtained and replicated in the left ear and suggest normal function. Responses were absent in the right ear. This suggests dysfunction in the pathway of the utricle and superior branch of the vestibular nerve.

evaluation and provides ear-specific information about the responsiveness of the horizontal semicircular canal. The test is administered by creating a convection current in the endolymph housed within the horizontal semicircular canal. The result is a nonphysiological response as the brain perceives movement at a very low and unnatural frequency (0.002–0.004 Hz), while the head remains stationary. In this case, the audiologist observed from the caloric test results that there was an asymmetry with the right ear unresponsive to caloric irrigation. The information the audiologist gained from the caloric test, however, is limited. While the caloric test contributes important lateralizing cues, the information it provides is limited to the function of the horizontal semicircular canal at a single frequency and does not indicate the extent of the loss or the status of other vestibular organs.

- **VEMP.** Development of the VEMP test began in the mid-1990s and resulted in the addition of two distinct tests of otolith function to the vestibular evaluation. When the active electrode is placed near the contralateral inferior oblique muscle (oVEMP), the resulting waveform is a reflection of the integrity of the pathway, which includes the utricle and the superior branch of the vestibular nerve (▶ Fig. 22.4). In contrast, when the active electrode is placed on the belly of the ipsilateral sternocleidomastoid muscle (cVEMP), the resultant waveform arises from the saccule and the inferior branch of the vestibular nerve (▶ Fig. 22.5). In this case, the patient had normal VEMP responses with the exception of the absent right oVEMP. This suggests that dysfunction is limited to the superior branch of the vestibular nerve, a common characteristic of vestibular neuritis.

- **vHIT.** One of the most recent additions to vestibular evaluation, the vHIT is performed via quick, passive movements of the head in the plane of semicircular canal pairs while the patient attempts to maintain his/her gaze on a fixed target. To perform the test, the examiner places his/her hands on the patient's head and quickly thrusts the head in the horizontal plane to the right or left, or diagonally, with equal components of pitch and roll, in the vertical plane. The head thrusts are small, quick, and unpredictable. Dysfunction is identified by the presence of corrective covert and/or overt saccades along with reduced gain values. During this test, the VOR is evaluated within the range of natural head movement (0.1–5 Hz). Recent research has suggested that the vHIT also provides clues concerning dynamic compensation following vestibular loss. In a study,[1] it was suggested that corrective saccades occur earlier in the head movement as the patient begins to compensate. When the insult is acute, the saccades are overt, occurring after the head movement. During the recovery process, as compensation begins to take place, the corrective saccades move temporally until they become covert, occurring during the head movement. In this case, the vHIT results revealed high-frequency dysfunction in the right horizontal semicircular canal. The absent overt saccades and present covert saccades suggest that at least partial compensation for the loss has already occurred.

These test results, along with the patient's case history of symptoms beginning with one severe vertigo attack lasting several hours, substantiated the diagnosis of vestibular neuritis in the right ear. Due to the patient's complaints, the audiologist knew that DT had not fully compensated from the loss of function in the right ear despite previous physical therapy.

3. What additional information would have rotational chair testing provided?

Rotational chair testing evaluates the vestibular system between 0.1 and 1 Hz. VOR gain, phase, and symmetry values, along with time constants, provide further insight regarding the status of dynamic compensation that has occurred following the initial vertigo attack. As compensation progresses, gain, phase, and symmetry values begin to normalize. Symmetry is often the first value to normalize, followed by gain and then phase. In some cases, neither gain nor phase will completely recover.

Time constants are defined as the time it takes for the vestibular response to decay to 37% of its peak amplitude and is a reflection of the integrity of the velocity storage mechanism.

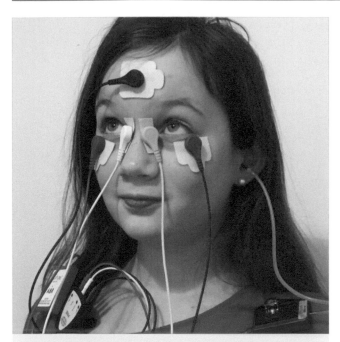

Fig. 22.4 Electrode configuration for recording a left ocular vestibular-evoked myogenic potential response. The active electrode is placed under the right (contralateral) eye near the inferior oblique muscle, the reference electrode is on the right side of the nasal bridge, and the ground electrode is on the forehead. The patient is instructed to gaze upward during sound presentation, to position the belly of the muscle closer to the electrode.

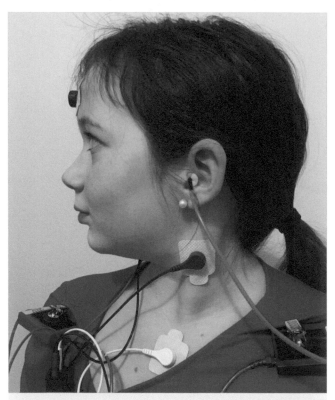

Fig. 22.5 Electrode configuration for recording a cervical vestibular-evoked myogenic potential (cVEMP) response. The active electrode is placed on the belly of the ipsilateral sternocleidomastoid muscle, the reference electrode is near the sternum, and the ground electrode is on the forehead. The cVEMP response is inhibitory in nature and requires the patient to adequately contract the sternocleidomastoid muscle during sound presentation.

Time constants of less than 7 seconds indicate disabling of central velocity storage. This is seen in uncompensated peripheral vestibular dysfunction.

If rotational chair study had been completed in this patient, the audiologist would have likely seen a pattern of reduced low-frequency VOR gain with phase lead and reduced time constants indicating uncompensated unilateral peripheral dysfunction.

4. **Why is an accurate diagnosis and quantitative assessment of remaining function important?**

An accurate diagnosis and quantitative assessment of remaining function is crucial to developing an effective treatment plan. Treatment options for patients experiencing dizziness and/or balance disorders vary depending on diagnosis, remaining vestibular function, and stability of the lesion. Treatment options include dietary changes, surgery, and physical therapy. In stable lesions such as vestibular neuritis, vestibular rehabilitation is the most effective treatment and provides a method to promote compensation in patients who have failed to do so naturally. Vestibular rehabilitation is often provided by a physical therapist (PT) who utilizes the quantitative information obtained from vestibular tests to customize exercises for the patient.

22.5 Diagnosis and Recommended Treatment

DT was diagnosed with incomplete compensation following a vestibular neuritis attack in the right ear. Physical therapy was recommended and DT was referred to a PT specializing in vestibular rehabilitation. The PT met with DT to determine goals and prescribe exercises. DT expressed that his primary desire was relief from his symptoms of dizziness and imbalance, improved tolerance of busy visual environments, and ability to drive at night and participate in recreational softball and golf. A physical therapy plan was created and included balance retraining and neuromuscular re-education.

22.6 Outcome

As the clinic was quite far from home, DT met with the PT twice a month and completed the majority of his therapy through home exercises over a period of 10 weeks. At discharge, the majority of his goals had been met. He reported less anxiety when driving, had returned to recreational sports, and reported an 85 to 90% improvement in balance. Tolerance of busy visual environments, however, continued to be difficult. Those goals he had not met were improving and the patient was instructed to continue his exercises at home.

22.7 Key Points

- Recent technological advances have led to new tests in the vestibular laboratory, allowing the audiologist to provide information regarding the integrity of the pathway between the otolith organs and individual branches of the vestibular nerve as well as the function of the six semicircular canals at a wide frequency range.

- Information gained from comprehensive vestibular evaluation along with a thorough case history allows for more accurate patient diagnoses.
- The results from these tests of vestibular integrity can lead to the creation of a customized treatment plan and improved outcome.

Reference

[1] Manzari L, Burgess AM, MacDougall HG, Curthoys IS. Vestibular function after vestibular neuritis. Int J Audiol. 2013; 52(10):713–718

Suggested Reading

[1] Colebatch JG, Halmagyi GM. Vestibular evoked potentials in human neck muscles before and after unilateral vestibular deafferentation. Neurology. 1992; 42(8):1635–1636

[2] Iwasaki S, Chihara Y, Smulders YE, et al. The role of the superior vestibular nerve in generating ocular vestibular-evoked myogenic potentials to bone conducted vibration at Fz. Clin Neurophysiol. 2009; 120(3):588–593

[3] Macdougall HG, Curthoys IS. Plasticity during vestibular compensation: the role of saccades. Front Neurol. 2012; 3(21):21

23 Vestibular Migraine Disease and Horizontal Canal Benign Paroxysmal Positional Vertigo in an Adult Patient

Andrea Gohmert

23.1 Clinical History and Description

JA is a 27-year-old female referred to our office for an evaluation of dizziness. JA reported waking in the middle of the night with vertigo approximately 6 weeks prior to the visit. She reported severe spinning each time she would lay down and was evaluated by her primary care physician who diagnosed her with bilateral ear infections and prescribed antibiotics. JA reported persistent "bobbing" sensations between episodes of vertigo and stated the vertigo was provoked by changes in head and body position. She also complained of symptoms of photophobia (sensitivity to light) and headaches and was evaluated by a neurologist for migraines. At the point of her visit, JA reported consistent dizziness that lasted for days. She noted no particular direction for her spinning sensation. She noted that the spinning is present whenever she lies down so she had been sleeping upright in a chair for several weeks. She also noted spinning whenever she turns her head. She could not identify the direction of her spinning. Medical history was also positive for bilateral tinnitus of 1-week duration, ear pain (otalgia) and fullness that began 6 weeks prior to the visit, and anxiety.

23.2 Clinical Testing

The initial audiological examination (▶ Fig. 23.1) was conducted by an audiologist from the referring otolaryngologist and was consistent with normal hearing bilaterally. The Speech Recognition Threshold (SRT) was in good agreement with the pure-tone average (PTA) bilaterally and revealed normal ability to receive

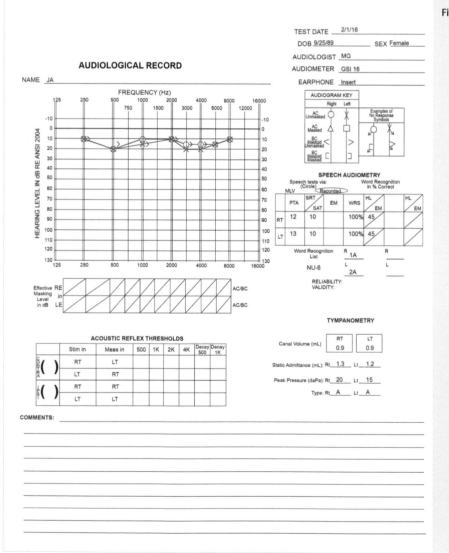

Fig. 23.1 Audiogram of first examination.

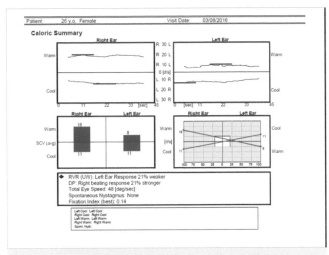

Fig. 23.2 Caloric test results reporting a 27% left unilateral weakness.

speech. The Word Recognition Score (WRS) at 35-dB sensation level indicated normal ability to receive speech. Tympanograms revealed normal ear canal volume, middle ear pressure, and static compliance. Acoustic Reflex Thresholds (ART) for contralateral and ipsilateral stimulation was not completed in either ear with no explanation as to why it was not completed.

Videonystagmography (VNG) testing (▶ Fig. 23.2) was completed and results were consistent with normal ocular motility. Dix–Hallpike testing (▶ Fig. 23.3) was unremarkable with the right ear in the downward position, but positive for horizontal left-beating nystagmus only in the head-down and head-left positions that had no torsional component. The nystagmus did not fatigue on repeat. Positional testing (▶ Fig. 23.4) was remarkable for geotropic direction-changing positional nystagmus in all positions with a torsional component in the head-left and body-left positions. The direction-changing nystagmus was very strong measuring up to 60 deg/s in the horizontal compo-

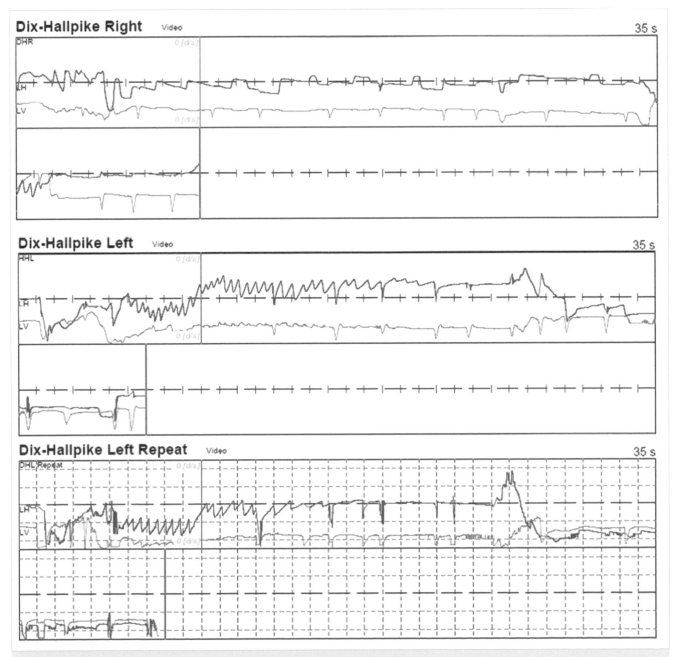

Fig. 23.3 Dix–Hallpike testing reporting left posterior canal benign paroxysmal positional vertigo.

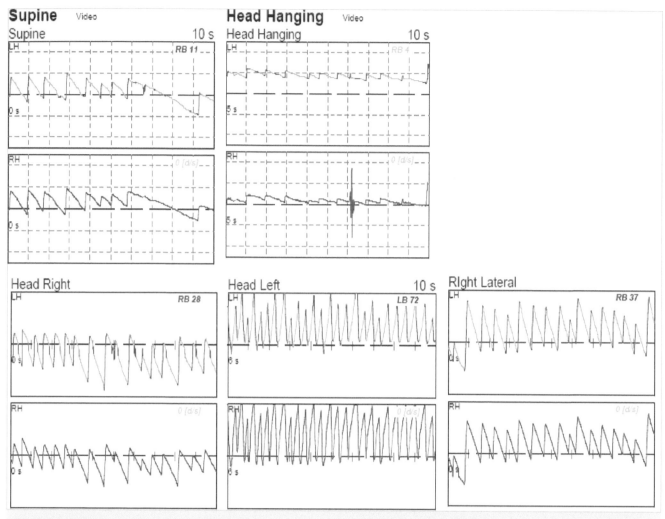

Fig. 23.4 Position testing reporting right-beating nystagmus in supine, head-hanging, head-right, and body-right positions; left-beating nystagmus in head-left and body-left positions. These are examples of geotropic direction-changing positional nystagmus.

nent and 30 deg/s in the vertical component. The patient was nauseated throughout testing. Caloric testing was consistent with a 21% left equivocal caloric weakness.

23.3 Questions for the Reader

1. Given the patient's initial medical history and audiological findings, what diagnosis would the reader suspect as the cause of her vertigo?
2. Based on the VNG results, what diagnosis can be confirmed and what disorders can be ruled out?
3. What further testing could be completed to reach a diagnosis for JA?

23.4 Discussion of Questions

1. **Given the patient's initial medical history and audiological findings, what diagnosis would the reader suspect as the cause of her vertigo?**

Given the fact JA had normal hearing and reported of dizziness that was sudden in onset and aggravated by head and body

movement, benign paroxysmal positional vertigo (BPPV) is a good hypothesis. This patient, however, reported her symptoms were constant and had not resolved. JA also reported bilateral tinnitus in addition to the vertigo. Based on those symptoms, vestibular neuritis could not be ruled out. Vestibular neuritis affects the branch of the vestibular nerve associated with balance, resulting in dizziness or vertigo, but no change in hearing. Vestibular neuritis is commonly caused by a viral infection. In addition, since JA was being evaluated for migraines, vestibular migraine disease could not be ruled out. The presentation of vestibular migraine varies. Symptoms include spontaneous and positional vertigo, head motion vertigo/dizziness, and ataxia of variable duration, ranging from seconds to days. Most episodes have no temporal relationship with the headaches. Therefore, audiologists need to rely on additional testing to reach a differential diagnosis.

2. **Based on the VNG results, what diagnosis can e confirmed and what disorders can be ruled out?**

The results from the VNG ruled out vestibular neuritis because there was no significant caloric weakness. Abnormal results for this clinic are a unilateral weakness greater than or equal to

25% difference between the caloric responses in each ear. Test results reported a positive Dix–Hallpike with horizontal nystagmus in the left ear down condition, the presence of geotropic direction-changing positional nystagmus, and the response fatiguing on repeat tests. These results would point to a positive indication of horizontal canal BPPV with the left semicircular horizontal canal affected. In addition, the presence of geotropic direction-changing positional nystagmus was present in head-right, head-left, body-right, and body-left positions. The strongest nystagmus was in the head-left position. Vestibular migraine is known to frequently cause geotropic direction-changing positional nystagmus, but will not cause nystagmus following a Dix–Hallpike maneuver that will fatigue on repeated testing. JA, however, reported photophobia, headache, tinnitus, otalgia, and anxiety. Therefore, audiologists still have two possible diagnoses: horizontal canal BPPV affecting the left semicircular canal and possible vestibular migraine.

3. **What further testing could be completed to reach a diagnosis for JA?**

Another test for horizontal canal BPPV not requiring additional equipment other than a chair that reclines or an exam table is the Supine Roll Test. In idiopathic cases with geotropic nystagmus, the "bad" ear is assigned to the side with the stronger nystagmus. This would be known as a canalithiasis. In JA's case, this was the left ear.

Video Head Impulse Test (VHIT) would report an abnormality toward the left ear. In this case, however, JA had such strong nystagmus when the head was turned to either side that the author believes JA would not have tolerated VHIT nor been able to focus on the fixation point.

Essentially, a good case history and a trial with medications and diet were used to diagnose the vestibular migraine component for JA. No additional audiological tests were necessary.

23.5 Diagnosis and Recommended Treatment

Based on the available test results, the neurotologist diagnosed JA with horizontal canal BPPV and vestibular migraine. The patient was treated with the Lempert roll maneuver by the physician. The Lempert Roll, also known as the "BBQ Roll," is a canalith repositioning maneuver used to treat horizontal canal BPPV. The following steps describe the Lempert Roll:

1. The patient should lie supine on the examination table, affected ear down. Quickly turn the patient's head 90 degrees toward the unaffected side.
2. Wait 15 to 20 seconds between each head turn.
3. Turn the patient's head 90 degrees so the affected ear is now up.
4. Have the patient tuck his/her arms to his/her chest and roll the patient to a prone position with his/her face down.
5. Have the patient turn on his/her side as the audiologist rolls his/her head 90 degrees (returning to original position, affected ear down).

6. Position the patient so he/she is face up and brought to a sitting position.

Following the procedure, JA was instructed to sleep in a semi-upright position for two nights following the procedure. In addition, the physician prescribed a migraine diet with keeping a food diary and a prescription of amitriptyline for her migraines. A follow-up appointment was scheduled in 2 weeks.

23.6 Outcome

At the follow-up appointment, JA reported her headaches improved 90%. JA still, however, reported some positional vertigo with some improvement since the previous visit. The Lempert Roll maneuver was performed again by the physician's assistant with instructions to sleep in the semi-upright position for two nights following the procedure and another follow-up appointment was scheduled in 1 month.

At the final follow-up appointment, JA was examined by the audiologist using VNG goggles and the Dix–Hallpike was negative in both directions. JA reported no further positional nystagmus and resolution of her headaches as a result of taking amitriptyline.

23.7 Key Points

- Patients with vestibular disorders present with a variety of symptoms, and diagnosis begins with a detailed case history and dizziness inventories. The Dizziness Handicap Inventory (DHI)[1] and Vestibular Disorders Activities of Daily Living (VADL)[2] are excellent dizziness inventories to assess the symptoms of a patient and aid in diagnosis. Prior to seeing JA, she completed a thorough dizziness inventory that was formulated for our clinic and a case history allowing the audiologist and physicians to begin to consider possible diagnoses prior to testing.[3]
- Many audiologists forget there are several diagnostic tests to diagnose BPPV and not all cases of BPPV result in a diagnosis of posterior canal BPPV. Although rare, horizontal or lateral canal BPPV can occur and a simple supine roll test or examination of positional testing results on VNG can aid in correct diagnosis.[4]
- Vestibular migraine is very common and is the second most common presentation for vertigo after BPPV. Vestibular migraine will mimic symptoms of Meniere's disease and BPPV, but there are a few key reports from the patient in the case history that are common to vestibular migraine and include photophobia, diplopia, tingling, and numbness along with headache. When a patient reports these symptoms along with vertigo, vestibular migraine should be suspected.[5]
- Finally, it is possible to reach more than one diagnosis for a patient reporting vertigo. Often, audiologists feel they are searching for a single diagnosis, but it is possible for a patient to have several disorders concurrently. It is import to remember that an incomplete diagnosis will lead to a patient continuing to experience vertigo.[6]

References

[1] Jacobson GP, Newman CW. The development of the Dizziness Handicap Inventory. Arch Otolaryngol Head Neck Surg. 1990; 116(4):424–427

[2] Cohen HS, Kimball KT. Development of the vestibular disorders activities of daily living scale. Arch Otolaryngol Head Neck Surg. 2000; 126(7):881–887

[3] Zhao JG, Piccirillo JF, Spitznagel EL, Jr, Kallogjeri D, Goebel JA. Predictive capability of historical data for diagnosis of dizziness. Otol Neurotol. 2011; 32(2): 284–290

[4] Balatsouras DG, Koukoutsis G, Ganelis P, Korres GS, Kaberos A. Diagnosis of single- or multiple-canal benign paroxysmal positional vertigo according to the type of nystagmus. Int J Otolaryngol. 2011; 2011(2):483965

[5] Chu C-H, Liu C-J, Lin L-Y, Chen TJ, Wang SJ. Migraine is associated with an increased risk for benign paroxysmal positional vertigo: a nationwide population-based study. J Headache Pain. 2015; 16:62

[6] Teggi R, Manfrin M, Balzanelli C, et al. Point prevalence of vertigo and dizziness in a sample of 2672 subjects and correlation with headaches. Acta Otorhinolaryngol Ital. 2016; 36(3):215–219

24 A Case of Central and Peripheral Vestibular Impairment

Steven M. Doettl and Devin L. McCaslin

24.1 Clinical History and Description

MM is a 64-year-old female referred from an otolaryngologist for a second opinion regarding intermittent episodic positional vertigo occurring only with changes in head position and persistent unsteadiness of gait. MM's primary concern was that her gait disturbance had become significantly worse over the last 6 years, but had been present for the past 25 years. At the time of the consultation, MM described two distinct forms of dizziness. First, MM reported a sensation of nausea and light-headedness with true vertigo provoked by changes in body position (e.g., looking up and bending over). Second, she described progressively worsening disequilibrium when walking or standing. During the direct patient interview, it was revealed that 6 years ago MM experienced a severe episode of true vertigo that lasted approximately 2 days. Of further note is MM had a history of persistent moderate alcohol intake (an average of 12 drinks per weekend) for the last 25 years. When questioned about her hearing, MM reported she had bilateral hearing loss and it had progressed slowly over the last 10 years. She denied any fluctuation in hearing, aural fullness, or tinnitus. At the time of presentation, she carried diagnoses of depression, restless leg syndrome, and Meniere's Disease (MD; diagnosed 28 years prior). Her management at the time of the appointment consisted of a low salt diet, diuretic for the MD, and pramipexole for restless leg syndrome.

24.2 Audiological Testing

The results from the initial audiological examination (▶ Fig. 24.1) were obtained with good reliability and revealed a mild sensorineural hearing loss (SNHL) at 250 to 2,000 Hz rising to normal hearing at 3,000 to 8,000 Hz for the right ear. Results

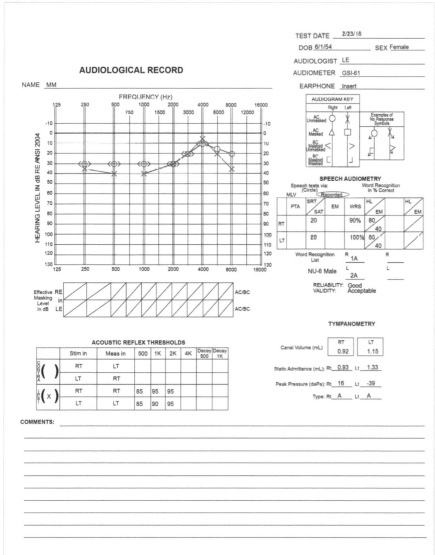

Fig. 24.1 Audiogram revealing a mild predominantly low-frequency SNHL (sensorineural hearing loss) bilaterally. Immittance testing indicated normal middle-ear pressure and middle-ear compliance bilaterally. Ipsilateral ARTs (acoustic reflex thresholds) were obtained at normal sensation levels bilaterally.

for the left ear indicated a mild SNHL at 250 to 2,000 and 8,000 Hz with normal hearing at 3,000 to 6,000 Hz. Her Speech Recognition Threshold (SRT) was 20 dB hearing level (HL) bilaterally, indicating a normal ability to receive speech. Word Recognition Scores (WRS) revealed normal ability to recognize speech bilaterally. Immittance testing indicated normal ear canal volume, middle ear pressure, and static compliance bilaterally. Ipsilateral Acoustic Reflex Thresholds (ARTs) were obtained at normal sensation levels bilaterally.

24.3 Otolaryngology Consultation

Evaluation by the otologist noted that MM's symptoms and history were not entirely consistent with MD. The possibility of migrainous dizziness was also discussed; however, MM did not

meet the diagnostic criteria for vestibular migraine, which include, but are not limited to, the following: (1) at least five episodes with vestibular symptoms (5 min to 72 hours), (2) history of migraine with or without aura, (3) one or more migraine features with at least 50% of the vestibular episodes, (4) headache with (at least two of) one-sided location, (5) pulsating quality, (6) moderate or severe pain intensity, (7) aggravation by routine physical activity, (8) photophobia, and/or (9) phonophobia.[1] While MM did experience several of the criteria for vestibular migraine, she did not have a history of migraines or headache with the significant qualities. Vestibular function testing consisting of Videonystagmography (VNG), Cervical Vestibular Evoked Myogenic Potentials (cVEMPs), and rotary chair testing (RCT) were subsequently ordered as well as magnetic resonance imaging (MRI) of the brain with and without contrast.

24.4 Clinical Vestibular Evaluation

MM was found to be positive for anxiety and depression via the Hospital Anxiety and Depression Scale (HADS).[2] The VNG evaluation revealed normal horizontal and vertical saccade latency, velocity, and accuracy with random frequency and amplitudes. Gaze testing at center gaze was positive for persistent Downbeat Nystagmus (DBN) that increased in intensity with lateral and downward gaze and decreased with upward gaze (▶ Fig. 24.2). Horizontal rebound nystagmus was also noted. Smooth pursuit tracking was abnormal with reduced gain values for right and left tracking at 0.2 to 0.5 Hz with saccadic intrusion throughout the recording (▶ Fig. 24.3). Additionally, optokinetic nystagmus revealed reduced gain bilaterally. Positional/positioning subtests were also positive for persistent DBN throughout all positions consistent with the gaze findings. Caloric testing was completed with a binaural bithermal technique indicating a total caloric response of 35 degrees/s with a 49% left unilateral weakness (i.e., > 25% is abnormal) and 49% right directional preponderance (i.e., > 35% is abnormal). RCT slow harmonic acceleration results indicated abnormal phase leads at 0.01 and 0.02 Hz with normal gain and symmetry across the frequencies evaluated. cVEMP testing was completed with normal N1-P1 latency and amplitude values bilaterally. No

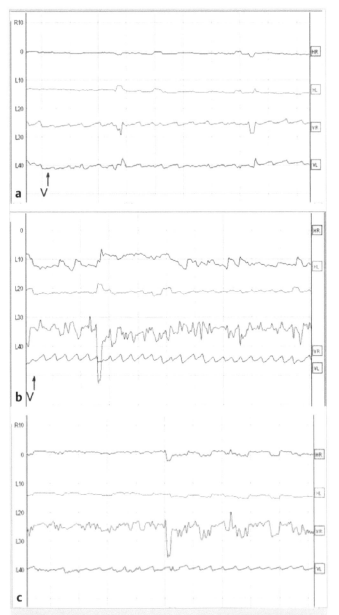

Fig. 24.2 Gaze testing at **(a)** center gaze revealing persistent DBN (downbeat nystagmus) that increased in intensity with **(b)** left gaze and **(c)** right gaze.

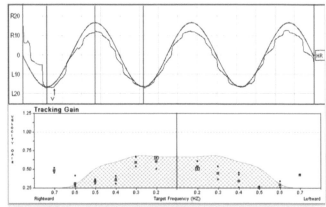

Fig. 24.3 Smooth pursuit tracking was abnormal with both reduced gain values for right and left tracking at 0.2 to 0.5 Hz with saccadic intrusion throughout the recording.

significant amplitude asymmetry or reduced thresholds were noted. RCT Vestibuloocular Reflex (VOR) suppression was abnormal at 0.04 and 0.08 Hz. The saccadic pursuit and abnormal RCT suppression suggested central vestibular involvement. Additionally, the presence of DBN is also highly suggestive of central vestibular pathology. DBN is most often associated with infarction, cerebellar and spinocerebellar degeneration syndromes, MS (multiple sclerosis), and developmental anomalies affecting the pons and cerebellum.[3] Based on these findings, specifically the presence of DBN, a referral to neuro-ophthalmology was requested.

24.5 Neuro-ophthalmology Consultation

Neuro-ophthalmology consultation included a cranial nerve exam and direct patient interview. The patient was noted to have a normal appearance and was alert and oriented with a normal affect. DBN was present with vision and vision denied and exacerbated on lateral gaze to either side, noted to be a positive Daroff sign (DBN with increased amplitude when looking down or laterally). Cranial nerves II to XII were evaluated with no indication of specific nerve involvement. It was also noted that she had slightly unusual speech, possibly subtle scanning speech (also referred to as explosive speech), which is a type of ataxic dysarthria resulting in separations or pauses between syllables of words.

24.6 Imaging

MRI, without and with gadolinium enhancement (GAD), requested along with the aforementioned vestibular evaluation indicated mild diffuse cerebellar and cerebral atrophy.

24.7 Questions to the Reader

1. Based on the combination of the audiological and vestibular results, neuro-ophthalmological evaluation, and MRI, what conclusions can be made with regard to the cause of MM's dizziness and unsteadiness?
2. What aspect(s), if any, of MM's reported history would be consistent with or possibly explain the cause of the above results?
3. What is the likely origin of the DBN observed for MM?
4. What is a potential consequence of having simultaneous cerebellar and peripheral vestibular system impairment?
5. What is the prognosis for this patient and what should be the recommendations for further evaluation, treatment, or management?

24.8 Discussion of Questions

1. Based on the combination of the audiological results, neuro-ophthalmological evaluation, and MRI, what conclusions can be made with regard to the cause of MM's dizziness and unsteadiness?

While audiometric results revealed low-frequency SNHL, it was bilateral and there were no other accompanying symptoms or findings that suggest MD. The vestibular evaluation was suggestive of both central and peripheral vestibular pathology. Caloric testing indicated unilateral peripheral vestibular hypofunction with a left caloric weakness. Positioning/positional testing was positive for DBN, which can be suggestive of anterior canal Benign Paroxysmal Positional Vertigo (BPPV). MM also reported a previous second event consistent with BPPV. She did not, however, report any current episodic symptoms of dizziness or vertigo that would be associated with BPPV and the noted nystagmus was persistent across positions and was consistent with gaze testing.

DBN was observed during central gaze with increased amplitude with lateral gaze. Reduced smooth pursuit gain with saccadic intrusion and reduced optokinetic gain were also noted. RCT results also indicated abnormal phase leads and VOR suppression. Abnormal pursuit function, reduced optokinetic gain, and abnormal VOR suppression have all been noted along with DBN in cases of cerebellar dysfunction.[3] The results of the neuro-ophthalmological evaluation, specifically the positive Daroff sign and noted scanning speech, were also highly suggestive of cerebellar dysfunction. The MRI indicated mild diffuse cerebellar and cerebral atrophy confirming the vestibular and neuro-ophthalmological evaluation findings, suggesting cerebellar dysfunction.

2. **What aspect(s), if any, of MM's reported history would be consistent with or possibly explain the cause of the above results?**

The previously reported 2-day episode of vertigo was consistent with caloric findings of a left unilateral peripheral weakness and was suggestive of a left vestibular neuritis. The vestibular, neuro-ophthalmological and MRI also suggested central vestibular pathology, specifically midline cerebellar dysfunction. Overall, the reported history appears benign for neurologic deficits; however, there is the reported social history including an average of 12 drinks per weekend over 25 years, which could qualify MM as a "moderate" drinker. Alcohol consumption has been found to be associated with both DBN and progressive cerebellar ataxia.[4,5,6] Cerebellar ataxia from moderate alcohol use has been noted.[7,8,9] Specifically, moderate alcoholic intake has been linked to a loss of Purkinje's cells, a decrease in the volume of the anterior vermis, and cerebellar atrophy.[7] Severe long-term alcohol abuses in cases of alcoholism have been specifically associated with cerebellar ataxia, Wernicke's encephalopathy, and other neuropathological problems.[5,6]

3. **What is the likely origin of the DBN observed for MM?**

DBN can occur in association with many different disorders and can often be observed in patients that have atrophy of the vestibulocerebellum. DBN is commonly present in central gaze and enhances with lateral gaze; thus, the optimal gaze position to observe DBN is down and lateral.[10] The slow phase velocities may increase in velocity (not linear) as is documented in this case. One theory regarding the origin of DBN is that impairment in the cerebellum has created a persistent asymmetry in the vertical VOR.[11] The flocculus of the cerebellum exerts inhibitory control over the electrical tone of the pathways running from anterior semicircular canal to the superior rectus (primary function is to elevate the eye). Posterior semicircular projections used to draw the eye down with the depressor extraocular muscles are not influenced by the flocculus. Consequently, when the flocculus of the cerebellum is impaired, the anterior canal pathway is released from inhibition and the superior rectus is slowly contracted, pulling the eye upward (i.e., slow phase of the DBN). The corrective fast eye movement downward resets the eye on the target (i.e., fast phase of the DBN). Patients manifesting DBN often complain of oscillopsia (unsteady visual field resulting in blurry/jumping vision) and postural instability.[3] It has been reported previously by several different groups that alcohol abuse can result in cerebellar degeneration and as a consequence these patients demonstrate DBN.[4,9,12]

One word of caution is that when evaluating a patient during positioning testing, it is important to remember that DBN can be enhanced when the patient is placed in a head-hanging or prone position. It is critically important that the clinician does not confuse this central pathology with what may at first appear to be a case of anterior BPPV.

4. **What is a potential consequence of having simultaneous cerebellar and peripheral vestibular system impairment?**

Following loss of function of one peripheral vestibular end organ, patients will experience acute vestibular syndrome. That is, these patients will describe true vertigo, nausea, and disequilibrium. Vestibular compensation is the central process that is invoked following a peripheral vestibular insult that works to resolve these symptoms. The efficiency of the process is governed by several factors including, age, level of activity, and the integrity of central nervous system. The central structures that facilitate vestibular compensation are well described and include the vestibular nuclei, the inferior olive, and the cerebellum. The cerebellum has several different areas that control a variety of different functions. Key to vestibular compensation is the flocculus, nodulus/uvula, and vermis. Of particular interest to this case is the finding of DBN in the presence of unilateral peripheral vestibular dysfunction. DBN as is described in question 3 can be localized to impairment of the uvula/nodulus or the flocculus. It has been demonstrated that rhesus monkeys generate increased phase leads (50%), impaired tracking, impaired VOR suppression, and DBN when the flocculus is lesioned.[13]

All of these findings were manifested by MM. This case represents an unfortunate set of events wherein a patient with an impairment of the cerebellum due to long-term moderate alcohol intake incurred a loss of peripheral vestibular function (e.g., viral) and now has the inability to compensate. The findings during the clinical vestibular examination that lend support to this finding are the multiple phase leads documented during RCT and the presence of a significant directional preponderance during VNG 6 years after the acute event. Evidence from experiments in animals supports this notion of impairment in the cerebellum disrupting vestibular compensation. For example, investigators reported that squirrel monkeys with lesions of the nodulus and uvula prevented the compensation of spontaneous nystagmus after a unilateral labyrinthectomy.[14] Overall, the clinical findings in this case suggest that the source of the DBN (i.e., vestibulocerebellum) is inhibiting central vestibular compensation.

5. **What is the prognosis for this patient and what should be the recommendations for further evaluation, treatment, or management?**

The patient reported herein exhibited findings expected in patients with unilateral peripheral vestibular loss that may, as a consequence of the cerebellar impairment, be lifelong. The prognosis for vestibular rehabilitation in patients with cerebellar impairment and concomitant peripheral vestibular dysfunction should be guarded as compensation will likely be compromised by the cerebellar involvement.[14]

Predominantly, the recommended treatment for cerebellar ataxia is centered on neurorehabilitative strategies.[15,16] These strategies may include physical therapy (PT), occupational therapy (OT), and speech therapy combined with the use of adaptive equipment, nutritional counseling, and medications. Medications such as amantadine, buspirone, and acetazolamide can be prescribed to improve balance and coordination. Gabapentin, baclofen, and clonazepam can be prescribed for cerebellar nystagmus.[15] Abstinence of alcohol has also been noted to result in reversal of some of the noted neuropathological effects.[9]

24.9 Final Diagnosis

A moderate left uncompensated peripheral vestibular hypofunction was noted most consistent with a left vestibular neuritis. The cerebellar atrophy realized by MRI and history of alcohol abuse explains the presence of the DBN as well as the uncompensated state of the peripheral impairment years after the event of vertigo. By history, MM likely had a short bout of BPPV, but there is none active at the present time. Overall results revealed no indication that MD was involved in the production of her symptoms.

24.10 Outcome

To address the DBN, MM was prescribed baclofen and she reported a reduction in the symptoms of oscillopsia with lateral gaze. Additionally, MM underwent vestibular and balance therapy for sensitivity to head movements and sensitivity to visual patterns to push the compensation process as much as possible considering the central impairment. The patient reported that she did notice a decrease in her symptoms following therapy. Safety issues (i.e., risk of falls) were also addressed with MM and an appointment was made for OT to visit the home.

24.11 Key Points

- DBN noted during gaze or positional testing, which increases with lateral or down gaze, is highly suggestive of central vestibular pathology. It is important, however, to differentiate central DBN from other causes of DBN, namely, anterior canal BPPV, by also investigating further and noting additional signs or symptoms of central vestibular pathology. Oculomotor and RCT testing may also be valuable diagnostic tools. Patients manifesting DBN also often complain of oscillopsia and/or postural instability
- DBN can occur in association with infarction, cerebellar and spinocerebellar degeneration syndromes, MS, and other anomalies affecting the pons and cerebellum. A prevailing theory regarding DBN suggests a persistent asymmetry in the vertical VOR resulting from inhibition of the superior rectus muscle, followed by fast corrective eye movement downward.

- Alcohol consumption has been found to be associated with DBN and progressive cerebellar ataxia. Moderate to severe alcohol use has been associated with cerebellar ataxia with loss of Purkinje's cells, decrease in the volume of the anterior vermis, cerebellar atrophy, Wernicke's encephalopathy, and other neuropathological problems.
- The prognosis in patients with cerebellar impairment should be guarded. The recommended treatment should include various neurorehabilitative strategies that may combine PT, OT, speech therapy, adaptive equipment, nutritional counseling, and medications. In cases of concomitant peripheral vestibular dysfunction, compensation using vestibular rehabilitation may be inhibited by the underlying cerebellar impairment.

References

[1] Lempert T, Olesen J, Furman J, et al. Vestibular migraine: diagnostic criteria. J Vestib Res. 2012; 22(4):167–172

[2] Zigmond AS, Snaith RP. The Hospital Anxiety and Depression Scale. Acta Psychiatr Scand. 1983; 67(6):361–370

[3] Yee RD. Downbeat nystagmus: characteristics and localization of lesions. Trans Am Ophthalmol Soc. 1989; 87:984–1032

[4] Zasorin NL, Baloh RW. Downbeat nystagmus with alcoholic cerebellar degeneration. Arch Neurol. 1984; 41(12):1301–1302

[5] Harper C. The neuropathology of alcohol-related brain damage. Alcohol Alcohol. 2009; 44(2):136–140

[6] Zahr NM, Kaufman KL, Harper CG. Clinical and pathological features of alcohol-related brain damage. Nat Rev Neurol. 2011; 7(5):284–294

[7] Karhunen PJ, Erkinjuntti T, Laippala P. Moderate alcohol consumption and loss of cerebellar Purkinje cells. BMJ. 1994; 308(6945):1663–1667

[8] Harper C, Kril J, Daly J. Does a "moderate" alcohol intake damage the brain? J Neurol Neurosurg Psychiatry. 1988; 51(7):909–913

[9] Sasa M, Takaori S, Matsuoka I, Miyazaki T, Miyazaki K. Peripheral and central vestibular disorders in alcoholics. A three-year follow-up study. Arch Otorhinolaryngol. 1981; 230(1):93–101

[10] Cogan DG. Down-beat nystagmus. Arch Ophthalmol. 1968; 80(6):757–768

[11] Ito M. Cerebellar flocculus hypothesis. Nature. 1993; 363(6424):24–25

[12] Costin JA, Smith JL, Emery S, Tomsak RL. Alcoholic downbeat nystagmus. Ann Ophthalmol. 1980; 12(10):1127–1131

[13] Zee DS, Yamazaki A, Butler PH, Gücer G. Effects of ablation of flocculus and paraflocculus of eye movements in primate. J Neurophysiol. 1981; 46(4):878–899

[14] Igarashi M, Ishikawa K. Post-labyrinthectomy balance compensation with preplacement of cerebellar vermis lesion. Acta Otolaryngol. 1985; 99(3–4):452–458

[15] Perlman SL. Cerebellar ataxia. Curr Treat Options Neurol. 2000; 2(3):215–224

[16] Brown KE, Whitney SL, Marchetti GF, Wrisley DM, Furman JM. Physical therapy for central vestibular dysfunction. Arch Phys Med Rehabil. 2006; 87(1):76–81

25 Importance of Audiologic and Vestibular Evaluation in the Diagnosis of Unilateral Vestibular Schwannoma

Alicia Restrepo and Gail M. Whitelaw

25.1 Clinical History and Description

AM is a 34-year-old male police officer who made an appointment with otolaryngology in July 2016. AM's medical history is significant for non-Hodgkin lymphoma, which is a malignancy of the lymphatic system. He was diagnosed when he was in his early 20s and was treated with chemotherapy and radiation therapy.

AM scheduled an appointment with otolaryngology due to reported sudden hearing loss and nonpulsatile tinnitus in the right ear beginning approximately 3 weeks prior. He also reported intermittent vertigo and imbalance as well as facial weakness on the right side. The dizziness and facial weakness began 2 days before scheduling an appointment with otolaryngology. An oral steroid was prescribed by the otolaryngologist due to the sudden onset of AM's hearing loss and he was referred to audiology for a comprehensive audiologic and videonystagmography (VNG) evaluation.

25.2 Audiological Testing

The results of the comprehensive audiologic evaluation revealed normal hearing sloping to a mild sensorineural hearing loss (SNHL) at 6,000 to 8,000 Hz for the right ear and normal hearing sloping to a slight SNHL at 6,000 to 8,000 Hz for the left ear. There was an interaural asymmetry of 15 to 25 dB hearing level (HL) at 2,000, 4,000, and 6,000 Hz, with the right ear being poorer than the left ear. A Speech Recognition Threshold (SRT) of 10 dB HL was found in the right ear and 5 dB HL in the left ear, indicating a normal ability to receive speech bilaterally. Word Recognition Scores (WRS) were performed using a full NU-6 (Northwestern University Auditory Test No. 6) word list and administered via monitored live voice (MLV) presentation using a female talker. Results revealed moderate difficulty in the ability to recognize speech for the right ear and normal ability for the left ear when presented at 40 dB SL (sensation level; re: SRT). When the presentation level was increased to 75 dB HL in the right ear, the WRS decreased to 16%. This is consistent with rollover, or a decrease in WRS, as the presentation level is increased. The calculated Rollover Index was 0.76, using the highest speech discrimination score (PBmax)—lowest speech discrimination score (PBmin)/PBmax formula (68−16/68)[1] and is suggestive of the presence of retrocochlear pathology in the right ear.

Tympanometry indicated normal middle ear pressure, ear canal volume, and compliance bilaterally. Ipsilateral Acoustic Reflex Thresholds (ARTs) were absent for the right ear and present for the left ear. Contralateral ARTs were not performed due to equipment limitations; however, elevated or absent contralateral ARTs would have been expected in the case of a unilateral vestibular schwannoma. Absent ipsilateral ARTs relative to the pure-tone thresholds for the right ear support a suspicion

of retrocochlear pathology. Distortion-Product Otoacoustic Emissions (DPOAEs) were present and robust at 1,600 to 7,100 Hz and absent at 8,000 Hz bilaterally. These results were consistent with the audiometric thresholds. ▶ Fig. 25.1 reports the results from the audiologic evaluation.

The Gans Sensory Organization Performance (SOP) test was administered. The Gans SOP is a test battery consisting of seven conditions that address postural stability and assists the audiologist to differentiate between central and vestibular pathology. The audiologist determines if the patient is able to remain standing with minimal sway in each condition or if he or she demonstrates excessive sway or loses balance and falls.[2] The seven conditions include the Fukuda stepping test and six static positions. AM's results revealed a vestibular pattern of abnormality because he fell on conditions 4 (standing with the feet in a tandem position and the eyes closed) and 6 (standing on foam with the eyes closed). Also, AM turned to the right during the Fukuda step test. See ▶ Fig. 25.2 for results from the Gans SOP test.

AM demonstrated left beating nystagmus post–high-frequency headshake and 83% reduced vestibular response (RVR) in the right ear. All additional measures from the VNG (oculomotor, Dix–Hallpike, gaze, and positional) were within normal limits and no spontaneous nystagmus was noted during testing. ▶ Fig. 25.3, ▶ Fig. 25.4, ▶ Fig. 25.5, ▶ Fig. 25.6, ▶ Fig. 25.7, ▶ Fig. 25.8 report the results from the VNG evaluation. Note that the evaluation titled "Repeat Spontaneous Nystagmus" is the high-frequency headshake.

25.3 Questions to the Reader

1. **Explain why the audiologist elected to test at two presentation levels during WRS testing in the right ear.**
2. **Compare the results of the DPOAEs and the audiogram for the right ear. Were these results expected?**
3. **Why would an audiologist expect to see left beating nystagmus following the high-frequency headshake with a right-sided RVR?**
4. **Why are ipsilateral ARTs absent on the affected side in vestibular schwannoma?**

25.4 Discussion of Questions

1. **Explain why the audiologist elected to test at two presentation levels during WRS testing in the right ear.**

The audiologist was examining the patient for Rollover, which can be a test result in patients with retrocochlear pathology. AM performed poorer than expected on the WRS test when the presentation level was 40 dB SL. Because of this unexpectedly poor WRS, the threshold asymmetry and the patient's reported symptoms, the audiologist increased the presentation level to 65 dB SL and the patient's WRS significantly decreased. An ear

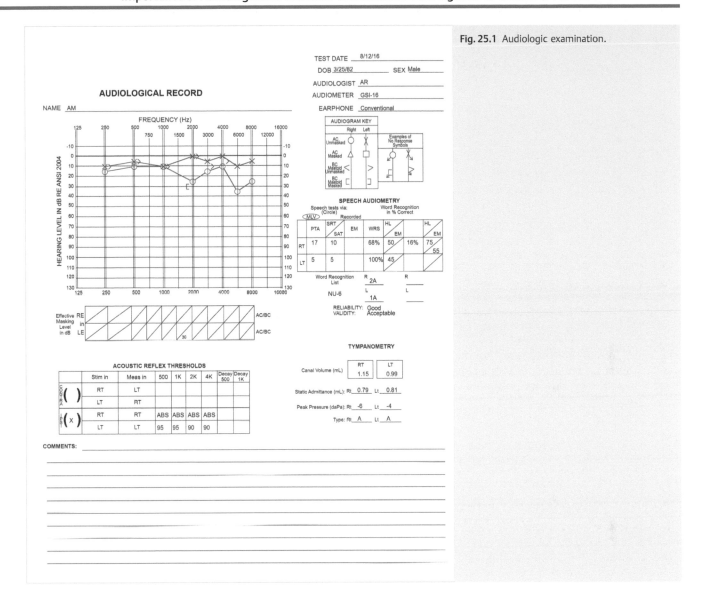

Fig. 25.1 Audiologic examination.

with cochlear pathology generally demonstrates little or no improvement in WRS when the presentation intensity level is increased. In contrast, an ear with retrocochlear pathology demonstrates poorer performance with an increase in presentation level. The calculated Rollover Index was 0.76, which is indicative of retrocochlear pathology. In addition, there was a clinically significant difference between the PBmax result (68%) and the PBmin result (16%).[3]

2. Compare the results of the DPOAEs and the audiogram for the right ear. Were these results expected?

The DPOAEs in the right ear were present and robust at 1,600 to 7,100 Hz and absent at 8,000 Hz. This finding was consistent with the audiometric thresholds in the right ear and therefore the results were not surprising. It is important, however, to recall the potential site of the lesion in this patient. The hearing loss is the result of a tumor pressing against the eighth cranial nerve. Therefore, a healthy cochlea may produce robust DPOAEs even if the patient demonstrated a greater degree of hearing loss. DPOAEs may provide important information when

determining possible site of lesion. This is rare, however, as only 20% of patients with moderate or greater hearing loss caused by vestibular schwannoma will demonstrate normal DPOAEs.[4]

3. Why would an audiologist expect to see left beating nystagmus following the high-frequency headshake with a right-sided RVR?

Patients with an uncompensated unilateral vestibular weakness may display nystagmus after a high-frequency headshake due to a mismatch within the velocity storage mechanism in the brainstem.[5] Nystagmus post–high-frequency headshake often beats away from the side of the lesion, assuming the lesion is peripheral rather than central. A vestibular schwannoma is considered a peripheral lesion.

4. Why are ipsilateral ARTs absent on the affected side in cases of vestibular schwannoma?

The ART occurs when an intense stimulus is introduced into a normal ear canal causing the stapedius muscles to contract bilaterally. This response is measured and provides important

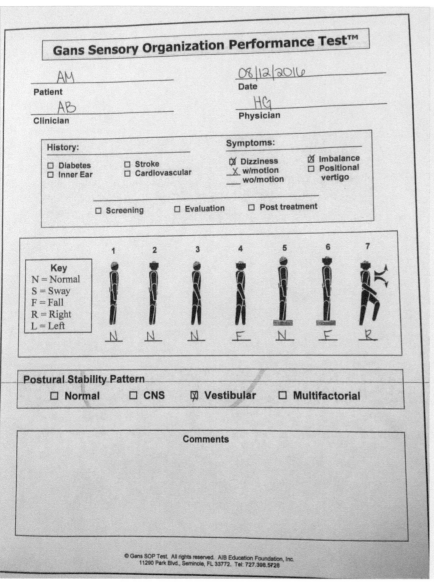

Fig. 25.2 Results from Gans Sensory Organization Performance (SOP) test.

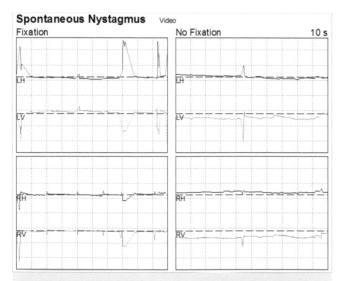

Fig. 25.3 Spontaneous nystagmus. AM had his eyes open with vision denied and is tasked throughout the recording. The audiologist is evaluating for spontaneous nystagmus. If spontaneous nystagmus occurs, the audiologist must note if the nystagmus suppresses with fixation. AM did not display spontaneous nystagmus.

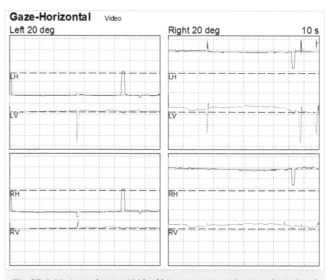

Fig. 25.4 Horizontal gaze. AM had his eyes open with vision denied and looked to the far right and far left. The audiologist is evaluating for nystagmus and to see if AM was able to maintain the gaze for 10 s. AM did not display nystagmus and was able to maintain his gaze for 10 s.

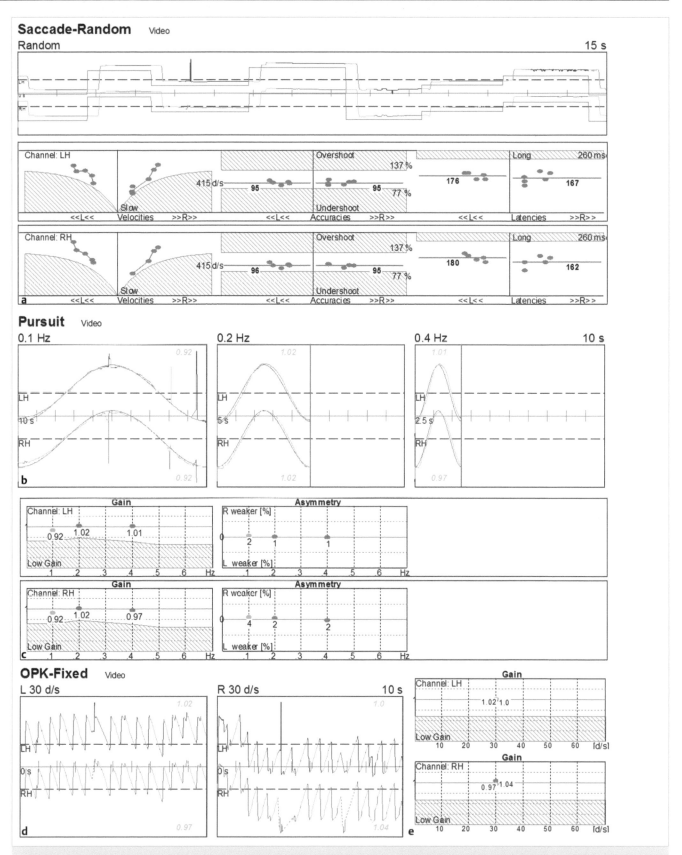

Fig. 25.5 Oculomotor evaluations. Saccades, smooth pursuit, and optokinetics. AM must follow a randomized target with his eyes, pursue a target back and forth with the eyes, and follow a series of targets, resulting in nystagmus. The audiologist evaluated AM for accuracy and timing, as well as the ability to complete the task appropriately. AM was within normal limits for all oculomotor evaluations.

Repeat Spontaneous Nystagmus Video

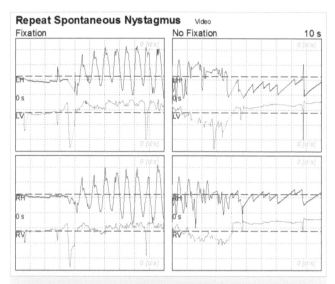

Fig. 25.6 High-frequency headshake. The audiologist shook AM's head in a horizontal motion for 30 s while AM kept his eyes open. The shaking is stopped abruptly. The audiologist is evaluating for nystagmus post headshake. AM displayed left beating nystagmus post headshake, which is considered a peripheral finding.

information for the differential diagnosis of retrocochlear pathology. A vestibular schwannoma will often result in elevated or absent ARTs, even with normal or near-normal hearing thresholds.[4] ART testing have a high degree of sensitivity (85%) and specificity (97%) in the detection of retrocochlear pathology.[6] In this patient, the authors would expect the right-sided contralateral ARTs (stimulus right, probe left) to be absent and the left-sided contralateral ARTs (stimulus left, probe right) to be present. In contrast, ARTs would be expected to be present with normal hearing acuity or in cochlear hearing losses with thresholds below 50 dB HL.[7]

25.5 Description of Disorder and Recommended Treatment

AM was scheduled to follow-up with the otologist the day after his comprehensive audiologic and VNG evaluation due to the concerning findings on these evaluations. The otolaryngologist ordered a magnetic resonance imaging (MRI) of the internal auditory canals with and without contrast. The MRI revealed a small 6-mm vestibular schwannoma within the right internal auditory canal that was protruding into the cerebellopontine

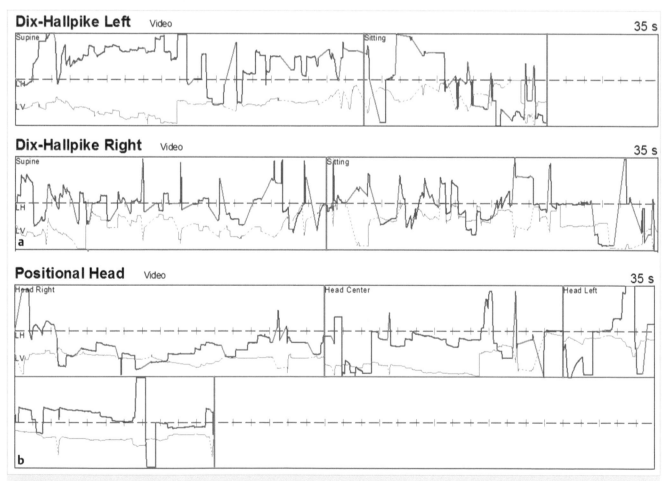

Fig. 25.7 Dix–Hallpike test. AM was moved from a seated position to a supine position with his head extended off the table. The audiologist is evaluating for nystagmus. AM did not display nystagmus or report subjective vertigo.

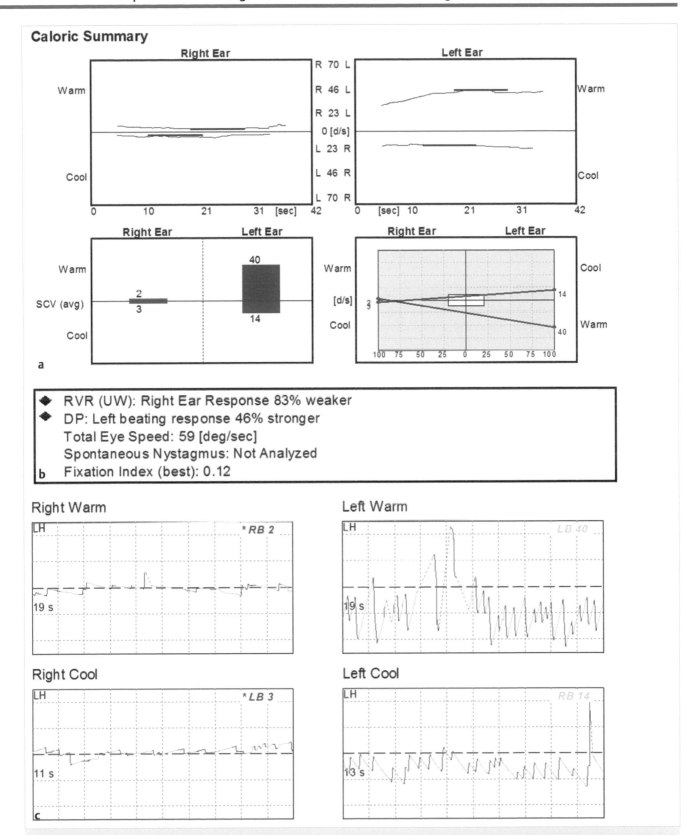

Fig. 25.8 Caloric evaluation. The audiologist irrigated AM's ears with cold and warm air or water. Each irrigation stimulates the horizontal semicircular canal and will produce nystagmus in a healthy vestibular system. The audiologist is evaluating for the strength of the nystagmus and is looking for an equal response from the two ears. AM demonstrated a significant weakness in the right ear as compared to the left ear.

angle and pressing on the seventh (facial) and eighth (vestibulo-cochlear) cranial nerves. A number of treatment options may be considered for a patient with a vestibular schwannoma, including watchful waiting.[8,9] The patient was scheduled to undergo Gamma knife radiosurgery, a type of stereotactic radiosurgery, 2 days following his MRI. Gamma knife radiosurgery utilizes radiation to damage the deoxyribonucleic acid (DNA) within the cells of the tumor, hindering its ability to reproduce and grow. Unlike traditional surgery, no incision is required. Stunting the growth of the tumor prevents further deterioration of the patient's hearing and does not pose the risk of destroying the hearing in the right ear as may occur using a traditional surgical approach.

A vestibular schwannoma, also known as an acoustic neuroma, is a benign tumor that originates from the Schwann cells of the eighth cranial nerve and is generally unilateral. Approximately 95% of patients with a vestibular schwannoma will experience some degree of hearing loss[2] and approximately 20% will experience sudden SNHL.[4] The majority of patients with vestibular schwannoma do not report dizziness; however, an RVR in AM's case suggests that the tumor is pressing on the superior vestibular nerve that innervates the horizontal semicircular canal.[6]

25.6 Outcome

AM completed gamma knife surgery in August 2016. His neurologist will continue to monitor the size of his tumor with serial MRIs. He will return for a follow-up audiometric evaluation in February 2017, which is 6 months following his initial audiometric evaluation. If no significant changes are noted from his initial audiometric evaluation, AM will return for annual audiologic evaluations. Hearing conservation strategies were discussed at AM's initial audiologic evaluation. This included using earplugs or earmuffs when in noisy situations, such as the firing range, and avoiding excessive noise exposure for extended periods of time. It is essential for AM to protect his hearing due to the reduced WRS in his right ear.

In addition, AM was referred for Vestibular Rehabilitation Therapy (VRT) to aid in central compensation of his unilateral vestibular weakness. VRT is essential for any patient; however, this patient's vocation as a police officer may make this even more imperative. Police officers must undergo annual physical evaluations that include hearing screening and tests to evaluate the officer's physical fitness. A police officer unable to pass the physical may be transitioned to an administrative position and no longer be able to work in the field.

25.7 Key Points

- A comprehensive audiologic evaluation plays an essential role in the differential diagnosis of retrocochlear pathology. The

audiologic findings in this case resulted in a rapid referral to neurology and timely surgical intervention.

- It is essential to utilize multiple diagnostic tools (i.e., Auditory Brainstem Response [ABR] audiometry, DPOAEs, Rollover, and ARTs) whenever possible, especially in instances of sudden SNHL. AM may not fit the referral criteria for asymmetrical hearing thresholds in many clinics; however, he displayed rollover as well as absent ipsilateral ARTs and unilateral vestibular weakness on the right side. An audiologist who did not employ the use of additional behavioral (i.e., ABR) and vestibular testing may have recommended an annual audiologic evaluation to monitor the asymmetry rather than a referral to the otolaryngologist. Timely and accurate diagnosis of vestibular schwannoma is also critical in hearing preservation. A strong audiology/otolaryngology partnership provided for a quick decision to treat the vestibular schwannoma based on the information obtained and the available treatment plan. Additionally, in AM's case, supporting his work performance and quality of life through vestibular rehabilitation was a critical factor in treatment.

References

[1] Jerger J, Jerger S. Diagnostic significance of PB word functions. Arch Otolaryngol. 1971; 93(6):573–580

[2] American Institute of Balance. Gans Sensory Organization Performance Test. Seminole FL: American Institute of Balance; 2011

[3] Thornton AR, Raffin MJ. Speech-discrimination scores modeled as a binomial variable. J Speech Hear Res. 1978; 21(3):507–518

[4] Valente M, Peterein J, Goebel J, Neely JG. Four cases of acoustic neuromas with normal hearing. J Am Acad Audiol. 1995; 6(3):203–210

[5] Huh YE, Kim JS. Patterns of spontaneous and head-shaking nystagmus in cerebellar infarction: imaging correlations. Brain. 2011; 134(Pt 12):3662–3671

[6] Olsen WO, Bauch CD, Harner SG. Application of Silman and Gelfand (1981) 90th percentile levels for acoustic reflex thresholds. J Speech Hear Disord. 1983; 48(3):330–332

[7] Silman S, Gelfand SA. The relationship between magnitude of hearing loss and acoustic reflex threshold levels. J Speech Hear Disord. 1981; 46(3):312–316

[8] Robinette M, Durrant J. Contributions of evoked otoacoustic emissions in differential diagnosis of retrocochlear disorders. In: Robinette M, Glattke T, ed. Otoacoustic Emissions: Clinical Applications. New York, NY: Thieme Medical Publishers; 1997:205–232

[9] Pogodzinski MS, Harner SG, Link MJ. Patient choice in treatment of vestibular schwannoma. Otolaryngol Head Neck Surg. 2004; 130(5):611–616

Suggested Readings

[1] Régis J, Pellet W, Delsanti C, et al. Functional outcome after gamma knife surgery or microsurgery for vestibular schwannomas. J Neurosurg. 2002; 97(5):1091–1100

[2] Sauvaget E, Kici S, Kania R, Herman P, Tran Ba Huy P. Sudden sensorineural hearing loss as a revealing symptom of vestibular schwannoma. Acta Otolaryngol. 2005; 125(6):592–595

[3] Takahashi S, Fetter M, Koenig E, Dichgans J. The clinical significance of head-shaking nystagmus in the dizzy patient. Acta Otolaryngol. 1990; 109(1–2):8–14

26 The Presentation of Cerebellar Disease in Vestibular Testing of an Adult Patient

Frederick E. Cobb and Kelly A. Sharpe

26.1 Clinical History and Description

TP is a 55-year-old male with normal hearing and a lifelong history of imbalance. There is also mild short and long term memory loss, slow ambulation, and a report of a mild traumatic brain injury (mTBI). These diagnoses were the result of an extensive evaluation completed by TP after he accessed healthcare in 2005. Recent evaluations documented a history of tobacco and alcohol dependence, multiple closed fractures of the head and extremities due to motor vehicular accidents, headaches, diplopia, depression, mood disorder, gait ataxia, chronic lower back pain, hypothyroidism, and most recently a diagnosis of rostral vermis syndrome (cerebellar disease) secondary to alcohol abuse. Audiometric assessments are well within normal limits bilaterally. Most recently, he was screened by a fall prevention and mTBI team that resulted in a request for a comprehensive vestibular assessment to rule out peripheral vestibular system disease due to TP's given history that "he gets dizzy if he turns too suddenly and if he changes position too quickly."

26.2 Clinical Testing

The initial working diagnosis was postural instability secondary to Benign Paroxysmal Positioning Vertigo (BPPV) given TP's history of head trauma. TP was scheduled for a balance assessment and was provided written instructions to follow in preparation for the assessment. Assessment of functional balance (computerized dynamic posturography) included Motor Control (MC) and Sensory Organization Testing (SOT). The MC composite score was within normal limits, but with a rightward weight symmetry. SOT, a nonclinical assessment of functional balance consisting of six conditions, was abnormal with poor use of vestibular system cues. That is, TB did not utilize input from his peripheral vestibular system to maintain balance. There were falls within 1 second for conditions 5 and 6, which depend a great deal upon good input from the peripheral vestibular system due to compromised visual and somatosensory input. All conditions were recorded as borderline normal (rightward) center of gravity (▶ Fig. 26.1).

Rotary Chair Testing (RCT) included oculomotor tests in the horizontal and vertical planes; calibration saccades, a search for spontaneous nystagmus, gaze testing, pseudorandom saccades, pursuit at increased target speeds, and optokinetic nystagmus; Sinusoidal Harmonic Acceleration (SHA); visual fixation suppression; and visual vestibuloocular reflex and step velocity testing (▶ Fig. 26.2). Generally, tests of the peripheral vestibular system were normal, while tests of the oculomotor system were abnormal.

A search for spontaneous nystagmus (vision denied with mental alerting) resulted in a 1 to 3 deg/s slow phase velocity (SPV) up-beating nystagmus. SHA testing was normal at 0.01, 0.04, and 0.16 Hz. Visual fixation suppression, tested at 0.04 Hz, was abnormal with high failure of visual fixation suppression gains of 0.36 to 0.40 upon repeated measures. Visual vestibuloocular reflex (0.16 Hz) and step velocity testing (100 deg/s) resulted in low gain values that remained within normal limits upon repeated measures. Horizontal and vertical gaze testing

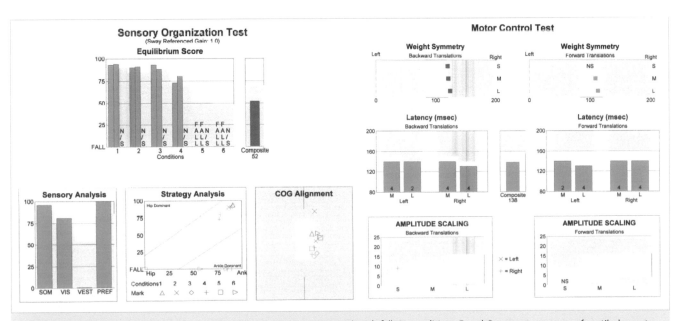

Fig. 26.1 Assessment of function balance. SOT (sensory organization testing) with falls in conditions 5 and 6 support poor use of vestibular system cues in maintaining balance and a rightward center of gravity that was repeated upon normal motor control testing.

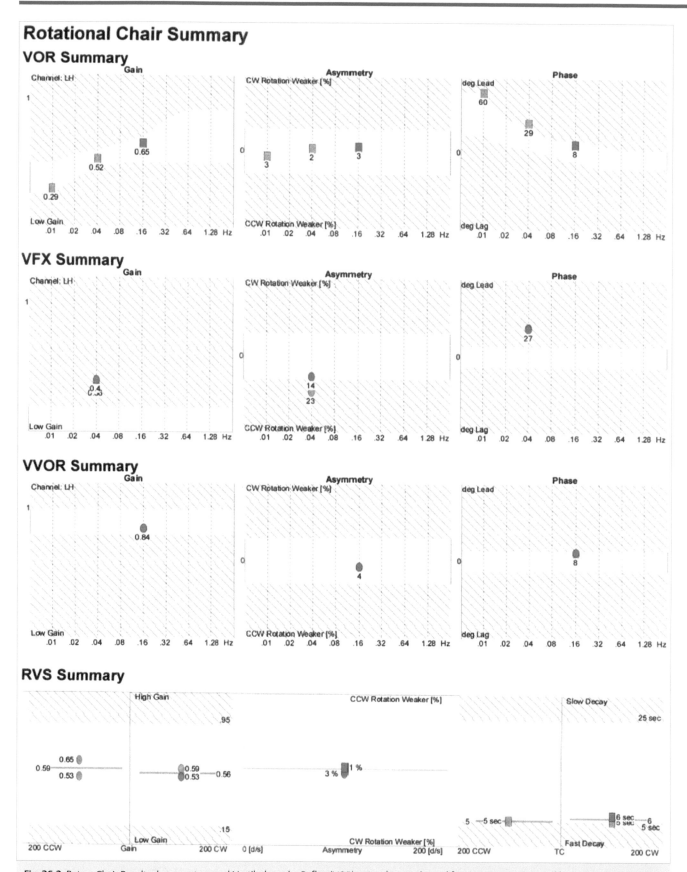

Fig. 26.2 Rotary Chair Results document normal Vestibuloocular Reflex (VOR) gain, abnormal visual fixation suppression, and low normal step velocity of the storage velocity mechanism.

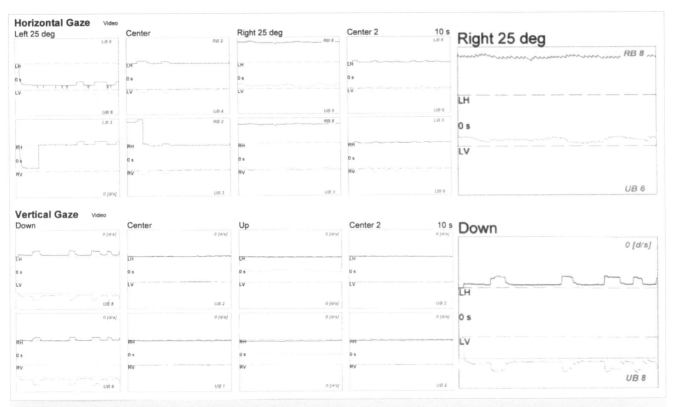

Fig. 26.3 Horizontal and vertical gaze testing with rebounding horizontal gaze-evoked nystagmus and vertical gaze testing with the greatest up-beating nystagmus recorded upon downward gaze.

was characterized by direction-changing gaze-evoked nystagmus upon the horizontal channel that measured 5 to 8 deg/s SPV and an up-beating nystagmus upon the vertical channel that measured 3 to 6 deg/s SPV. Upon changing from a lateral gaze to center gaze, "rebounding" was noted that changed the direction of the horizontal nystagmus. That is, from a rightward gaze holding, there is a right- and up-beating nystagmus that changed to a left and up beating nystagmus upon a return of the gaze to the center position. Upon vertical gaze testing, the up-beating nystagmus was greatest for downward gaze at 6 deg/s SPV and was eliminated upon an upward gaze (▶ Fig. 26.3).

Continuing with oculomotor system testing, pseudorandom horizontal and vertical saccades were normal (▶ Fig. 26.4). Horizontal and vertical pseudorandom saccades present with mild inaccuracies: leftward undershooting and upward undershooting. Horizontal pursuit demonstrated a distinct "cogwheeling" with rightward-directed targets and with low, but normal pursuit gain at 0.10 and 0.20 Hz. At 0.40 Hz, the gain was abnormally low. Vertical pursuit also produced "cogwheeling" and abnormal gain values bidirectionally becoming poorer (worse) with an increase in target speed (▶ Fig. 26.5). Horizontal optokinetic nystagmus was essentially absent with mental alerting despite repeated testing (▶ Fig. 26.6). Vertical optokinetic nystagmus could not be tested due to equipment limitations.

Medication(s), lack of patient cooperation, patient motivation, and mental alertness can adversely affect eye movement test outcomes. Medication complications were minimized by using the clinic's pretest instructions. These instructions request that all recently prescribed medications for "dizziness" and/or vertigo be stopped 2 days prior to testing and that all other long-term medications be continued as usual. TP was a very cooperative, motivated, and alert test subject. Mental alerting, simple verbal reciting tasks said aloud were employed during the search for spontaneous nystagmus, SHA testing, optokinetic nystagmus testing, positioning and positional tests, and caloric testing. Mental alerting maintains a calm and comfortable test environment during subtests that involve a turning sensation, occupies the person being tested, and keeps him/her alert to maximize the successful recording of eye movements.

Results from Videonystagmography (VNG) that included calibration saccades, positioning tests (Dix–Hallpike and head-roll maneuvers), positional tests (static head positions), and binaural bithermal open-water calorics (6% unilateral weakness, 6% directional preponderance) were clinically normal; however, there was failure of visual fixation suppression for right-beating nystagmus (left cool and right warm) that measured 78% for the left cool water irrigation and 67% for the right warm irrigation (▶ Fig. 26.7). Cervical and ocular vestibular evoked myogenic potentials were without repeatable waveforms.

26.3 Questions to the Reader

1. **Why was TP's functional balance so good?**
2. **Why are only selected eye movements abnormal?**
3. **What other audiology tests could be considered in TP's case?**

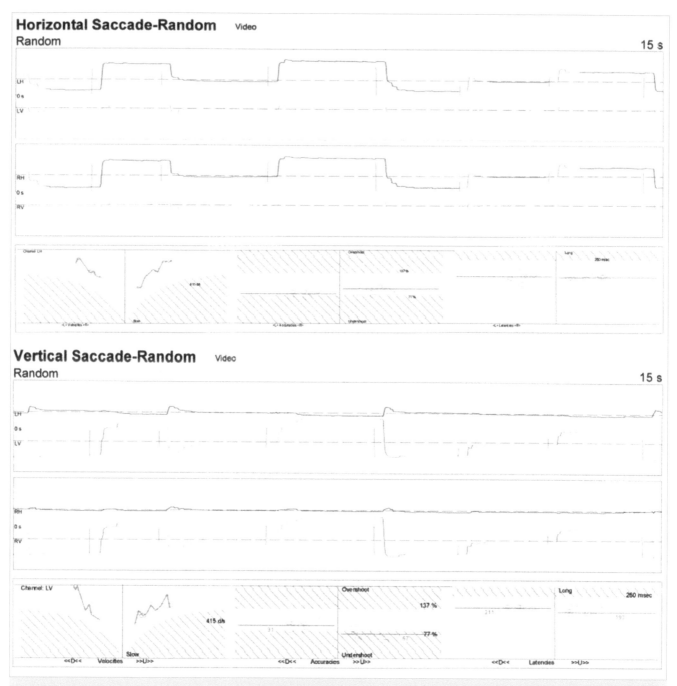

Fig. 26.4 Horizontal and vertical pseudorandom saccades with mild leftward accuracy (undershooting) and mild upward accuracy (undershooting) aberrations. There is sparing of velocity and latency capabilities bidirectionally.

26.4 Discussion of Questions

1. Why was TP's functional balance so good?

Typically, with a patient report of "imbalance" an experienced clinician will not expect test results that support unilateral peripheral vestibular system disease or disorder. This report of "imbalance" might cause the clinician to be wary of the functional status of the lower extremities, the brain, and the possibility of a bilateral vestibular weakness. It is possible this finding could be the result of all three. On the other hand, TP

most recently reported, "I get dizzy if I turn too suddenly and if I change position too quickly," which may lead a clinician to consider a positioning vertigo condition or a peripheral vestibular weakness, which is why TP was scheduled for balance testing.

In this case, a middle-aged male with a lifelong history of poor balance has abnormal functional balance. The SOT results obtained were not uncommon for patients having unilateral peripheral vestibular disease. Cerebellar syndromes supported from previous workup may or may not affect the lower extrem-

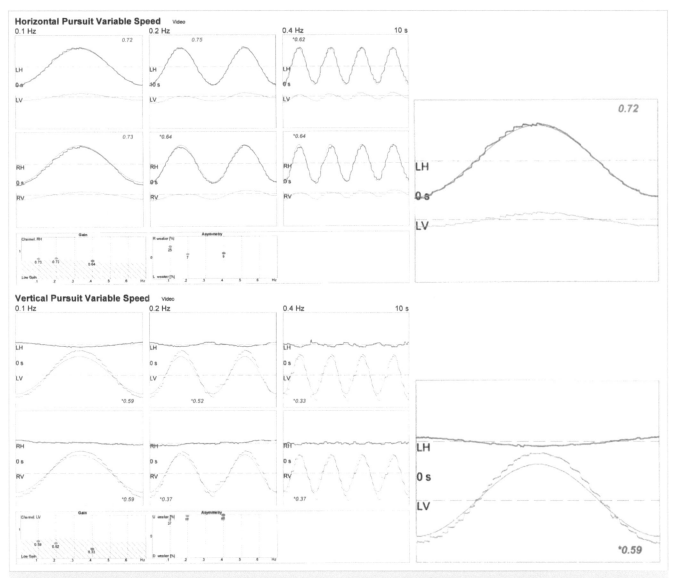

Fig. 26.5 Horizontal with low-normal horizontal pursuit gains and "cogwheeling" (especially tracking rightward targets). Vertical pursuit with abnormally low gain.

ities depending upon where the lesion is located. Disorders of the caudal vermis have little or no limb ataxia. Hemispheric and rostral cerebellar syndromes carry noticeable and clinically significant limb and fine motor coordination deficits. In this case, there are numerous oculomotor aberrations that would suggest a disorder of the caudal cerebellum. These vestibulocerebellar lesions often cause disequilibrium. TP fell within 1 second for SOT conditions 5 and 6 and displayed a rightward center of gravity alignment. This is a common finding in patients with peripheral disease; however, for TP no peripheral vestibular system disorder was clinically found. Thus, in this case it is presumed that good MC and relatively good functional balance remain because rostral cerebellar structures were spared damage, whereas the caudal cerebellum appear impaired.

2. Why are only selected eye movements abnormal?

In this case, some eye movements were normal such as horizontal and vertical saccades, whereas horizontal and vertical pursuit eye movements were mildly impaired. Direction-changing gaze-evoked nystagmus was present in horizontal and vertical gaze holding tests. Horizontal optokinetic nystagmus was nearly absent. Generally, with eye-movement difficulties to one side or one direction, an ipsilateral cerebellar lesion(s) may be present. Global cerebellar lesion(s) result in generally poor and symmetrically disordered eye movements. Disorders of the vestibulocerebellar region, the caudal (posterior) cerebellar lobe, have a devastating effect upon the clinical optokinetic response. Electrophysiologic and clinical evidence supports a common neural network that integrates all conjugate eye movement commands. In this case, there appeared to be a disorder of that

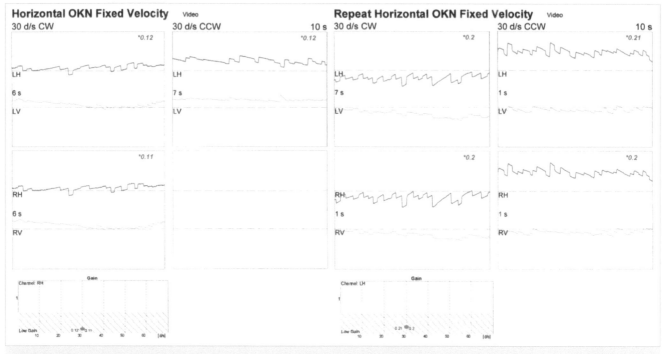

Fig. 26.6 Repeated horizontal optokinetic nystagmus with abnormally low gains bidirectionally.

neural integrator resulting in very poor optokinetic, gaze-holding, pursuit eye movement and visual fixation suppression of the vestibuloocular reflex with relative sparing of other eye movement functions.

3. **What other audiology tests could be considered in TP's case?**

To rule out a progressive disorder, a follow-up visit was scheduled for a year later. The result of that testing was equivalent to the initial exam. The marginally normal saccadic inaccuracies improved (i.e., became more normal), but remained asymmetric upon repeated testing with undershooting to the left. The findings for other tests previously discussed remained unchanged. Since TP's hearing is normal and his peripheral vestibular system is normal, further assessments of peripheral systems (i.e., auditory brainstem response [ABR] testing) would not add any new information to the diagnosis.

26.5 Description of Disorder and Recommended Treatment

A magnetic resonance imaging (MRI) series of the brain was ordered prior to TP's balance assessment due to the reported head injuries. This examination revealed minimal cerebellar atrophy. Upon physical examination, there was a diagnosis of rostral vermis syndrome secondary to alcohol abuse. There were three or four cerebellar syndromes that were considered to be possible. In TP's case, there is normal MC. There is no functional evidence of disorder of the extremities. There was oculomotor test evidence of a functional disorder of the vestibulocerebellum. There was repeated and a clinically signifi-

cant reduction in reflexive eye movements such as the generation of optokinetic nystagmus and successful visual fixation suppression of vestibular-induced nystagmus with relative sparing of cortically generated eye movements such as gaze holding, saccades, and pursuit. As a result, the balance assessment suggested a caudal (posterior) cerebellar syndrome, as opposed to a rostral (anterior) cerebellar syndrome, which was the original diagnosis. A caudal cerebellar syndrome presents with eye movement aberrations and nystagmus while sparing the extremities. A rostral cerebellar syndrome presents in just the opposite fashion.

TP's functional balance is problematic in two areas: (1) the poor use of vestibular system cues to maintain balance and (2) a rightward center of gravity. Because of this, it was recommended that TP be referred to physical therapy for a balance rehabilitation assessment with possible treatment options provided. It was also recommended that TP be referred to a recreational therapy program that provides education and counseling in addition to strength and conditioning training that does not affect TP's current physical disabilities. Finally, it was recommended that TP return to the clinic in 1 year's time to rule out any progressive component.

26.6 Outcome

TP lives a long distance from the clinic, has several pressing personal life issues, and additional health concerns. An initial consultation for balance rehabilitation was recommended, but not completed. TP returned to the clinic in a year and the results ruled out any progressive component of the initial findings.

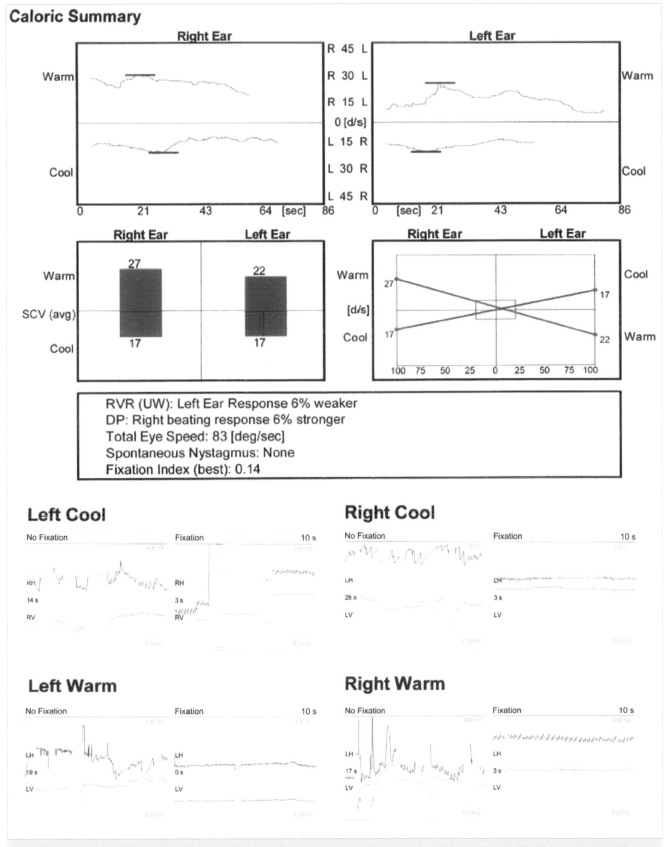

Fig. 26.7 Normal open water caloric testing with failure of visual fixation suppression for right-beating nystagmus (left cool and right warm) that measured 78% for the left cool water irrigation and 67% for the right warm irrigation.

26.7 Key Points

- Medications and/or a lack of patient cooperation, patient motivation, and mental alerting can adversely affect eye movement testing outcomes.
- Consistent, repeatable, and carefully collected clinical evidence of poor and/or abnormal eye movements can lead to a cogent diagnosis of central vestibular system disease.
- Disorders of the cerebellum may be present despite normal peripheral vestibular system function.
- There can be significant differences in the clinical findings of volitional versus reflexive eye movement tests.
- Different cerebellar syndromes can affect balance, a patient's extremity movements, and a patient's eye movements differently.

26.8 Disclaimer

The lead author of this chapter is an employee of the Department of Veterans Affairs. However, the views expressed in this chapter are the authors' personal views. They do not necessarily represent the views of the Department of Veterans Affairs or of the U.S. government.

26.9 Acknowledgments

We thank Ms. Sharpe, BS, and Dr. John "Jack" King, PhD, for reviewing the manuscript and for inspiration. We also thank Linda, Anne, Dick, Jo, and Go Bearcats.

Suggested Reading

[1] Leigh RJ, Zee DS. Disorders of ocular motility due to disease of the brainstem, cerebellum and diencephalon. In: Leigh RJ, Zee DS, eds. The Neurology of Eye Movements. 5th ed. New York, NY: Oxford Press; 2015:844–858

27 The Role of an Inciting Event Causing Vertigo

Andrew Schuette and Nsangou Ghogomu

27.1 Clinical History and Description

LK is a 48-year-old female referred to otolaryngology with right-sided hearing loss, otalgia, and vertigo that began abruptly 5 months ago while she was scuba diving. At the time of the dive, LK was recovering from an upper respiratory tract infection (URI) and had significant difficulty auto-insufflating (using the Valsalva maneuver to equalize while diving). In addition to her symptoms, which began during the dive, she noticed increased autophony (hearing one's own voice abnormally loud) after the dive. At the time of presentation to the clinic, LK's primary complaint was autophony. The otalgia and vertigo appeared to have resolved. Her physical examination was normal with no evidence of middle ear fluid or a nasopharyngeal mass. An audiologic evaluation was recommended to further investigate LK's symptoms.

27.2 Audiologic Testing

The audiologic examination revealed a slight conductive hearing loss in the right ear and slight sensorineural hearing loss (SNHL) in the left ear (▶ Fig. 27.1). Results for the right ear report a slight conductive hearing loss (20 dB air–bone gap) at 250 Hz with normal hearing from 500 to 8,000 Hz. The Speech Recognition Threshold (SRT) for the right ear indicated normal ability to receive speech, while results for the left ear revealed a slight loss in the ability to receive speech. The Word Recognition Score (WRS) was obtained using a half-list of the Northwestern University Auditory Test No. 6 (NU-6) with a recorded female talker at a presentation level of 60 dB hearing level (HL) with 30 dB HL of contralateral speech masking. Results revealed normal ability to recognize speech in the right and left ears. Immittance audiometry revealed normal ear canal volume, middle ear pressure, and static admittance. Ipsilateral and contralateral Acoustic Reflexes Thresholds (ARTs) were present

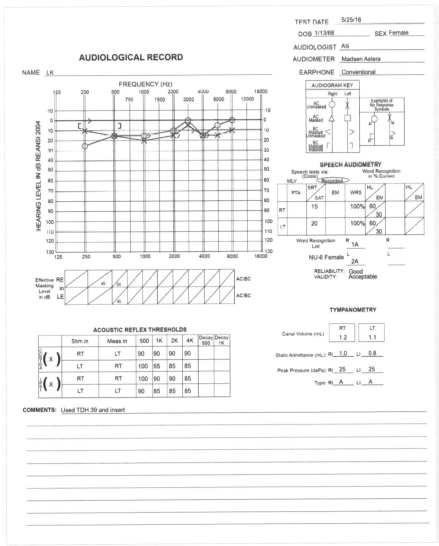

Fig. 27.1 Audiometric results of LK.

bilaterally and at normal sensation levels. Interestingly, LK reported vertigo during ART testing at 500 and 1,000 Hz for the right and left ears.

27.3 Questions to the Reader

1. **Given LK's medical history and the results of the initial audiological evaluation, what impression can be drawn with respect to potential cause(s) of her slight hearing loss?**
2. **What is the next best diagnostic test to confirm a clinician's suspicion?**
3. **Explain how scuba diving may have incited vertigo.**
4. **Would the impressions be similar if the bone-conduction thresholds were not measured at 250 Hz (as is often the case in common clinical practice)?**

27.4 Discussion of Questions

1. **Given LK's medical history and the results of the initial audiological evaluation, what impression can be drawn with respect to potential cause(s) of her slight hearing loss?**

The initial audiological evaluation revealed two significant findings that result in an impression of potential causes of her hearing loss: (1) the 250-Hz air–bone gap with normal tympanometry and (2) vertigo during ART testing.

The presence of an air–bone gap with normal tympanometry and vertigo during the measurement of ARTS raises suspicion of third-window pathology. Third-window pathologies include Superior Semicircular Canal Dehiscence (SSCD), Enlarged Vestibular Aqueduct (EVA), and, less frequently, otic capsule deficits due to an erosive process (e.g., tumor). The air–bone gap seen in third-window pathology is a result of loss of air-conduction energy through a "third-window." The first and second windows are the oval and round window of the cochlea.

LK reported vertigo during ART testing at 500 and 1,000 Hz. The vertigo appears to be triggered by loud sounds (presentation levels used to obtain thresholds: 80–105 dB HL) and is referred to as Tullio's phenomenon, discovered in 1929 by the Italian biologist Prof. Pietro Tullio (1881–1941).[1,2] He drilled holes in the semicircular canals of pigeons, which resulted in balance problems when the birds were exposed to loud sounds. Tullio's phenomenon is associated with fistulas (openings) in the middle and inner ears.

LK's audiometric findings and medical history were discussed with LK's otolaryngologist. SSCD was suggested to the referring otolaryngologist as a possible cause of LK's symptoms.

2. **What is the next best diagnostic test to confirm the clinician's suspicion?**

A noncontrast temporal bone computed tomography (CT) scan is used to diagnose SSCD. If a clinician is specifically concerned about SSCD, the CT scan should be completed in the plane of the superior canals to increase sensitivity. Vestibular Evoked Myogenic Potential (VEMP) testing can also be utilized in diagnosis of SSCD with 91% sensitivity.[3] A CT scan, however, is considered the gold standard in SSCD diagnosis and was ordered for LK.

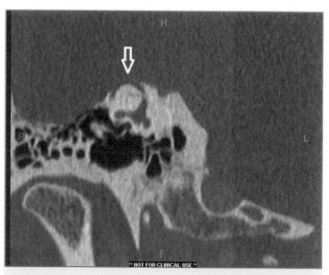

Fig. 27.2 Right temporal bone CT (computed tomography) scan. Arrow points to right semicircular canal dehiscence.

LK's CT scan (▶ Fig. 27.2) reveals the presence of bilateral SSCD. However, the CT scan shows no evidence of EVA, erosion of the ossicles or otic capsule, masses, fracture, or infection in the temporal bone. SSCD was first described by Lloyd Minor in 1998.[4]

3. **Explain how scuba diving may have incited vertigo.**

The bone surrounding the superior semicircular canal is thinnest at its superior extent where the canal lies directly below the brain, separated by a thin layer of bone. In some patients, that bone is extremely thin either at birth (congenital) or as a result of elevated intracranial pressure (acquired).

Regardless of the cause for the thinning, when the bone becomes sufficiently thin, events such as head trauma, significant changes in intracranial pressure, or significant changes in middle ear pressure can be sufficient to disrupt the narrow remaining bony barrier and create a third window in the otic capsule at the superior end of the superior semicircular canal. A single event is attributed to the onset of symptoms for SSCD in approximately 37% of patients.[5]

For LK, negative middle ear pressure was building as she was simultaneously performing a Valsalva maneuver (auto-insufflation), which was increasing her intracranial pressure. This combination is likely what led to the disruption of the very thin barrier during her dive.

4. **Would the impressions be similar if the bone-conduction thresholds were not measured at 250 Hz (as is often the case in common clinical practice)?**

It is critical to consider the patient history prior to completing audiological evaluation. If the assumption was that the right-sided hearing loss at 250 Hz was sensorineural, then Meniere's disease would have likely been suspected. Presence of the inciting event and careful review of the history suggested that bone conduction thresholds were needed to seek an air–bone gap and suprathreshold levels at 250 Hz.

Not testing bone conduction at 250 Hz appears to be a common clinical practice. One reason why a clinician may not perform the test may be due to a concern that the noise floor in the sound booth may mask bone conduction and elevate (increase) thresholds. Also, the presence of a computer in a sound booth may have the same affect due to the internal fan.

27.5 Diagnosis, Recommended Treatment, and Outcome

The results from the initial audiological evaluation (air–bone gap with normal immittance and Tullio's phenomenon) and CT scan were consistent with bilateral SSCD. LK's symptoms were quite mild and she does not routinely have noise-induced vertigo as seen during ART assessment or significant autophony. The otolaryngologist consulted an otologist and together they did not recommend surgical intervention because they felt the risks outweighed the benefits. Additionally, it was recommended LK discontinue scuba diving due to the concern about exacerbating symptoms. LK will follow up with the otologist if her symptoms worsen and surgical intervention may be considered.

27.6 Key Points

- The presence of a conductive hearing loss with normal immittance is not an error, but may be indicative of possible third-window pathology (e.g., SSCD and EVA) that needs to be evaluated by an otologist to confirm the diagnosis.
- SSCD is common in a clinical population. Three percent of patients in a retrospective study who had received a temporal bone CT scan, regardless of the reason, had SSCD. Only 20% of patients with SSCD, however, were symptomatic.[6] An inciting event (e.g., intracranial pressure, head injury) can often lead to this disorder becoming symptomatic. A positive CT scan without symptoms is considered a nonclinical SSCD. In order

to diagnose SSCD, both a positive CT scan and symptoms are required. LK has both symptoms and a positive CT scan.
- Bone conduction thresholds should always be measured at 250 Hz for its diagnostic value in differentiating conductive from sensorineural or mixed hearing losses. If bone conduction was not performed for LK, it is possible a different diagnosis (e.g., Meniere's disease) would have been considered, resulting in unnecessary testing, delayed diagnosis, and subsequently increased health care costs.

27.7 Acknowledgments

The authors thank Jonathan Law, MD, otolaryngology resident at Washington University in St. Louis, for his help in obtaining and creating ▶ Fig. 27.2 for LK's CT scan.

References

[1] Pietro T. Das Ohr und die Entstehung der Sprache und Schrift. Berlin: Urban and Schwarzenberg; 1929

[2] Tullio Pietro. Some experiments and considerations on experimental otology and phonetics: a lecture delivered at the meeting of the "Società dei cultori delle scienze ... e naturali" of Cagliari on July 1, 1929: L. Cappelli 1929 ASIN: B0008B2T6Y

[3] Minor LB, Solomon D, Zinreich JS, Zee DS. Sound- and/or pressure-induced vertigo due to bone dehiscence of the superior semicircular canal. Arch Otolaryngol Head Neck Surg. 1998; 124(3):249–258

[4] Zhou G, Gopen Q, Poe DS. Clinical and diagnostic characterization of canal dehiscence syndrome: a great otologic mimicker. Otol Neurotol. 2007; 28(7): 920–926

[5] Niesten ME, McKenna MJ, Grolman W, Lee DJ. Clinical factors associated with prolonged recovery after superior canal dehiscence surgery. Otol Neurotol. 2012; 33(5):824–831

[6] Masaki Y. The prevalence of superior canal dehiscence syndrome as assessed by temporal bone computed tomography imaging. Acta Otolaryngol. 2011; 131(3):258–262

28 Benign Paroxysmal Positional Vertigo Lateral Canal Conundrum

Belinda C. Sinks

28.1 Clinical History and Description

Although Benign Paroxysmal Positional Vertigo (BPPV) is the most common cause of vertigo, lateral canal BPPV accounts for 10 to 20% of those cases. Lateral canal BPPV is rare compared to posterior canal BPPV and can be more difficult to diagnose. Compared to posterior canal BPPV, lateral canal or horizontal canal BPPV is diagnosed by a side-lying position from the sitting position, a head rotation, or a roll test while the patient is supine. The remission rate for lateral canal BPPV is lower than that for posterior canal BPPV. This is most likely due to the difficulty in identifying the side affected by the lateral canal BPPV.[1] This case report summarizes how the **bow and lean test (BLT)** can help improve diagnosis in patients with lateral canal BPPV when the offending ear is unclear.

HC, a pleasant 62-year-old woman, reported a 2-year history of severe vertigo spells and a recent history of severe vertigo spells triggered by moving her head in certain positions. Two years ago, HC reported she went to a spa and had a whole-body vibration. That night she awoke with a violent vertiginous episode that caused nausea and vomiting that lasted for days. HC slowly recovered only to have it recur several days later after a very turbulent flight. This episode lasted for 2 days. Since that time, HC has had episodic sensations of vertigo whenever she would lie flat on her back, and upon rolling over (she could not recall left vs. right). HC reported these bursts of dizziness would last a few seconds, but were very debilitating. HC saw a physician who laid her down and told her she had positional vertigo and referred her to physical therapy, but HC reported no relief. HC scheduled an appointment at our facility to determine whether or not the clinical staff could provide additional insight in diagnosing and treating her symptoms.

HC saw a neuro-otologist at our clinic. HC's clinical examination was normal with the exception of a brisk upbeat geotropic (toward the ground) torsional nystagmus when her head was hanging left, which is consistent with left posterior canalithiasis. The nystagmus lasted approximately 15 to 20 seconds after a 2- to 3-second latency. An Epley maneuver was performed with gentle vibration and was successful. HC returned for follow-up a week later with no complaints. Because HC travels abroad extensively for her work and is often away from developed areas, she was shown how to do the repositioning maneuver in the event she experienced difficulty. HC was also instructed to stay off her left side while sleeping in order to avoid recurrence.

Two years later, HC returned from a visit abroad specifically due to symptoms of increasing and debilitating vertigo that had been increasing over the last few weeks. Triggers for the vertiginous episodes were rolling over in bed and any tipping movement of her head. Upon her physician's examination, a left Dix–Hallpike resulted in a brisk geotropic horizontal nystagmus with minimal rotation, consistent with lateral canalithiasis.

When testing for lateral canal BPPV utilizing the roll test, rolling her onto her right side eye movement seemed to be stronger than when she rolled to her left. Thus, her physician started the maneuver progressing right to left using a log roll procedure; however, the eye movement on the left side markedly increased, as did her symptoms of acute vertigo. At this point, her physician switched directions making the assumption that it was indeed the left lateral canal that was involved and rolled her from left to right in a log roll maneuver. The nystagmus extinguished and she felt better upon sitting up.

HC returned in 1 week with continued symptoms of positional vertigo. Her physician examination revealed a very brisk geotropic horizontal nystagmus in the right and left side-lying positions. Her physician referred HC to the vestibular laboratory at this clinic for positional testing to help differentiate the offending canal.

28.2 Vestibular Testing

Spontaneous, gaze-evoked, and positional nystagmus testing was performed. There was a 1 deg/s rightward-beating spontaneous nystagmus when vision was denied. There was no gaze nystagmus in any direction with or without fixation. Positional nystagmus results revealed robust geotropic (toward the ground) horizontal nystagmus. As seen in ▶ Fig. 28.1 when lying in the right Dix–Hallpike position, there is a robust horizontal rightward-beating nystagmus. ▶ Fig. 28.2 reveals a robust, but less intense horizontal leftward-beating horizontal nystagmus. Neither of these responses included a torsional component suggesting horizontal canal involvement or posterior canal like what was seen in the clinical examination. In the supine body right position (▶ Fig. 28.3), the reader can see the robust rightward-beating geotropic nystagmus and in the supine body left position (▶ Fig. 28.4) another robust, but less intense geotropic

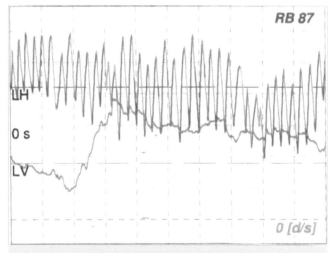

Fig. 28.1 Dix–Hallpike head hanging right nystagmus.

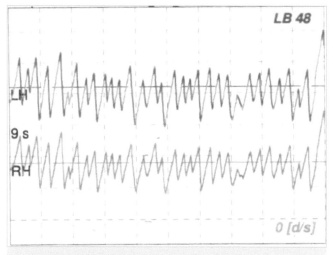

Fig. 28.2 Dix–Hallpike head hanging left nystagmus.

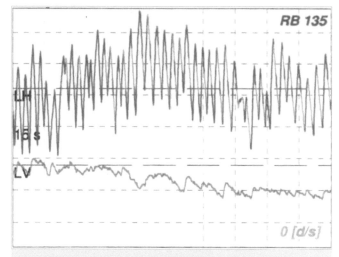

Fig. 28.3 Side-lying right positional nystagmus.

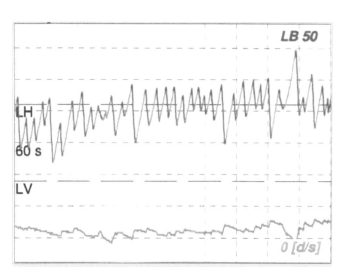

Fig. 28.4 Side-lying left positional nystagmus.

Table 28.1 Degree and direction of nystagmus in each position

Position	Nystagmus
Sitting head right	No nystagmus
Sitting head left	No nystagmus
Dix–Hallpike right	87 deg/s rightward
Dix–Hallpike left	48 deg/s leftward
Supine body right	135 deg/s rightward
Supine body left	50 deg/s leftward

Table 28.2 Degree and direction of nystagmus in the bow and lean positions

Position	Nystagmus
Bow	97 deg/s rightward
Lean	65 deg/s leftward

leftward-beating nystagmus. Using infrared video cameras and computer software, it is not difficult to determine which ear is creating the more robust response (▶ Table 28.1); however, with the naked eye during the clinical examination it would be very difficult to determine because the eye is moving extremely rapidly in all of these positions. In this case, due to the history of multiple-canal BPPV involvement, the bilateral brisk geotropic response witnessed by her physician and the overall difficulty in ascertaining the site of lesion, a **BLT** was added to the battery of positional testing and revealed robust horizontal nystagmus in both positions (▶ Table 28.2 and ▶ Fig. 28.5). The response in the bow position was beating rightward. This indicates that the offending ear is the right ear in horizontal canalithiasis.

28.3 Questions for the Reader

1. **Why did HC's physician conclude it was the left lateral canal that was involved?**

2. **How does a clinician perform the BLT?**
3. **How does the direction of the nystagmus differ between canalithiasis and cupulolithiasis?**

28.4 Discussion of Questions

1. **Why did HC's physician conclude it was the left lateral canal that was involved?**

HC's physician concluded HC had a disorder with her left lateral canal because HC had previously been treated for posterior canal BPPV in the left ear. He had given HC the maneuvers to perform while HC was away in the event the vertigo recurred and most likely assumed HC had converted, or inadvertently moved, the otoconia from the left posterior canal to the left lateral canal. This was an understandable conclusion especially after he began to treat HC for right lateral canalithiasis and the leftward nystagmus became stronger than the rightward nystagmus and her symptoms were much more severe when rolling HC onto her left ear than onto her right ear. Her physi-

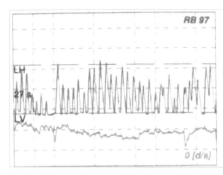

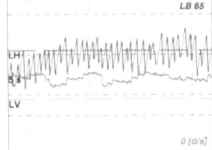

Fig. 28.5 Bow nystagmus/lean nystagmus.

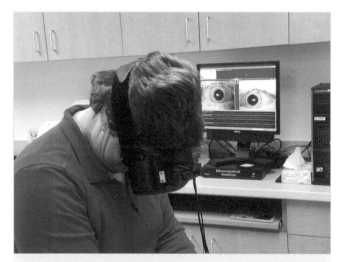

Fig. 28.6 Demonstration of the bow position.

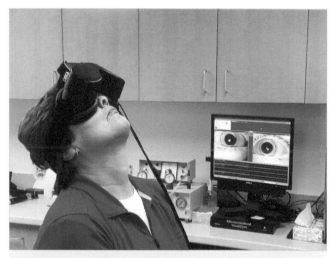

Fig. 28.7 Demonstration of the lean position.

cian then switched treatment plans and treated the left lateral canal. After the treatment, HC's symptoms improved.

When a "brisk" nystagmus appears during both lateral positions and the patient is symptomatic, it becomes difficult to differentiate which ear to treat. During a clinical examination, the physician does not have high-speed cameras to assist in measuring the nystagmus to determine if one side is stronger than the other. Physicians often have to rely on the previous history of the patient and the severity of the symptoms to differentiate which ear to treat. Also, nystagmus intensity can be variable upon repeated positional maneuvers.

2. How does a clinician perform the BLT?
The BLT is performed with the patient sitting upright and with the cover on the goggles so that vision is denied and the patient cannot fixate. The patient leans forward with head downward or "bows" head forward at least 90 degrees (▶ Fig. 28.6). This is followed by the patient leaning the head back at least 45 degrees[1,2] (▶ Fig. 28.7).

3. How does the direction of the nystagmus differ between canalithiasis and cupulolithiasis?
In canalithiasis, the otoconia moves within the lateral canal in response to movement of the head and the nystagmus will resolve within 60 seconds. When the otoconia adheres to the cupula that prolongs the nystagmus and symptoms, this is considered cupulolithiasis.

The literature assumes a clinician will have determined canalithiasis from cupulolithiasis prior to performing the BLT. Canalithiasis is more common than cupulolithiasis in lateral canal BPPV not unlike posterior canal BPPV. It is not always necessary to rely on the ear that has the most "robust" nystagmus when doing a side-lying test especially if high-speed cameras are not available and knowing the nystagmus intensity can be variable. A study reported that the BLT could correctly identify the affected ear for lateral canal BPPV more efficiently than when head rotation testing was used alone, making this very short and well-tolerated test a good addition to the test battery.[1]

For canalithiasis, the nystagmus will beat in the same direction as the affected or offending ear during the "bow" segment and away from the affected ear in the "lean" segment.[1,2] For cupulolithiasis, the nystagmus will beat toward the opposite ear or the unaffected ear during the "bow" segment and the same direction as the "lean" segment.[1,2]

28.5 Diagnosis and Recommended Treatment

A diagnosis of right horizontal canalithiasis was made. HC was treated with a 360-degree log roll from right to left. It was recommended HC sleep on her left side with her head propped up a little.

28.6 Outcome

HC remains to be symptom free for 20 months to date. She has been instructed to return if her symptoms recur.

28.7 Key Points

- Site of lesion of lateral canalithiasis can be difficult to differentiate even for experienced physicians and audiologists.
- The BLT test is helpful in differentiating which ear to treat in lateral canalithiasis and lateral cupulolithiasis.

References

[1] Lee JB, Han DH, Choi SJ, et al. Efficacy of the "bow and lean test" for the management of horizontal canal benign paroxysmal positional vertigo. Laryngoscope. 2010; 120(11):2339–2346

[2] Choung YH, Shin YR, Kahng H, Park K, Choi SJ. "Bow and lean test" to determine the affected ear of horizontal canal benign paroxysmal positional vertigo. Laryngoscope. 2006; 116(10):1776–1781

Suggested Readings

[1] Schuknecht HF. Cupulolithiasis. Arch Otolaryngol. 1969; 90(6):765–778

[2] Schuknecht HF, Ruby RR. Cupulolithiasis. Adv Otorhinolaryngol. 1973; 20: 434–443

29 Adult Patient with Chronic Otitis Media and Recurrent Benign Paroxysmal Positional Vertigo

Katie Barnhouse

29.1 Clinical History and Description

ES was referred for audiologic testing by his primary care physician due to ES's reports of hearing difficulties. These reports included difficulty hearing, "no right eardrum," and occasional dizziness. A report from a previous otolaryngology visit indicated that ES had a history of chronic otitis media with malodorous otorrhea and this condition is aggravated when he has upper respiratory infections (URI) that occur four to five times a year. ES was also previously evaluated by neurology for severe dizziness and stroke. At that time, ES underwent magnetic resonance imaging (MRI) and magnetic resonance angiography (MRA) of his head because of his history of a stroke and to rule out retrocochlear pathology as a cause of his dizziness. The imaging studies reported no acute infarct, hemorrhage, or vestibular schwannoma. Through additional questioning and administration of the Dix–Hallpike maneuver, neurology determined ES's dizziness was positional in nature (i.e., Benign Paroxysmal Positional Vertigo [BPPV]). As a result of this diagnosis, several canalith repositioning maneuvers (i.e., Epley maneuvers) were performed in the neurology clinic that reduced ES's dizziness. ES also reports a long history of exposure to noise having been employed at a welding factory for 5 years. He also reports constant bilateral tinnitus that is long-standing, yet manageable. Finally, ES reports additional pertinent health conditions that include hypertension, Hepatitis C, and expressive aphasia secondary to his stroke.

29.2 Audiologic Testing

Initial audiologic testing was obtained with good reliability (▶ Fig. 29.1). Results indicated slight to a gradually sloping moderate-severe Sensorineural Hearing Loss (SNHL) in the left ear and slight steeply sloping to severe mixed hearing loss in the right ear. Air–bone gaps in the right ear ranged from 15 to 30 dB HL across test frequencies. Otoscopy revealed a large central perforation in the right tympanic membrane (TM) without obvious drainage. The left TM was intact and normal in appearance. The right 226-Hz tympanogram indicated a flat tympanogram and a large ear canal volume (4.5 mL), which was consistent with the TM perforation. The left 226-Hz tympanogram indicated significant negative middle ear pressure (–155 daPa), normal ear canal volume, and normal compliance. Due to the finding of negative pressure in the left ear, a 678-Hz B/G tympanogram was performed. Multifrequency tympanometry, specifically two-component 678-Hz B/G tympanograms, can be helpful in differential diagnosis when TM or middle ear pathology is suspected.[1] A 678-Hz B/G tympanogram produces two curves: susceptance (B) and conductance (G). The resulting pattern of the two curves will indicate whether the middle ear system is mass or stiffness controlled. The 678-Hz B/G tympanogram will also indicate whether the middle ear is abnormally mass dominated, in which case a flaccid TM, fluid, or ossicular disarticulation is likely.[1] If the curve pattern indicates an abnormally stiffness-dominated middle ear system, otosclerosis. or tympanosclerosis is more likely.[1] ES's left 678-Hz B/G tympanogram revealed an abnormally mass-dominated middle ear system, which was consistent with his previous diagnosis of chronic otitis media. Right Acoustic Reflex Thresholds (ARTs) were not measureable due to the TM perforation. Left ARTs were absent to ipsilateral and contralateral stimulation. Speech Recognition Thresholds (SRTs) indicated a moderate loss in the ability to receive speech in the right ear and a mild loss in the left ear. Both SRTs were in good agreement with respective Pure-Tone Average (PTA). Word Recognition Scores (WRS) were performed using recorded Maryland Consonant-Nucleus-Consonant (CNC) 50-word lists. Results revealed moderate difficulty in the ability to recognize speech in the right ear and slight difficulty in the left ear. At this appointment, ES also completed the Hearing Handicap Inventory for Adults – Screening (HHIE-S), which is a 10-item screening questionnaire estimating the subjective handicap a patient perceives due to his or her hearing loss.[2] ES's score was 28/40, indicating a severe perceived handicap as a result of his hearing loss.

29.3 Diagnosis and Treatment

ES arrived at his otolaryngology appointment later that day. Microscopic otoscopy confirmed a large central perforation in the right TM with otitis media. Surgical risks associated with surgically repairing the right TM (i.e., tympanoplasty) were discussed with ES. Risks included bleeding, infection, persistent perforation, damage to facial nerve, taste disturbances, and need for further surgical procedures. ES decided to proceed with surgery and was advised to follow strict dry ear precautions, which meant he needed to keep the right ear as dry as possible. For showering, ES needed to pack his right ear with a large cotton ball and create an airtight seal with petroleum jelly. Using a postauricular approach, the otologist used cartilage palisades to patch the right TM. During the surgery, the ossicular chain was confirmed to be intact and mobile. Recovery from surgery was unremarkable and ES was given medical clearance for bilateral amplification.

29.4 Additional Testing

ES returned for postoperative audiologic testing (▶ Fig. 29.2) and discussion of hearing aids. Results indicated a slight hearing loss sloping to severe SNHL in the right ear and a slight hearing loss sloping to moderate-severe SNHL in the left ear. All air-bone gaps previously observed in the right ear had been effectively resolved. Right and left audiometric configurations were essentially symmetric. The right 226-Hz tympanogram was consistent with hypocomplaint TM movement (i.e., static compliance of 0.2 mL); however, ear canal volume and middle ear

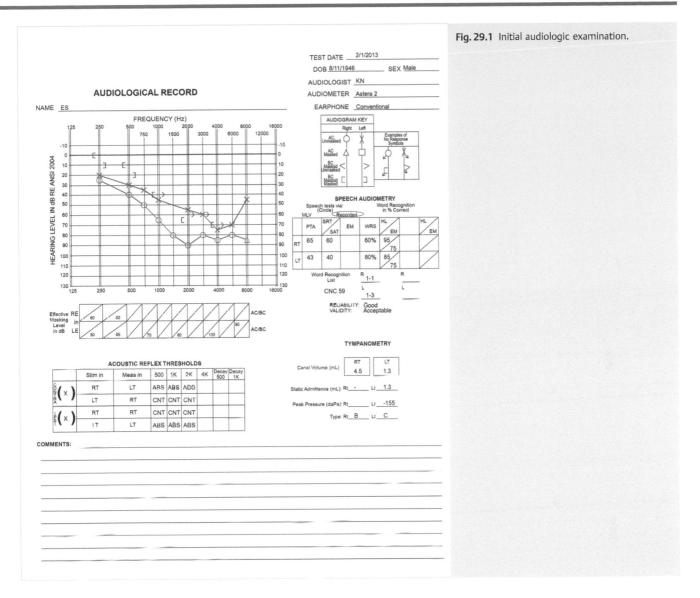

Fig. 29.1 Initial audiologic examination.

pressure were within normal limits. The left 226-Hz tympanogram was within normal limits. SRTs were in good agreement with the PTAs, bilaterally. WRS testing was consistent with moderate difficulty bilaterally. ARTs were absent in both ears for ipsilateral and contralateral stimulation. Given ES's history of chronic otitis media and right ear surgery, ES was scheduled for annual audiometric examinations. Since ES was medically cleared by otolaryngology, amplification options were discussed. After a thorough review of style options, the clinician and ES decided to trial bilateral wireless Behind-The-Ear (BTE) devices with acrylic earmolds and number 13 thick tubing. The earmolds were ordered with large vents to maximize air flow within the ear canals and the hearing aids fit to National Acoustics Laboratories' nonlinear fitting procedure, version 2 (NAL-NL2) using real-ear measures. At the fitting appointment, output of each hearing aid was verified using the Audioscan Verifit2. Speech mapping was performed using input levels of 55, 65, and 75 dB SPL (sound pressure level) and revealed excellent matches to the NAL-NL2-prescribed targets. ES reported the aforementioned speech levels to be "comfortable" (65 dB SPL),

"loud, but OK" (75 dB SPL), and "soft but audible" (55 dB SPL), respectively. At the fitting, ES also reported recurrence of episodic vertigo. He reported that episodes occur daily, last 10 to 20 seconds, and are triggered primarily when turning over to his right side in bed. Due to ES's history of positional vertigo, he was referred to a physical therapist (PT) for further workup. The PT report indicated ES displayed a strong subjective response to the right Dix–Hallpike maneuver, and objectively mild nystagmus was observed. Vertigo fatigued with repetitions of repositioning maneuvers and ES was provided at-home instruction for the Epley Maneuver. At ES's hearing aid follow-up 4 weeks later, ES completed the HHIE-S, and results revealed a score of 8/40, indicating no subjective hearing handicap. Verbally, ES reported a high degree of satisfaction and benefit with his hearing aids.

29.5 Questions for the Reader

1. **Other than URI, what other factors or health conditions can exacerbate recurrent otitis media?**

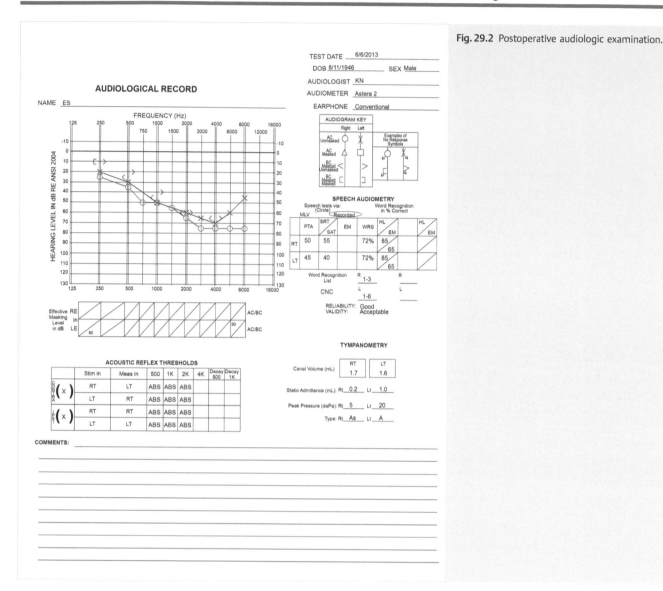

Fig. 29.2 Postoperative audiologic examination.

2. **Is there a preferred style of hearing aids that a patient with a history of chronic otitis media or ear surgery should be fitted with? Should any "special" programming be considered?**

3. **Based on ES's description of dizziness and previous success using the Epley maneuver to fatigue his symptoms, reoccurring BPPV is very likely. If repositioning maneuvers had proved ineffective, what other conditions might be considered and what tests might be necessary?**

29.6 Discussion of Questions

1. **Other than URI, what other factors or health conditions can exacerbate recurrent otitis media?**

Radiation of the head or neck, Eustachian tube dysfunction,[3] direct or indirect exposure to tobacco smoke or other environmental allergens,[4] sinusitis,[5] and autoimmune disorders[5] can increase the likelihood of recurrent otitis media.

2. **Is there a preferred style of hearing aids that a patient with a history of chronic otitis media or ear surgery should be fitted with? Should any "special" programming be considered?**

Patients with recurrent otitis media or a history of otologic surgery should be fitted with hearing aids allowing for maximum air ventilation while meeting the prescribed gain/output of the hearing loss. The prescribed targets should also take into consideration any air–bone gaps in the case of conductive or mixed hearing loss (i.e., add 20–25% of the air–bone gap to the prescribed targets). Optimal ventilation is critical as excessive moisture in the ear canal can promote further infection. Fortunately, current hearing aid platforms have advanced feedback managers allowing for increased venting and more open-fit options than previously available. For patients with Eustachian tube dysfunction, he/she may experience fluctuations in hearing. For this reason, independent volume controls would be recommended.

3. **Based on ES's description of dizziness and previous success using the Epley maneuver to fatigue his symptoms, reoccurring BPPV is very likely. If repositioning maneuvers had proved ineffective, what other conditions might be considered and what tests might be necessary?**

If repositioning maneuvers did not fatigue ES's symptom of dizziness, a unilateral or bilateral peripheral vestibular weakness might be present and a comprehensive vestibular evaluation should be recommended. Tests including videonystagmography (VNG), rotary chair, and caloric testing would help identify any potential peripheral weakness. Given ES's history of stroke, the possibility of a central etiology should also be investigated. Tests to assess central etiology include vestibular evoked myogenic potential and oculomotor testing, which includes saccades, gaze holding, optokinetics, and smooth pursuit. If a peripheral weakness was identified, ES would be referred to physical therapy for vestibular rehabilitation. If central abnormalities were identified, ES would be referred to otolaryngology for additional workup.

29.7 Outcome

ES is 66-year-old man with a known history of chronic otitis media who underwent right-sided tympanoplasty to surgically repair a large central perforation in his TM. Prior to surgery, audiologic testing indicated a slight sloping to severe mixed hearing loss in the right ear. Postoperative testing demonstrated significant improvements in right hearing thresholds and resolved air–bone gaps. ES was subsequently fitted with binaural BTE devices and reported a high level of perceived benefit at his follow-up. ES also presented with recurrent BPPV, which was effectively treated with the Epley maneuvers. Due to ES's history of middle ear pathology and right ear surgery,

ES will return for annual audiologic and otolaryngology appointments.

29.8 Key Points

- In cases of recurrent otitis media and TM perforation, medical management is essential not only to maximize hearing ability but also to minimize risk of systemic infection, erosion of canal bone or middle ear bones, or cholesteatoma.
- Oftentimes, the cause of dizziness is multifactorial and cannot be qualified into one diagnosis, such as BPPV. When conducting a case history, questioning should be thorough in order to provide as much detail pertaining to dizziness as possible (i.e., date of onset, frequency, severity, duration, and triggers). The clinician should also inquire regarding any recent head trauma, illnesses, new or increased stress, or changes in medications.

References

[1] Shanks JE, Wilson RH, Cambron NK. Multiple frequency tympanometry: effects of ear canal volume compensation on static acoustic admittance and estimates of middle ear resonance. J Speech Hear Res. 1993; 36(1): 178–185

[2] Lichtenstein MJ, Bess FH, Logan SA. Validation of screening tools for identifying hearing-impaired elderly in primary care. JAMA. 1988; 259(19):2875–2878

[3] Bluestone CD. Eustachian tube function: physiology, pathophysiology, and role of allergy in pathogenesis of otitis media. J Allergy Clin Immunol. 1983; 72(3):242–251

[4] Gaur K, Kasliwal N, Gupta R. Association of smoking or tobacco use with ear diseases among men: a retrospective study. Tob Induc Dis. 2012; 10(1):4

[5] Corren J, Rachelefsky G. Sinusitis and Otitis Media. In: Liberman P, Anderson JA, eds. Allergic Diseases Diagnosis and Treatment. Totwana, NJ; Humana Press Inc.; 2007:167–180

30 A Case of "Definite" Meniere's Disease: Unilaterally Abnormal Caloric Test with Bilaterally Normal Video Head Impulse Testing Test

Kathryn F. Makowiec and Gary P. Jacobson

30.1 Clinical History and Description

DM is a 28-year-old female referred for audiologic evaluation with a long-standing history of disequilibrium and headaches. DM reported episodes of vertigo lasting 8 to 10 hours. The vertiginous spells were accompanied by tinnitus, aural fullness, and fluctuating hearing loss on the left side. DM also reported a history of headaches along with the vertiginous episodes. Further, DM reported visual aura before, and photophobia and phonophobia during the headaches. An MRI was completed and was found to be normal. An audiogram completed prior to the consultation with otology revealed normal hearing in the right ear and a moderate to severe slightly rising fluctuating Sensorineural Hearing Loss (SNHL) from 250 to 4,000 Hz and then falling in configuration at 6,000 to 8,000 Hz in the left ear. Speech Recognition Thresholds (SRT) revealed normal ability to receive speech in the right ear and a moderate loss in the ability to receive speech in the left ear. Word Recognition Scores (WRS) revealed normal ability to recognize speech in the right ear and very poor ability to recognize speech in the left ear. Immittance audiometry revealed normal ear canal volume, static compliance, and middle ear pressure in each ear. Acoustic Reflex Thresholds (ART) was attempted but could not be completed due to an inability to maintain a hermetic seal. Ipsilateral acoustic reflexes were screened at 1,000 Hz and were absent bilaterally (▶ Fig. 30.1).

30.2 Additional Clinical Testing

A balance function test battery consisting of Videonystagmography (VNG), Sinusoidal Harmonic Acceleration (SHA) testing, Cervical Vestibular Evoked Myogenic Potential (cVEMP) testing, Ocular Vestibular Evoked Myogenic Potential (oVEMP) testing, and Video Head Impulse Testing (vHIT) was conducted.

Bithermal water caloric testing revealed a clinically significant 42% unilateral weakness on the left side (▶ Fig. 30.2). Ocular motility was normal. Results from static positional and dynamic positioning testing (i.e., Dix–Hallpike and the Roll test) were normal. SHA testing revealed normal phase, gain, and symmetry at 0.02, 0.04, 0.08, 0.16, and 0.32 Hz. The patient revealed an isolated phase lead at 0.01 Hz (▶ Fig. 30.3). Taken together with the caloric test findings, the SHA results were consistent with a compensated unilateral peripheral vestibular system impairment. cVEMP and oVEMP examinations (see ▶ Fig. 30.4 and ▶ Fig. 30.5, respectively) revealed normal symmetrical responses for both ears. This is consistent with normal peripheral vestibular system function for the saccules, utricles, and the superior and inferior vestibular nerves. The vHIT was completed for the left and right lateral canals (▶ Fig. 30.6). Vestibuloocular Reflex (VOR) gains were normal and there were no overt or covert saccades. When taken together, results from the vestibular test battery were consistent with a left peripheral vestibular system impairment in a static and dynamically compensated state. This impairment affected at least the horizontal semicircular canal on the left side.

30.3 Questions to the Reader

1. **What could be the potential cause of the reduced caloric response in the presence of normal vHIT?**
2. **Given the normal vHIT examination and abnormal caloric test, should vHIT be used as a stand-alone test of vestibular function in a diagnostic setting?**
3. **Since rotary chair testing revealed that DM has compensated for the unilateral impairment, should Vestibular Rehabilitation Therapy (VRT) be recommended?**

30.4 Discussion of the Questions

1. **What could be the potential cause of the reduced caloric response in the presence of normal vHIT?**

There are two primary theories why this patient would present with a normal horizontal canal vHIT examination and an abnormal caloric response. Researchers have suggested that the difference in responses such as this is due to the differences in the stimuli used in each test.[1] That is, vHIT testing uses angular acceleration, which is a "physiological" stimulus for the semicircular canals (i.e., a stimulus that is experienced in everyday life), while caloric testing uses a thermal stimulus that is "nonphysiological" (i.e., a stimulus that is not normally encountered in everyday life). In a normal ear, a warm caloric stimulus produces a thermal gradient in the ipsilateral horizontal semicircular canal such that the warmed endolymph becomes less dense and rises pushing the horizontal canal cupula toward the utricle (i.e., utriculopetal movement). This results in a depolarization of the ipsilateral horizontal canal neurons and an increase in neural firing rate. On the other hand, cooling the endolymph results in a utriculofugal deflection of the horizontal canal cupula and a hyperpolarization of the ipsilateral horizontal canal neurons and a reduction in their firing rates. In a system with "definite" Meniere's disease, however, histopathological studies have shown a swelling of the membranous labyrinth occurs, introducing the possibility of local endolymph flow within the labyrinth and multiple local, smaller convection currents.[1] These multiple lower currents would be insufficient to create the hydrostatic pressure required to deflect the cupula and initiate the caloric response. The overall diameter of the labyrinth does not change in Meniere's disease and so vHIT testing would not be impacted since the angular acceleration is

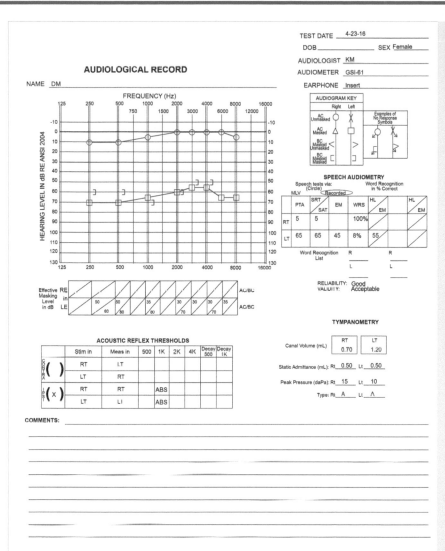

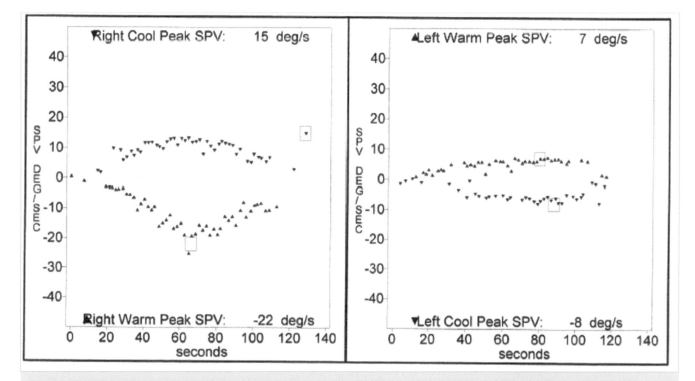

Fig. 30.2 Bithermal caloric test "pods." Results revealed a 42% unilateral weakness on the left side. The directional preponderance was 15%.

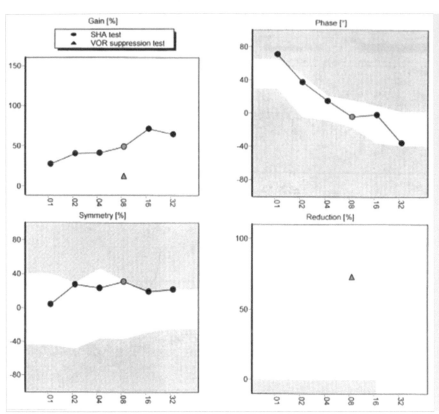

Fig. 30.3 Sinusoidal Harmonic Acceleration examination measuring the gain, phase, and symmetry of the Vestibuloocular Reflex response from 0.01 to 0.32 Hz.

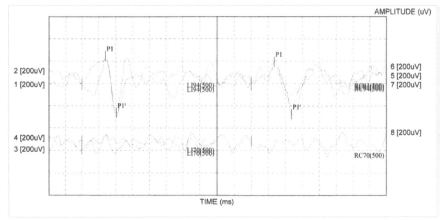

Fig. 30.4 **(a)** Cervical Vestibular Evoked Myogenic Potential (cVEMP) response for the left ear following a 500-Hz tone burst stimulation presented at 95 dB nHL. The peak-to-peak amplitude was 508.63 μV. The latency of the response was 13.9 ms. **(b)** cVEMP response for the right ear following a 500-Hz tone burst stimulation presented at 95 dB nHL. The peak-to-peak amplitude was 468.34 μV. The latency of the response was 13.57 ms.

dependent on the diameter of the labyrinth rather than the cross-sectional area.

Additional research has proposed an alternate hypothesis as to why a patient with Meniere's disease could have a normal vHIT response and abnormal caloric response.[2] These researchers proposed the difference is due to the neurophysiology of the crista. The crista consists of afferent nerve fibers in the peripheral zones that possess regular firing rates, and, afferent nerve fibers in the central zone that possess irregular firing rates. These afferent nerve fibers synapse on hair cells within the vestibular system, of which there are type I and II cells. The hair cells within the vestibular system respond to different stimulation rates. The nerve fibers from the peripheral zones of the crista primarily synapse on type II hair cells, whereas nerve fibers from the central zone of the crista primarily synapse on type I hair cells. The regularly firing nerve fibers are believed to drive the VOR in response to low-frequency stimulation (i.e., the caloric response). The irregularly firing nerve fibers are believed to drive the VOR in response to high-frequency transient acceleration and deceleration (i.e., the vHIT response). Histopathological evidence has shown that in patients with "definite" Meniere's disease there can be a significant loss of type II (regularly firing, peripheral zone) hair cells. Type I (irregularly firing, central zone) hair cells, however, remain intact. This could result in an abnormal response for the caloric test (i.e., since it is a low-frequency stimulus driven by type II hair cells), with a normal vHIT response (which is a high-frequency stimulus that is driven by type I hair cells).[2]

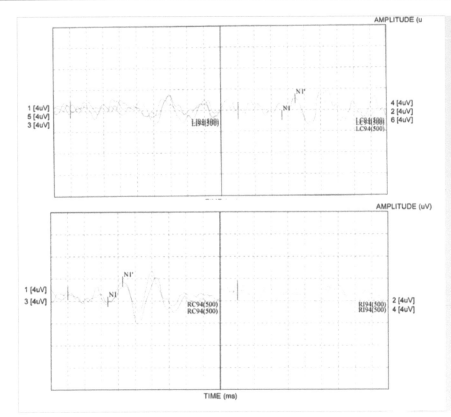

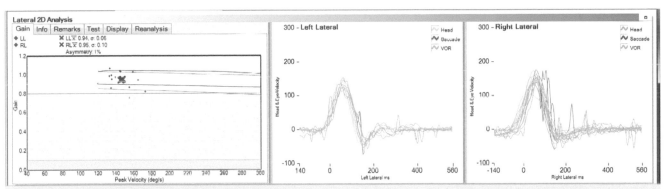

Fig. 30.5 **(a)** Ocular Vestibular Evoked Myogenic Potential (oVEMP) response for the right ear following a 500-Hz tone burst stimulation presented at 95 dB nHL. The peak-to-peak amplitude was 3.60 µV. The latency of the response was 11.93 ms. **(b)** oVEMP response for the left ear following a 500-Hz tone burst stimulation presented at 95 dB nHL. The peak-to-peak amplitude was 3.14 µV. The latency of the response was 12.09 ms.

Fig. 30.6 Summary screen of the Video Head Impulse Testing gains for the lateral semicircular canals. The Vestibuloocular Reflex gains were normal and no overt or covert saccades were noted.

Which theory prevails will need to explain the discordance between vHIT and caloric test results with the presence of the fluctuating, flat, or rising moderately severe SNHL often observed in patients with "definite" Meniere's disease.

2. **Given the normal vHIT examination and abnormal caloric test, should vHIT be used as a stand-alone test of vestibular function in a diagnostic setting?**

Because the vHIT test is designed to evaluate a different portion of the spectrum than the caloric response, only using the vHIT clinically would not allow for an assessment of the low-frequency function of the vestibular system. The caloric response mimics a natural stimulus of approximately 0.003 Hz.[3] The vHIT response mimics a head oscillation in the range of 4 to 7 kHz.[4] Using the caloric and the vHIT tests concurrently would allow

for evaluation of the vestibular system across its range of frequencies. As such, if only the vHIT examination was administered and the caloric examination was omitted, it would be possible to miss a low-frequency impairment impacting the peripheral vestibular system.

3. **Since rotary chair testing revealed that DM has compensated for the unilateral impairment, should Vestibular Rehabilitation Therapy (VRT) be recommended?**

A referral for VRT might be recommended based on DM's symptoms and her report of continued unsteadiness once Meniere's disease was managed with medications and/or diet changes. For example, DM may have developed maladaptive strategies such as an overdependence on visual information that could lead to unsteadiness when the patient was exposed to active visual environments. In this situation, VRT could address these maladaptive strategies.

30.5 Diagnosis and Recommended Treatment

A diagnosis of "definite" Meniere's disease requires the patient to experience the following symptoms: fluctuating, usually low-frequency SNHL, repeated attacks of vertigo, unilateral tinnitus, and unilateral aural fullness.[5] Meniere's disease may occur at any age, but typical onset is between 20 and 50 years of age. Episodes of decreased hearing, vertigo, aural fullness, and tinnitus can occur at different intervals from weeks to years apart and typically the patient is symptom free in the interim. "Probable" Meniere's disease may be diagnosed if the patient experiences the same vestibular symptoms as with "definite" Meniere's disease, but reports fluctuating aural symptoms.[5]

There are multiple theories for the cause of Meniere's disease with the most accepted theory being that Meniere's disease results from either an increased production or abnormally reduced resorption of endolymph in the inner ear.[5] A diagnosis of Meniere's disease requires the patient to have experienced at least two episodes of vertigo lasting longer than 20 minutes, but less than 24 hours, fluctuant SNHL documented via audiometry, unilateral tinnitus or aural fullness, and exclusion of any other cause for the above symptoms.[5] The following assessments are typically included in a diagnostic test battery for Meniere's disease: an audiometric evaluation including puretone audiometry, speech, and immittance audiometry, VNG, rotational chair testing, VEMP, vHIT, and, in many clinics, tympanic or transtympanic electrocochleography (ECochG).[1,2,5]

Treatments for Meniere's disease are targeted at reducing the frequency and intensity of the vertigo episodes and other symptoms because currently there is no cure for Meniere's disease. Treatments range from conservative to definitive. Conservative options include (1) diuretics to reduce fluid retention, (2) low sodium diet, (3) low caffeine diet, (4) VRT if a significant balance impairment is caused by Meniere's disease, (5) a hearing aid fitted to the affected ear to improve hearing and help relieve tinnitus, or (6) a contralateral routing of signal (CROS) amplification system if the ear with Meniere's disease has word recognition that is too poor to amplify.[6] More aggressive treatments are typically employed when conservative methods are not managing the symptoms well. These methods can include transtympanic injections of steroids (e.g., dexamethasone), or vestibulotoxic antibiotics (e.g., gentamicin).[5] Surgical options are often the last resort and represent "definitive treatments." These treatments include endolymphatic sac decompression, vestibular nerve section, or a chemical or surgical labyrinthectomy.[6]

30.6 Outcome

It was recommended that DM begin a low-sodium, low-caffeine diet. Further, DM was placed on a diuretic. It was also recommended that DM follow up with her neurologist for management of the headaches. At that time, DM was not interested in taking prescription medications and preferred holistic, herbal remedies.

DM was re-evaluated by her otologist 2 months later. At that time, DM reported continued "drop" attacks (i.e., sudden spontaneous falls when walking or standing). The otologist prescribed a diuretic (Maxzide) and encouraged DM to continue with the sodium and caffeine restrictions. Further, DM was evaluated by a neurologist who diagnosed DM with migrainous vertigo in addition to Meniere's disease. DM was scheduled to return for re-evaluation in 6 months with an accompanying audiogram. At this time, no amplification was recommended because DM was not interested in pursuing amplification until the vertiginous symptoms resolved.

30.7 Key Points

- It is possible for patients with "definite" Meniere's disease to demonstrate a unilaterally abnormal caloric test and bilaterally normal horizontal semicircular canal vHIT test.
- Typical symptoms for "definite" Meniere's disease include fluctuating unilateral low-frequency hearing loss, vertigo episodes lasting longer than 20 minutes, but less than 24 hours, aural fullness, and unilateral (ipsilesional) tinnitus.
- Meniere's disease symptoms can be successfully managed through conservative treatments including diuretics, low sodium diet, and caffeine restrictions.

References

[1] McGarvie LA, Curthoys IS, MacDougall HG, Halmagyi GM. What does the dissociation between the results of video head impulse versus caloric testing reveal about the vestibular dysfunction in Ménière's disease? Acta Otolaryngol. 2015; 135(9):859–865

[2] McCaslin DL, Rivas A, Jacobson GP, Bennett ML. The dissociation of video head impulse test (vHIT) and bithermal caloric test results provide topological localization of vestibular system impairment in patients with "definite" Ménière's disease. Am J Audiol. 2015; 24(1):1–10

[3] Hamid M, Hughes G, Kinney S. Criteria for diagnosing bilateral vestibular dysfunction. In: Graham MD, Kemink JL, eds. The Vestibular System: Neurophysiologic and Clinic Research. New York, NY: Raven Press; 1987:115–118

[4] Weber KP, MacDougall HG, Halmagyi GM, Curthoys IS. Impulsive testing of semicircular-canal function using video-oculography. Ann N Y Acad Sci. 2009; 1164:486–491

[5] Committee on Hearing and Equilibrium guidelines for the diagnosis and evaluation of therapy in Meniere's Disease. American Academy of Otolaryngology-Head and Neck Foundation, Inc. Otolaryngol Head Neck Surg. 1995; 113(3):181–185

[6] Foster CA. Optimal management of Ménière's disease. Ther Clin Risk Manag. 2015; 11:301–307

31 Superior Semicircular Canal Dehiscence Syndrome

Gary P. Jacobson, Alejandro Rivas, and Richard A. Roberts

31.1 Clinical History and Description

KA is a 32-year-old male with primary complaints of pulsatile tinnitus, noise-induced nystagmus, and autophony. He also reported that he became dizzy when exposed to loud sound, and when he strained during a bowel movement. The patient reported he could hear a 250-Hz tuning fork placed on his left lateral malleolus. Interestingly, the patient complained he could hear his eyes move, and further that the environment would move and he would become dizzy if he hummed loudly.

His past medical history was significant for anxiety, pulmonary embolism, morbid obesity, and hypercoagulability disorder. KA reported his medications were limited to Zoloft. A 10-point review of systems was conducted and was negative with the exception of the patient's balance and hearing disorders. KA's computed tomography (CT) scan showed that the superior semicircular canal (SSC) walls were thin, but intact. Despite the previous normal CT scan, it was felt that KA's history and primary complaints were suggestive of Superior Semicircular Canal Dehiscence Syndrome (SSCDS).

A "dehiscence" is an abnormal thinning, or complete absence of bone, and this can occur in different areas of the body including the bone overlying the semicircular canal system. The thinning of the bone overlying the SSC can be associated with a constellation of symptoms[1,2] including any of the following auditory and/or vestibular complaints: enhanced bone conduction auditory thresholds that can produce a spurious air–bone gap (i.e., air–bone gap with normal Acoustic Reflex Thresholds [ART]), Tullio's phenomenon (i.e., dizziness evoked by loud sound), Hennebert's sign (i.e., dizziness provoked by increasing pressure in the external auditory canal), dizziness during a Valsalva maneuver (i.e., dizziness provoked by increasing intracranial pressure), autophony (i.e., the ability to hear one's eye movements, neck muscle movements, and/or one's own voice louder in the affected ear), and, finally, the abnormal ability to hear a tone when a bone vibrator or tuning fork is placed on the lateral malleolus (i.e., the ankle bone).

These symptoms are accompanied by stereotypical electroneurodiagnostic test results including the following: an abnormally enhanced summating potential/action potential amplitude ratio (i.e., SP/AP ratio) in electrocochleographic (ECochG) testing,[3,4] abnormally reduced Cervical Vestibular Evoked Myogenic Potential (cVEMP) thresholds (usually 70 dB nHL or less), abnormally augmented Ocular Vestibular Evoked Myogenic Potential (oVEMP) amplitudes with stimulation delivered to the impaired side, and, most recently, it has been reported that patients with SSCDS demonstrate oVEMP at tone-burst frequencies that normally do not produce an oVEMP (e.g., 4,000-Hz tone burst).[5]

Treatment of SSCDS can range from counseling without treatment to intracranial surgery designed to create the missing anatomy (i.e., artificially manufacture a bony roof over the affected semicircular canal), or "deactivate" the errant SSC (i.e., "plugging" the superior canal). The choice in large part is dependent on the self-reported severity caused by the impairment.

31.2 Clinical Tests

The audiometric evaluation for KA revealed a slight conductive hearing loss for the right ear and a mild, predominately low and mid frequency, mixed hearing loss for the left ear (▶ Fig. 31.1). Speech Recognition Thresholds (SRT) revealed a slight loss in the ability to receive speech in the right ear and a mild loss in the left ear. Word Recognition Scores (WRS) revealed normal ability to recognize speech in each ear. Immittance audiometry revealed normal ear canal pressure, static compliance, and ear canal volume. Acoustic Reflex Thresholds (ART) were present at normal sensation levels bilaterally in the presence of the conductive hearing loss.

KA's Dizziness Handicap Inventory (DHI)[6] total score was 64/100 points representing severe, self-report, dizziness handicap. Additionally, the Hospital Anxiety and Depression Scale (HADS)[7] anxiety subscale score was 18/21 points (i.e., upper limit of normal is 10 points), suggesting the presence of significant self-report anxiety. Further, the depression subscale score was 7/21 points, which was normal (i.e., the upper limit of normal is 10 points).

Video Head Impulse Testing (vHIT) revealed normal Vestibuloocular Reflex (VOR) gains for the horizontal plane and for the left anterior/right posterior (RALP) and left posterior/right anterior (LARP) planes (▶ Fig. 31.2).

On Videonystagmography (VNG) testing, ocular motility subtests were normal, as were tests for the identification of positional and positioning (i.e., Benign Paroxysmal Positioning Vertigo [BPPV]) nystagmus. As previously noted, KA reported he could hear his eyes move and images moved any time he hummed loudly. Video recording of KA's eye movements revealed a downbeating nystagmus that occurred when he hummed loudly. The downbeating nystagmus suggested that the SSC crista was activated by the humming.

▶ Fig. 31.3 reports the caloric test summary. The total caloric response was 111 degree/s, indicating there was no evidence of a bilateral caloric weakness. The caloric test was normal, showing an 8% unilateral weakness (i.e., upper limit of normal 22%) and a 19% directional preponderance (i.e., upper limit of normal 27%). VOR suppression (fixation suppression) was normal.

The cVEMP test revealed that KA had symmetrical cVEMP latencies and amplitudes (i.e., the amplitude asymmetry was 29%; the upper limit of normal is 47%). The cVEMP threshold was reduced to 65 to 70 dB nHL on the (normal) right side and normal (70–75 dB nHL; ▶ Fig. 31.4, ▶ Fig. 31.5) on the (affected) left side. Further, a cVEMP could be recorded in response to a 4,000-Hz tone burst on the left side (i.e., the affected side), but not on the right side.

The right and left oVEMP demonstrated normal N1 latencies; however, the N1–P1 amplitude was 12.23 μV for the right ear and 198.71 μV for the left ear (▶ Fig. 31.6, ▶ Fig. 31.7). The latter value exceeded the upper limit of normal for absolute oVEMP

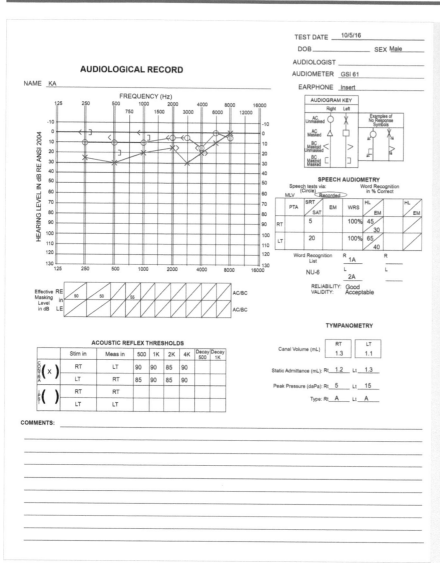

Fig. 31.1 Pure-tone audiometry showing the spurious conductive hearing impairment on the left side (i.e., air–bone gap in the presence of normal Acoustic Reflex Thresholds bilaterally).

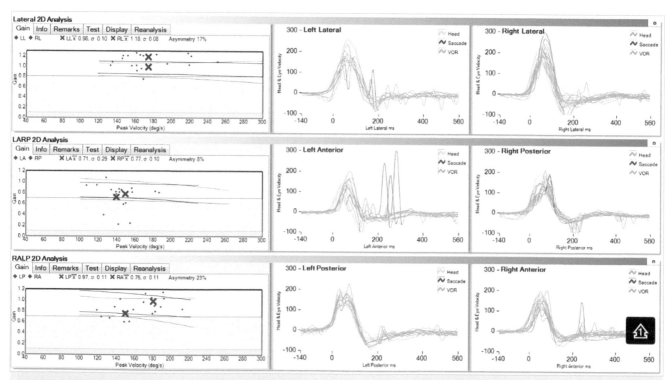

Fig. 31.2 Summary screen of Video Head Impulse Testing gains for horizontal as well as right anterior/left posterior (RALP) and left anterior/right posterior planes (LARP). The Vestibuloocular Reflex gains were all normal.

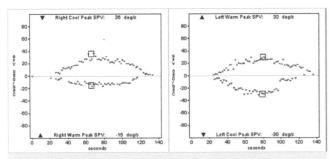

Fig. 31.3 Bithermal caloric test "pods." The patient showed an 8% right unilateral weakness and a 19% left directional preponderance. Laboratory upper limit for unilateral weakness is 22% and for directional preponderance is 27%.

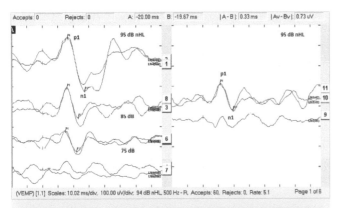

Fig. 31.5 Left panel: Cervical Vestibular Evoked Myogenic Potential (cVEMP) threshold for the left ear occurs at 70 to 75 dB nHL (trace 6). Notice that there is a P1 present in response to a 4,000-Hz tone burst (right panel, traces 10 and 11) that would not occur for normal subjects. The latency of the cVEMP in response to a 500-Hz tone burst presented at 94 dB nHL was 14.90 ms. The peak-to-peak amplitude of this response was 261.96 μV.

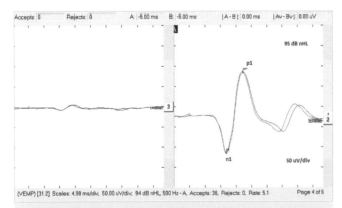

Fig. 31.7 Right panel: Ocular Vestibular Evoked Myogenic Potential for the left ear in response to a 500-Hz tone burst of 94 dB nHL. The peak-to-peak amplitude of n1-p1 was 198.71 μV. This resulted in a significant amplitude asymmetry of 88% (upper limit of normal is 35%). The n1 peak latency was 11.68 ms.

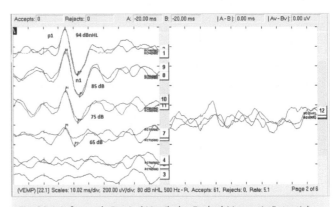

Fig. 31.4 Left panel: Cervical Vestibular Evoked Myogenic Potential (cVEMP) threshold for the right ear occurs at 65 to 70 dB nHL (trace 7). Notice that P1 is absent in response to a 4,000-Hz tone burst (right panel) where a response was present for the left ear. The latency of the cVEMP in response to a 500-Hz tone burst presented at 94 dB nHL was 14.57 ms. The peak-to-peak amplitude of this response was 475.83 μV. This created a nonsignificant amplitude asymmetry of 29% (upper limit of normal is 47%).

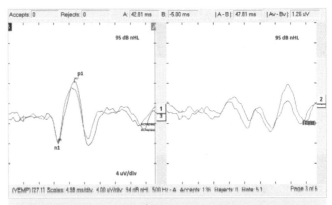

Fig. 31.6 Left panel: Ocular Vestibular Evoked Myogenic Potential for the right ear in response to a 500-Hz tone burst of 94 dB nHL. The peak-to-peak amplitude of n1-p1 was 12.23 μV. The n1 peak latency was 11.27 ms.

amplitude by greater than 10 standard deviations. This created an amplitude asymmetry of 88.46% favoring the left side. Further, while it was impossible to evoke an oVEMP in response to a 4,000-Hz tone burst for the right ear (▶ Fig. 31.8), a clear oVEMP could be recorded following stimulation of the left ear with the 4,000-Hz tone burst (▶ Fig. 31.9). Finally, ▶ Fig. 31.10 and ▶ Fig. 31.11 report CT imaging illustrating the normal right nondehiscent superior canal and the abnormal dehiscent left SSC.

31.3 Questions for the Reader

1. **What is the cause of KA's spurious conductive hearing loss?**
2. **Why is the recording of an oVEMP for a 4,000-Hz stimulus a significant finding for patients suspected of having SSCDS?**
3. **What causes the vertigo when the patient hums loudly?**
4. **What are potential surgical treatments for SSCDS?**

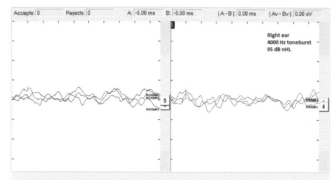

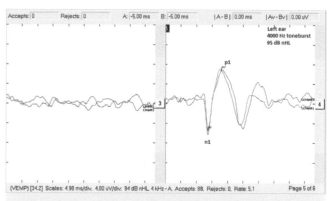

Fig. 31.8 Absent contralateral Ocular Vestibular Evoked Myogenic Potential in response to a 4,000-Hz tone burst following stimulation of the right ear (left panel).

Fig. 31.9 The Ocular Vestibular Evoked Myogenic Potential in response to a 4,000-Hz tone burst following stimulation of the left ear. Notice that there is a clear response present recorded from the contralateral infraorbital electrode (right panel).

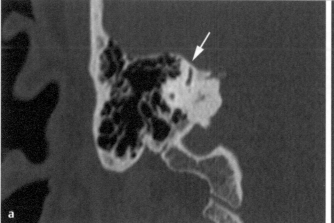

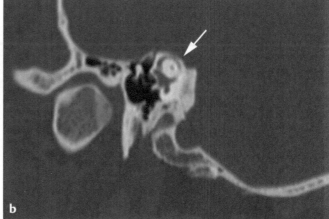

Fig. 31.10 Coronal views of high-resolution CT scans showing the normal, nondehiscent superior semicircular canal on the right side (see arrow).

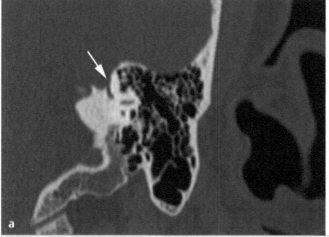

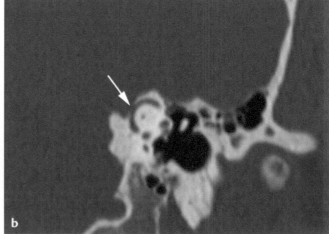

Fig. 31.11 Coronal views of high-resolution CT scans showing the dehiscent superior semicircular canal on the left side (see arrow).

31.4 Discussion of the Questions

1. What is the cause of KA's spurious conductive hearing loss?

The presence of a mobile third window (i.e., the dehiscence) causes pressure changes that vary from the normal two-window system (i.e., oval and round windows). This causes a portion of air-conducted sound energy to be shunted away from the cochlea to the area of the dehiscence that worsens the air-conduction threshold. The same pressure changes actually work to augment the displacement of the basilar membrane for bone-conducted sound that improves the bone-conduction threshold. These pressure changes affect the lower audiometric test frequencies and create an air–bone gap (i.e., conductive hearing loss) even though measures of middle ear function are unremarkable. Interestingly, the magnitude of air-conduction threshold at 250 Hz ($r = 0.25$), air–bone gap at 500 Hz ($r = 0.27$), as well as cVEMP amplitude ($r = 0.62$) and oVEMP amplitude ($r = 0.61$) have been shown to be significantly correlated with the magnitude of the SSCD.[8]

2. Why is the recording of an oVEMP for a 4,000-Hz stimulus a significant finding for patients suspected of having SSCDS?

Previous research[5] has reported that the presence of an oVEMP that occurs in response to a 4,000-Hz tone burst (i.e., a frequency that normally would not yield an oVEMP) has 100% sensitivity and 100% specificity for the detection of an SSCDS. This finding suggests that where a response to a 4,000-Hz tone burst is present, time-intensive threshold testing for oVEMP and/or cVEMP may be unnecessary.

3. What causes the vertigo when the patient hums loudly?

Humming mimics a low-frequency vibratory stimulus. In a left-sided SSCDS, humming results in an asymmetrical activation of the SSC (i.e., electrical output of the left superior semicircular canal is greater than the output of the right posterior semicircular canal). This produces increased electrical output to the contralateral superior rectus and ipsilateral inferior oblique muscles that draws the eyes upward (with a torsional component). That eye movement is followed by a saccade and that sequence in repetition is the origin of the excitatory downbeating nystagmus.

4. What are potential surgical treatments for SSCDS?

A common treatment for patients with minimal symptoms is observation. The primary decision to proceed with a surgical repair is dependent on whether or not symptoms cause alterations in the patient's activities of daily living and quality of life. The surgical treatments for SSCDS are designed to either repair the defect in the SSC (referred to as "resurfacing") or take the offending semicircular canal "offline" (referred to as "plugging" the SSCC). Both of these techniques can be achieved through a middle fossa approach, where a small craniotomy is made above the ear and the dura and brain are mildly elevated. Once the dehiscent SSC is identified to resurface the canal, bone pate, bone wax, and/or bone cement are used to create a new roof, thus replacing the dehiscence. Alternately, when canal plugging is performed, bone wax, fascia, and/or bone pate are placed inside the lumen of the canal, followed by bone chips to create a total obstruction to the flow of endolymph through the superior canal. The advantage of plugging is that it is a more definitive treatment with less risk of recurrence, but the disadvantage is increased risk of sensorineural hearing loss.

Two other procedures have been described to treat SSCDS surgically. An option that has been proven to provide similar results in selected patients is the transmastoid approach with plugging of the SSC. This option avoids the need for a craniotomy. After the mastoid bone is drilled and the SSC identified in order to plug the canal, two small holes are made at each end of each limb of the canal. Then the lumen of each limb is plugged, as previously described, bypassing the actual dehiscence and disconnecting the SSC.[9] The last surgical option is plugging the round window. This procedure has been described for patients with minimal auditory symptoms without dizziness or for patients with significant comorbidities where a larger operation is contraindicated. Primarily, this is a procedure attempting to provide symptomatic relief without treating the dehiscence. By plugging the round window with fascia, followed by small pieces of cartilage, it is postulated that the deflection of energy away from the cochlea, caused by the dehiscence, improves by increasing the resistance of the round window. This technique has only been seen to provide symptomatic relief in less than 50% of patients.[10]

31.4.1 Description of the Disorder and Recommended Treatment

There is agreement that the disorder represents a thinning (i.e., near dehiscence)[11] or complete absence of bone over the SSC. The loss of bone over that part of the membranous labyrinth results in a mobile third window. This window provides a route for acoustical energy to escape while enhancing bone-conducted energy. This produces the audiometric air–bone gap. Additionally, the mobile third window produces a system that moves with a greater magnitude than it would normally move when the entire membranous system is encased in solid bone. The increased motion "amplifies" the hydromechanical energy imparted by the tone burst, mechanical tap, or vibration, and this produces the abnormally large VEMP at supramaximal stimulus intensities that can be recorded at very soft intensities, as well as a response that can be recorded at threshold (i.e., low-intensity thresholds).

There are three primary approaches to the treatment of SSCDS. The first is counseling and waiting. For many patients with SSCDS, understanding the mechanism that causes the troublesome symptoms is sufficient to satisfy the patient (by demystifying the problem) and makes it possible for the patient to continue with their lives. A second approach is otologic surgery designed to either create a false roof over the SSC or disable the canal entirely. In the case of the former, a left middle fossa approach is used to gain exposure to the SSC. Once the canal is identified, a roof can be created with a number of materials including bone wax, bone pate, and/or bone cement. Once the canal has been identified, the second approach is to "plug" the SSC using fascia, bone pate, or bone wax, followed by very small pieces of bone chips effectively disconnecting the SSC. The patient usually is mildly dizzy postoperatively; however, the dizziness disappears after vestibular compensation has occurred. In the current case, the treatment was a canal resurfacing procedure.

KA underwent a left-sided middle fossa approach with a repair of the SSCDS. Intraoperatively, the surgeons encountered the SSC located in the anterior limb of a prominent arcuate eminence. The SSC could not be visualized with the surgical microscope and could only be visualized with the use of a 70-degree endoscope. The dehiscence was under the superior petrosal sinus at the level of the anterior limb and ampulla. The distorted anatomy made the operation complex. Plugging the canal was impossible due to the severe angulation and accordingly the canal was resurfaced instead with bone pate, bone wax, bone chips, bone cement, and fascia. Immediately postoperatively KA reported that all of his symptoms had abated. KA was discharged 2 days after surgery without complications.

31.5 Outcome

Immediately after surgery, KA did very well and the symptoms resolved. One month postoperatively, KA reported a new onset of disequilibrium, particularly when turning his head rapidly to the left. KA also reported decreased hearing. The patient was placed on a steroid taper and was evaluated in the neurotology clinic. On examination, the patient had a positive head-thrust test when turning the head rapidly to the left. The Weber lateralized to the right side. The patient was started on vestibular rehabilitative therapy (VRT) and this was accomplished at home.

After completing the steroid taper and VRT, 2 months after surgery, KA reported that all symptoms had completely resolved. On vestibular examination, KA showed no spontaneous nystagmus, no headshake nystagmus, no head-thrust nystagmus, and no nystagmus on hyperventilation or Valsalva maneuvers. The Dix–Hallpike maneuver was negative bilaterally.

Postoperative cVEMP and oVEMP tests are shown in ▸ Fig. 31.12 and ▸ Fig. 31.13. It can be observed that the oVEMP amplitude asymmetry disappeared. Further, the left ear no longer generated an oVEMP in response to a 4,000-Hz tone

burst. The patient did not report any symptoms of SSCDS. Postoperative audiometry (▸ Fig. 31.14) showed pure-tone thresholds to be within normal limits.

31.6 Key Points

- The diagnosis of SSCDS is established when patients complain of all, or some, of the vestibular and auditory symptoms that have been described herein. The gold standard assessment is the high-resolution CT scan with Pöschl and Stenvers' views (0.5-mm collimated helical CT scan with reformation in the plane of the superior canal).
- The thinning or absence of bone over the SSC can produce a mobile third window that creates a low-impedance route for acoustical energy to dissipate resulting in a spurious air–bone gap and for hydromechanical energy to be amplified resulting from the hypermobility in the membranous labyrinth.
- There is variability in the clinical presentation of SSCDS. That is, not all patients demonstrate all of the symptoms. In this case, the patient showed an augmented n1 amplitude on the left oVEMP test, and oVEMP and cVEMP were present in response to a 4,000-Hz tone burst. However, the patient did not demonstrate a unilaterally augmented cVEMP amplitude.
- The treatment for SSCDS may be watchful waiting if the symptoms can be tolerated. Alternately a middle fossa approach followed by either a plugging of the superior canal (i.e., with bone chips, bone pate, and bone paste) or resurfacing of the canal (i.e., with bone pate, bone chips, bone wax, and fascia) may be chosen by the patient if the symptoms negatively impact the patient's quality of life. If canal plugging is desired, a transmastoid approach also is an option.
- Should surgery be chosen as the treatment, it is important to be aware that tympanic electrocochleography (tECochG) may be utilized as a neuromonitoring modality to help guide the surgeon through to a successful outcome.[4]

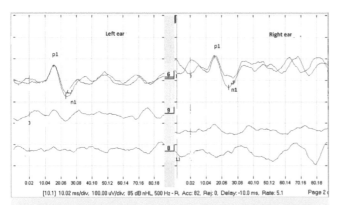

Fig. 31.12 Postoperative Cervical Ocular Vestibular Evoked Myogenic Potential (cVEMP) showing the left and right ear responses are equally scaled and there is no amplitude asymmetry. The VEMP threshold is approximately 85 dB nHL (i.e., middle traces in each panel).

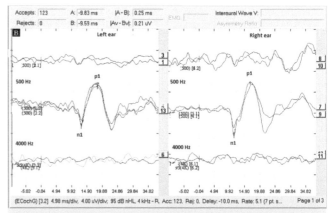

Fig. 31.13 Postoperative Ocular Vestibular Evoked Myogenic Potential examination. The left and right ear responses are equally scaled. Now there is no amplitude asymmetry, nor is there a response recorded to a 4,000-Hz tone burst on the left side.

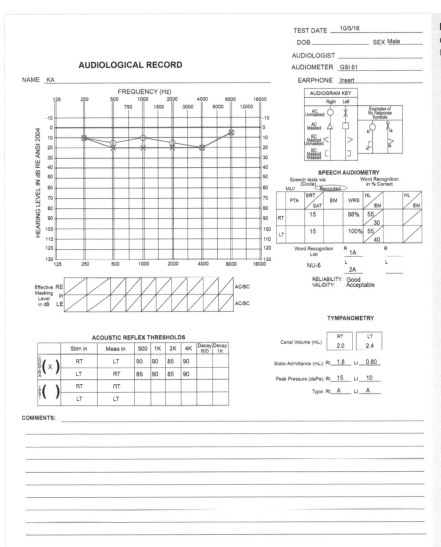

Fig. 31.14 Postoperative audiometric examination reporting normal pure-tone thresholds in each ear.

References

[1] Minor LB. Superior canal dehiscence syndrome. Am J Otol. 2000; 21(1):9–19

[2] Minor LB. Clinical manifestations of superior semicircular canal dehiscence. Laryngoscope. 2005; 115(10):1717–1727

[3] Arts HA, Adams ME, Telian SA, El-Kashlan H, Kileny PR. Reversible electrocochleographic abnormalities in superior canal dehiscence. Otol Neurotol. 2009; 30(1):79–86

[4] Wenzel A, Ward BK, Ritzl EK, et al. Intraoperative neuromonitoring for superior semicircular canal dehiscence and hearing outcomes. Otol Neurotol. 2015; 36(1):139–145

[5] Manzari L, Burgess AM, McGarvie LA, Curthoys IS. An indicator of probable semicircular canal dehiscence: ocular vestibular evoked myogenic potentials to high frequencies. Otolaryngol Head Neck Surg. 2013; 149(1):142–145

[6] Jacobson GP, Newman CW. The development of the Dizziness Handicap Inventory. Arch Otolaryngol Head Neck Surg. 1990; 116(4):424–427

[7] Snaith RP. The hospital anxiety and depression scale. Health Qual Life Outcomes. 2003; 1:29

[8] Hunter JB, O'Connell BP, Wang J, et al. Correlation of superior canal dehiscence surface area with vestibular evoked myogenic potentials, audiometric thresholds, and dizziness handicap. Otol Neurotol. 2016; 37(8):1104–1110

[9] Agrawal SK, Parnes LS. Transmastoid superior semicircular canal occlusion. Otol Neurotol. 2008; 29(3):363–367

[10] Silverstein H, Van Ess MJ. Complete round window niche occlusion for superior semicircular canal dehiscence syndrome: a minimally invasive approach. Ear Nose Throat J. 2009; 88(8):1042–1056

[11] Ward BK, Wenzel A, Ritzl EK, et al. Near-dehiscence: clinical findings in patients with thin bone over the superior semicircular canal. Otol Neurotol. 2013; 34(8):1421–1428

32 Endolymphatic Sac Tumor: Audiometric and Vestibular Considerations

Amy K. Winston

32.1 Clinical History and Description

KL is 25-year-old male who was referred by his neurotologist for audiometric testing and Videonystagmography (VNG) to investigate the etiology of KL's reported intermittent vertigo, dizziness, and hearing loss in his left ear.

KL reported decreased hearing sensitivity in the left ear that has progressed in severity since first noted at 17. KL stated the hearing in his left ear decreased suddenly approximately 3 years ago and he is now unable to hear anything from his left side. KL described significant communication difficulties in most listening conditions as well as an inability to localize sounds.

Also, KL noted episodes of "true" spinning vertigo with significant residual dizziness. These vestibular symptoms reportedly developed 7 months ago with no identifiable precipitating event. According to KL, true vertiginous episodes last from 1 to 2 hours and are accompanied by severe diaphoresis (abnormal, excessive sweating) and intense nausea and vomiting. KL stated he experiences residual symptoms for several days after each episode of vertigo and, during this time, quick head and body movements, particularly to the left side, generate intense dizziness. KL stated he has had five vertiginous episodes within the last 2 months, with the most recent occurring 1 week ago.

32.2 Audiologic Examination

KL was evaluated on two separate days. A comprehensive audiometric evaluation and immittance audiometry (tympanometry and Acoustic Reflex Thresholds, ARTs) were performed on the first day. KL returned approximately 1 week later for VNG evaluation.

Cursory otoscopy completed prior to testing revealed clear ear canals bilaterally. A bright red mass was visualized behind the left tympanic membrane. This otoscopic observation supported the referring physician's working diagnosis of a left glomus tympanicum tumor.

Results from the comprehensive audiometric examination revealed normal hearing sensitivity at 250 to 8,000 Hz in the right ear and a profound sensorineural loss in the left ear (▶ Fig. 32.1). As expected, the Speech Recognition Threshold (SRT) was normal in the right ear and could not be measured in the left ear when applying contralateral masking. Word Recognition Scores (WRS) were within normal limits in the right ear and could not be measured in the left ear. Tympanometric findings for ear canal volume, middle ear pressure, and static admittance were within normal limits bilaterally. ARTs were at normal sensation levels in the ipsilateral right test condition only; absence of measurable ARTs in the contralateral right test condition was unexpected and was considered to be inconsistent with audiometric findings.

VNG testing was completed and results were abnormal. No spontaneous gaze, post-headshake, or positional nystagmus was noted. Findings from oculomotor studies, including smooth pursuit, random saccades, and optokinetic tests were within normal limits. Dix–Hallpike testing yielded normal results in the right and left test conditions. Cool- and warm-air caloric irrigations in the right ear evoked robust nystagmus (cool: 21% per second; warm: 35% per second). Cool-air irrigation in the left ear yielded no measurable response. Ice-water irrigation in the left ear evoked a brisk (10% per second) right-beating nystagmus (▶ Fig. 32.2a) that slowed and was abolished as the patient moved from the standard 30-degree supine caloric test position to a sitting position (▶ Fig. 32.2b). The nystagmus then reversed to left-beating nystagmus when the patient assumed a sitting position with his head tilted down by 30 degrees (▶ Fig. 32.2c). The finding of a significant (100%) left unilateral weakness on standard air caloric testing strongly suggest a peripheral etiology to account for KL's episodic vertigo and dizziness.

32.3 Questions to the Reader

1. **Why does the right-beating nystagmus evoked by the ice-water caloric in the left ear reverse when the patient is moved to a sitting position with his head tilted downward?**
2. **What does the presence of a caloric response to ice water indicate about the status of KL's left peripheral vestibular system?**

32.4 Discussion of Questions

1. **Why does the right-beating nystagmus evoked by the ice-water caloric in the left ear reverse when the patient is moved to a sitting position with his head tilted downward?**

In most clinical settings, caloric irrigation testing is performed with the patient lying supine with the head elevated to 30 degrees. In this standard caloric position, the horizontal canal is essentially vertical and thus aligned with the gravitational plane. Introduction of a cool stimulus causes the endolymph on the side of the canal closest to the irrigation to become heavier (more dense) and sink. In the standard caloric test position, this generates an ampullofugal endolymph flow, or movement of the endolymph away from the utricle. Ampullofugal endolymph flow is inhibitory in the horizontal canal, triggering a reduction in neural activity from the baseline. The result is horizontal nystagmus that beats away from the irrigated ear. When the patient is moved to a sitting position with the head tilted downward at 30 degrees, the horizontal canal is again in the vertical plane, but the position of the crista ampullaris, the sensory end organ in the semicircular canal, relative to the irrigation side is reversed. With this, the same cooling effect and resultant sinking of the endolymph now generates an ampullopetal endolymph flow, or movement of the endolymph toward

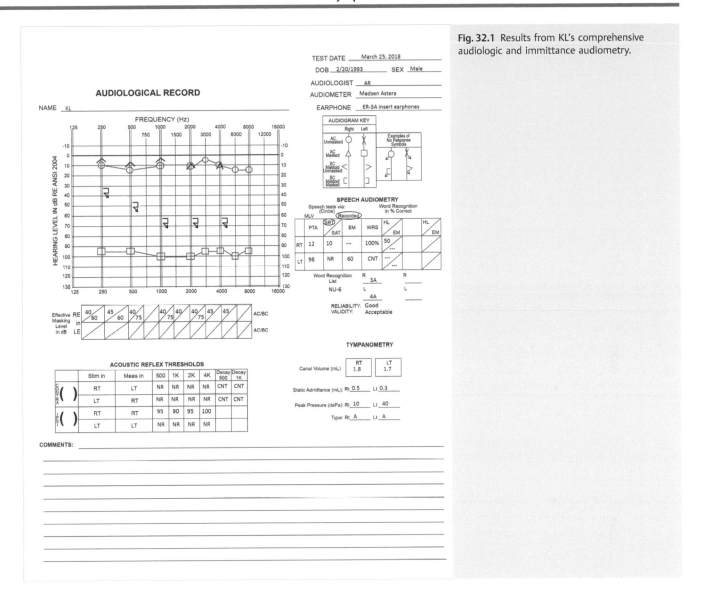

Fig. 32.1 Results from KL's comprehensive audiologic and immittance audiometry.

the utricle. Ampullopetal endolymph flow is excitatory in the horizontal canal, triggering an increase in the neural activity from the baseline. The result, then, of a cool irrigation in the sitting position is horizontal nystagmus that beats toward the irrigated ear. This reversal in nystagmus direction with the change in position clearly differentiates a caloric-induced nystagmus from peripheral-based spontaneous nystagmus, which would remain fixed in direction regardless of body position.

2. **What does the presence of a caloric response to ice water indicate about the status of KL's left peripheral vestibular system?**

Just as the auditory system responds to different frequencies, so, too, does the peripheral vestibular system. Normal head movements fall within the range of 0.1 to 10 Hz. The standard caloric stimulus (air or water) approximates a very low-frequency head rotation of approximately 0.002 to 0.004 Hz. With that, absence of a caloric response to a standard air or water stimulus should only be interpreted to reflect a loss of function within this very limited, and very low, frequency range. This

finding does not provide information about how the system responds to higher frequencies. Ice water is a stronger stimulus than standard air or water stimuli and approximates a higher-frequency rotation. The fact that KL's vestibular system responded to ice water in the left ear supports the presence of residual high-frequency peripheral vestibular function in that ear. Note that this could be confirmed through the use of rotational chair testing or the Video Head Impulse Test (vHIT), both of which evaluate higher-frequency vestibular function.

32.5 Diagnostic Imaging

32.5.1 Magnetic Resonance Imaging

KL underwent FLAIR (Fluid Attenuation Inversion Recovery) Magnetic Resonance Imaging (MRI) testing. MRI findings revealed a large (2.4 cm × 2.7 cm) enhancing mass centered along the posterior surface of the left petrous temporal bone (► Fig. 32.3).

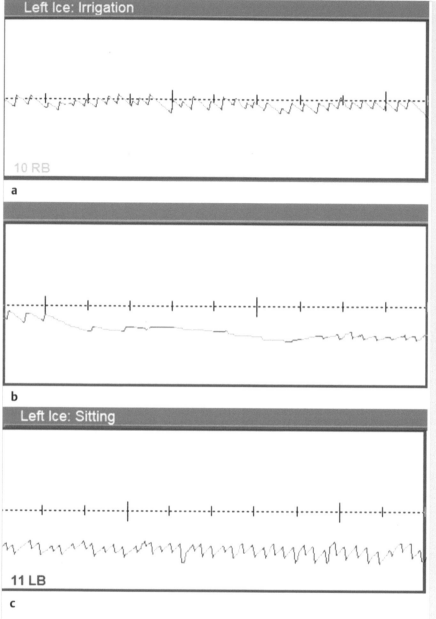

Fig. 32.2 Ice-water caloric tracings **(a)** in the standard caloric test position, **(b)** as the patient moves from supine to sitting, and **(c)** in a sitting position with the head tilted downward by 30 degrees. Note the reversal of the nystagmus direction.

32.5.2 Computed Tomography

A Computed Tomography (CT) scan of KL's temporal bones confirmed the presence of the mass and revealed that it extended into the cerebellopontine angle (CPA), internal auditory canal, and tympanic cavity. The CT also documented tumor encasement of the oval window, stapes, long process and lenticular process of the incus, and handle of the malleus.

32.6 Treatment

KL was provided three management options: observation, surgery, and radiation. Given the size and invasive nature of the tumor, the neurotologist recommended surgical removal. Ultimately, KL opted for surgical removal of the tumor via a transotic approach with left ear canal overclosure and packing of the left eustachian tube orifice. The transotic surgical approach, which can be used in cases of CPA tumors when there is no serviceable hearing, has been shown to be superior to other options, including the translabyrinthine approach, at preserving facial nerve function.[1]

32.7 Additional Questions to the Reader

1. **In light of the CT scans how would a clinician interpret the hearing loss and ART findings?**
2. **What are the implications of the ice-water caloric findings for KL's presurgical counseling?**

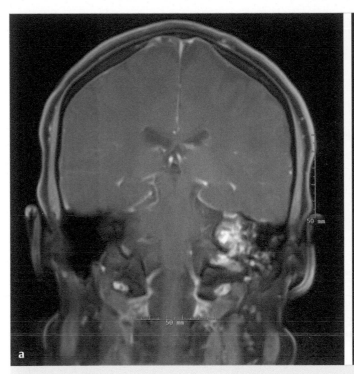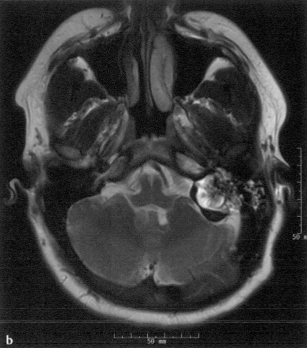

Fig. 32.3 KL's MRI findings, with **(a)** coronal and **(b)** axial views of the enhancing mass.

32.8 Discussion of Additional Questions

1. **In light of the CT scans how would a clinician interpret the hearing loss and ART findings?**

Recall that KL presented with a profound, presumably sensorineural loss in the left ear and ARTs were measured at normal sensation levels in the ipsilateral right test condition only. At the time of audiometric testing, these results were interpreted as inconsistent because measurable ARTs would have been expected to be present in the ipsilateral and contralateral right test conditions in the presence of a profound sensorineural loss in the left ear. The subsequent CT scan, however, revealed that KL's tumor extended into the left middle ear space and encased all three ossicles to a varying extent. Given this, it is probable that the left ear hearing loss is probably mixed, but the conductive component could not be "captured" on the audiogram due to the output limits of the bone oscillator. ART findings were consistent with the stimulus left ear responses being absent due to middle ear involvement and the severity of the hearing loss. The right ART contralateral response was absent due to the ossicular chain and oval window encasement, which would alter the ability to measure the change in static admittance in the left (probe) ear.

2. **What are the implications of the ice-water caloric findings for KL's presurgical counseling?**

Ice-water caloric test findings established the presence of residual high-frequency vestibular function in KL's left ear. The planned surgical intervention will eliminate all peripheral function on that side. Given this, KL is likely to experience postsurgical dizziness and/or vertigo as the loss of left-ear end organ activity will create an asymmetry in peripheral vestibular function. KL should be counseled on this likelihood as well as on the need for vestibular therapy after surgery to facilitate central compensation for the peripheral vestibular loss.

32.9 Diagnosis

As noted earlier, the large red mass behind KL's left tympanic membrane prompted the neurotologist's initial working diagnosis of a glomus tympanicum. Diagnostic imaging results, however, were strongly suggestive of an endolymphatic sac tumor (ELST). Postsurgical histopathologic evaluation of the tumor confirmed the ELST diagnosis.

ELSTs are rare, slow-growing tumors that originate from the tissues of the endolymphatic sac and duct. These epithelial neoplasms are benign and do not metastasize, but are very destructive and can erode the bone and surrounding tissues.[2,3] Symptoms of ELST include progressive hearing loss and tinnitus. As the tumor enlarges, symptoms may include aural fullness, vertigo, and facial paresis.[2,3,4] Onset of all symptoms is typically slow and reflects tumor growth. Note that this is consistent with KL's experience.

Imaging and operative findings suggest that the likely origin of ELSTs is epithelial tissues in the area of the distal endolymphatic duct and proximal endolymphatic sac which lies within the dura of the posterior cranial fossa.[4,5,6] Given the location of the endolyphatic sac, erosion of bony structures in the petrous portion of the temporal bone and posterior cranial fossa is common.[2,3,4] The growth and progression pattern of ELSTs from this originating location varies considerably from patient to patient. Researchers have documented tumor extension from the posterior cranial fossa into the CPA; progression into the tympanic cavity and external auditory canal; and involvement of the middle cranial fossa, cavernous sinus, and sigmoid sinus.[2,3] ELSTs are often highly vascularized and macroscopically appear red or brown.[2,5] As seen with KL, an ELST may invade the tympanic cavity and can be visualized via otoscopy as a red mass behind the eardrum, similar to a glomus tympanicum.[6]

ELSTs can occur spontaneously but are more prevalent in individuals with von Hippel–Lindau (VHL) Syndrome, an inherited, autosomal-dominant condition characterized by the development of cysts and benign and cancerous tumors throughout the body.[5,6,7] The incidence of ELSTs in the general adult population is estimated at 1:30,000, and tumor occurrence in this group is typically unilateral.[7] In contrast, approximately 10 to 16% of those with VHL will develop an ELST, and of those, it is estimated that 30% will develop bilateral tumors.[7] Although genetic testing has not been performed, KL's tumor is presumed to be spontaneous in origin given that it is unilateral and no additional tumors or cysts have been identified in diagnostic imaging.

The destructive nature of ELSTs necessitates surgical resection, regardless of size, in the majority of cases. Surgical approach will vary depending on the size of the tumor, which structures are involved, and on the presence or absence of residual auditory function.[2,6] Special consideration for hearing preservation is made in the VHL population given the propensity to develop ELSTs bilaterally.[2,7] In patients for whom surgery is not considered a viable option—for example, due to extensive cranial nerve involvement—and in instances of subtotal resection, radiation therapy may be recommended.[2,3] All patients who have had an ELST will require diagnostic imaging to monitor recurrence.[3]

32.10 Outcome and Rehabilitation

KL's surgical intervention was successful in removing more than 90% of his ELST. Subtotal resection was required due to the proximity of the tumor to KL's sigmoid sinus. Intraoperative monitoring indicated preservation of function of the left facial nerve. As anticipated, KL reported postsurgical dizziness and postural unsteadiness. These symptoms are currently being addressed through vestibular therapy, which has focused on functional balance, safety, and exercises designed to facilitate central vestibular compensation through stimulation of the vestibulo–ocular reflex. Over time, it is expected that KL's dizziness will resolve. KL has not yet returned to Audiology for postsurgical evaluation and counseling. Rehabilitative options for his unilateral hearing loss include a left osseointegrated hearing device or a Contralateral Routing Of the Signal (CROS) hearing

system. Both of these options would utilize the normal hearing in KL's right ear to provide him with access to sounds being presented to his left side. Note that neither of these options, however, would resolve his difficulties with sound localization. A cochlear implant, which could offer some improvement in localization, is not an option because the transotic surgical approach involves removal of the cochlea, and thus KL would not be a candidate.

32.11 Key Points

- Standard caloric stimuli approximate a very low-frequency head rotation and only evaluates a small portion of the functional frequency range of the peripheral vestibular system. Ice-water calorics, vHIT, and rotational chair can be used to assess higher-frequency vestibular function.
- Moving a patient from the standard caloric test position to sitting with the head tilted downward at a 30-degree angle will reverse a true caloric response due to repositioning of the crista ampullaris relative to the caloric-induced endolymph flow.
- ELSTs are rare, benign tumors that are locally destructive and can invade and erode structures in the posterior and middle cranial fossa, tympanic cavity, and external auditory canal.
- ELSTs are more common in individuals with VHL syndrome and are more likely to occur bilaterally in this population.
- In the majority of cases, treatment for ELSTs involves surgical resection with radiation therapy to follow in cases of subtotal resection.

References

[1] Xia Y, Zhang W, Li Y, Ma X, Liu Q, Shi J. The transotic approach for vestibular schwannoma: indications and results. Eur Arch Otorhinolaryngol. 2017; 274 (8):3041–3047

[2] Mendenhall WM, Suárez C, Skálová A, et al. Current treatment of endolymphatic sac tumor of the temporal bone. Adv Ther. 2018; 35:887–898

[3] Folker RJ, Meyerhoff WL, Rushing EJ. Aggressive papillary adenoma of the cerebellopontine angle: case report of an endolymphatic sac tumor. Am J Otolaryngol. 1997; 18(2):135–139

[4] Lonser RR, Baggenstos M, Kim HJ, Butman JA, Vortmeyer AO. The vestibular aqueduct: site of origin of endolymphatic sac tumors. J Neurosurg. 2008; 108 (4):751–756

[5] Corrales CE, Mudry A. History of the endolymphatic sac: from anatomy to surgery. Otol Neurotol. 2017; 38(1):152–156

[6] Diaz RC, Amjad EH, Sargent EW, Larouere MJ, Shaia WT. Tumors and pseudotumors of the endolymphatic sac. Skull Base. 2007; 17(6):379–393

[7] Ferri E, Amadori M, Armato E, Pavon I. A rare case of endolymphatic sac tumour: clinicopathologic study and surgical management. Case Rep Otolaryngol. 2014; 2014:376761

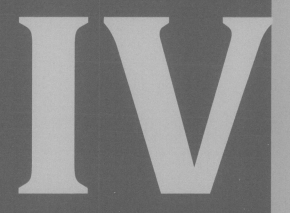

Part IV

Amplification—Hearing Devices

IV

33 Transcranial Contralateral Routing of Signal for Single-Sided Deafness

Lori Rakita

33.1 Clinical History and Description

CR is a 40-year-old female who reported removal of an acoustic neuroma in the left ear 3 years ago. Since surgery, CR has normal hearing in the right ear and a profound hearing loss in the left ear. She denies tinnitus, noise exposure, and a family history of hearing loss. Currently, CR reports fatigue from trying to understand speech, particularly in noisy situations, and expresses difficulty with localizing sound sources. She has not seen an audiologist since her postoperative evaluation following the removal of the acoustic neuroma. She is interested in receiving a current audiologic evaluation and discussing possible amplification options.

33.2 Audiological Testing

A comprehensive audiometric evaluation was completed. The comprehensive audiometric examination (▶ Fig. 33.1) revealed a unilateral hearing loss with normal hearing in the right ear and a profound sensorineural hearing loss in the left ear. The Speech Recognition Threshold (SRT) was 15 dB hearing level (HL) for the right ear and a 95 dB HL Speech Awareness Threshold (SAT) for the left ear. These results are in good agreement with pure-tone average (PTA) and indicate normal ability to receive speech in the right ear and a profound loss in the left ear. Word Recognition Scores (WRS) were obtained using recorded CD with a male talker at a 50 dB HL presentation level for the right ear. A full list of NU-6 (Northwestern University Auditory Test Number 6) words was presented and results revealed a WRS of 100% for the right ear, indicating normal ability to recognize speech. Word recognition testing was not completed for the left ear. Immittance audiometry revealed normal middle ear pressure (daPa), static compliance (mL), and ear canal volume (mL), bilaterally. Ipsilateral Acoustic Reflex Thresholds (ARTs) were present at normal hearing thresholds for the right ear and present at normal hearing thresholds for the right contralateral condition. As expected, left ipsilateral and contralateral ARTs were absent. Acoustic reflex decay at 500 and 1,000 Hz for contralateral presentation was normal for the right ear and not measured for the left ear.

33.3 Recommended Treatment

The audiologist recommended a right Contralateral Routing of Signal (CROS) system.[1] CR, however, reported she pursued a trial with CROS at an earlier date and was not pleased with the sound quality. She felt the sound quality was very tinny and made speech understanding difficult. She also did not like wearing devices on both ears and felt it interfered with her better hearing right ear. CR asked if she could pursue a trial with a transcranial CROS hearing aid in her left poorer hearing ear.[2,3,4]

The audiologist recommended a left behind-the-ear (BTE) transcranial CROS to ensure sufficient power to stimulate the better hearing cochlea across the head.

33.4 Questions to the Reader

1. **What are the benefits and limitations of a CROS system and what would be important information to convey to a CROS user during counseling?**
2. **What are potential benefits and limitations of a transcranial fitting?**
3. **What are the important audiologic criteria to meet when considering transcranial fittings?**

33.5 Discussion of Questions

1. **What are the benefits and limitations of a CROS system and what would be important information to convey to a CROS user during counseling?**

A CROS system can be an appropriate recommendation for patients who have normal, or near normal, hearing in one ear and no hearing (or minimal hearing) in the other ear. Original research on CROS suggests that some degree of high-frequency hearing impairment may improve acceptance of the CROS.[1] CROS can eliminate the "head shadow effect" or the reduction of the intensity of sound to the opposite ear when sound approaches one side. CROS eliminates the head shadow effect with the use of a transmitter microphone on the poorer hearing ear, sending the signal wirelessly to a hearing aid with a receiver in the better hearing ear. In quiet, CROS can be very effective in transmitting "wanted" information from the poorer ear to the better ear and can be especially effective when noise is on the better hearing side and the signal of interest is on the poorer hearing side. However, in situations where noise is on the poor side (i.e., transmitting microphone side), this unwanted signal is forwarded and amplified to the better ear and can be detrimental for speech understanding in noise. This situation has improved in CROS hearing aids with the fairly recent introduction of automatic adaptive multichannel directional microphones on the transmitter and receiver devices. In addition, multichannel digital noise reduction is currently available on the receiver and transmitter sides that can act to help reduce the annoyance of noise. It is, however, important for CROS users to understand the challenges of the CROS (i.e., noise arriving at the transmitter side and mixing with the speech arriving on the better ear side).

2. **What are potential benefits and limitations of a transcranial fitting?**

The benefits of a transcranial fitting include the use of only one device instead of two, and improved good sound quality.[2] The drawbacks may include the following:

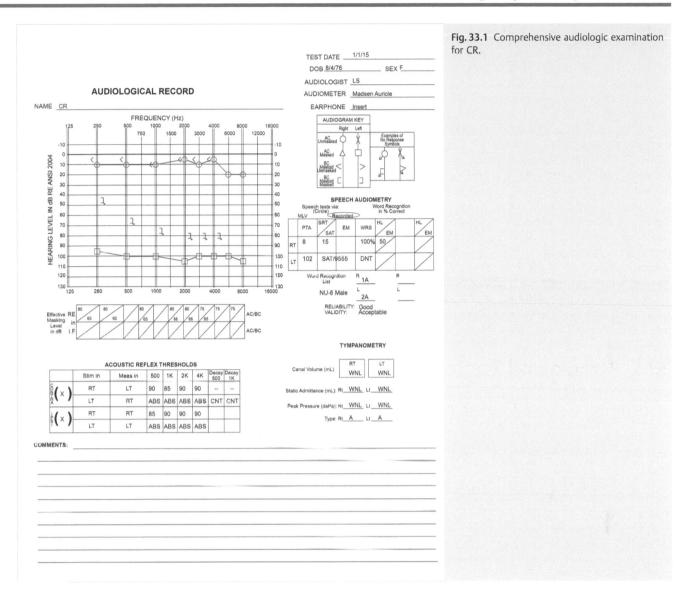

Fig. 33.1 Comprehensive audiologic examination for CR.

- **Comfort issues**. Owing to the nature of conducting sound via bone conduction in the bony portion of the ear canal, it is necessary for the hearing aid (completely-in-the-canal [CIC] fitting) or earmold (BTE fitting) to fit deeply and tightly in the ear canal of the poorer ear. This could lead to pain or discomfort in the ear canal of the poorer ear and result in the inability of the patient to adjust to this type of fitting.

- **Retention**. This fitting sends acoustical and mechanical vibrations through the bony portion of the ear canal of the poorer ear. Due to the required tight fit for the effective transmission of sound to the opposite inner ear with no feedback, retention is extremely important. This involves a well-made deeply seated earmold to provide excellent retention. This also involves increased maintenance to ensure that the hearing aid continues to provide a good fit over time.[2] This may include appointments with the audiologist to ensure there are no sores in the ear caused by the deeply seated device, and asking the patient if he or she is experiencing feedback due to an improper fit.

- **Feedback**. Issues related to feedback are another potential limitation of the transcranial CROS since high output levels (i.e., > 130 dB SPL for most patients) are needed to reach the cochlea of the better ear across the head. A pressure vent is recommended to reduce the possibility of leakage and feedback. With minimal venting, occlusion may be reported by the patient. This can be minimized with a deep insertion of the hearing aid or earmold into the bony portion of the ear canal.

- **Power limitations**. Owing to the small size of the receiver in a CIC device, power may be limited. Since high output levels are needed to reach the cochlea of the better ear, sufficient power may not be achievable. For this reason, bone conduction thresholds on the better hearing ear need to be as close to 0 dB HL as possible. A transcranial fitting of a BTE hearing aid would allow for greater amplification and could be used with bone conduction thresholds no poorer than 20 to 25 dB HL in the better hearing ear. It is essential that the audiologist be aware of the Tullio effect that may occur due to high output levels. The Tullio effect is when a patient experiences dizziness to loud sounds. If a patient reports dizziness when wearing a transcranial fit, then this approach no longer becomes a viable option.

3. What are the important audiologic criteria to meet when considering a transcranial fitting?

It is essential that bone conduction thresholds in the better hearing ear be as close to 0 dB HL through 2,000 Hz.[2,3,4] Also, interaural attenuation (IA) needs to be as low as possible. Both factors are important for the bone conduction signal to be heard by the cochlea of the better ear.

33.6 Additional Testing

Testing of unaided and aided transcranial thresholds using earphones can be valuable in verifying the potential success with a transcranial aid and assist in programming the hearing aid. Unaided crossover thresholds were measured by sending pure-tone signals via an insert earphone at 250 to 4,000 Hz to the left ear with a probe tube from a real ear analyzer in place.[4] These pure-tone signals were increased in signal level until it is heard

(i.e., heard by cochlea of the right ear). It is assumed that the crossover to the better hearing cochlea occurs at this presentation level in dB HL (audiometer dial) and dB sound pressure level (SPL; as measured by the real ear analyzer). These measures of transcranial thresholds directly reflect the patient's bone conduction threshold on the better hearing ear and IA of that patient.

To verify the transcranial fitting, real ear measures (REM) are used to verify that the real ear aided response (REAR in dB SPL) in the left ear to a speech-shaped signal presented at 50, 65 and 75 dB SPL exceeds the unaided transcranial threshold levels that was measured in dB SPL as described earlier.[4]

33.7 Diagnosis and Recommended Treatment

Based on research performed,[1] CR's unaided transcranial thresholds suggest (▶ Fig. 33.2) a high likelihood for success with a transcranial aid.[1] Measuring transcranial thresholds are essential for ensuring the fit of the hearing aid because REAR

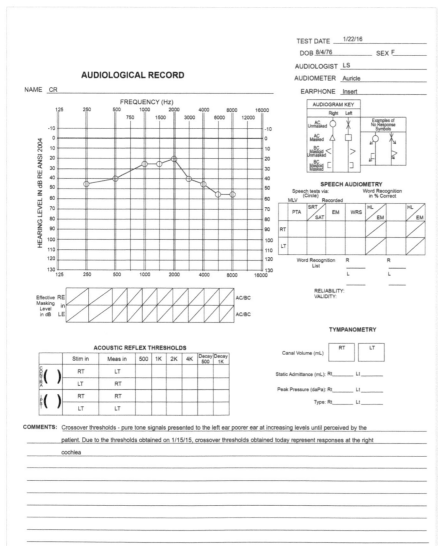

Fig. 33.2 Transcranial thresholds obtained by presenting pure-tone signals to the left ear at increasing levels until perceived by the right cochlea.

measures must exceed these levels to verify that the aided signal has crossover and is being heard by the right cochlea.[3] It was also essential that a deep ear impression was taken, that is, past the second bend to reach the bony portion of the ear canal. An open-mouth impression with a bite block ensured the earmold impression captured the important parts of the ear canal.

Finally, counseling is imperative, particularly in regard to noisy situations where noise is arriving from the side of the hearing aid. In this case, the presence of the hearing aid could be detrimental to speech understanding. An option for a "mute" button on the hearing aid and counseling of this program could be an option for situations in which noise is directed toward the poorer (aided) ear.

33.8 Outcome

CR was extremely pleased with the left transcranial hearing aid. She prefers this fitting to the right CROS system she previously tried and finds her speech understanding to be improved using the left transcranial CROS.

33.9 Key Points

- Counseling is an integral component of any hearing aid fitting, particularly in regard to situations where the user may find difficulty.

- A deep earmold impression, past the second bend, is essential for a successful transcranial fit.
- There is no "one size fits all" when interacting with patients that appear to have a predictable outcome (i.e., CROS is not the only option for single-sided deafness). It is essential to remember a variety of fitting approaches to determine which approach may provide the best outcome for an individual patient.

References

[1] Harford E, Dodds E. The clinical application of CROS. A hearing aid for unilateral deafness. Arch Otolaryngol. 1966; 83(5):455–464

[2] Hayes DE, Chen JM. Bone-conduction amplification with completely-in-the-canal hearing aids. J Am Acad Audiol. 1998; 9(1):59–66

[3] Hayes D. You want to put that CIC where?? A primer on CROS fittings using CICs. Audiology Online, 2001; Article 1572. www.audiologyonline.com/articles/article_detail.asp?article_id=1572. Accessed October 24, 2016

[4] Valente M, Oeding K. Transcranial contralateral routing of the signal as a fitting option for patients with single-sided deafness. Semin Hear. 2010; 31(4): 366–377

Suggested Reading

[1] Valente M, Oeding K. Evaluation of a BICROs system with a directional microphone in the receiver and transmitter. J Am Acad Audiol. 2015; 26 (10):856–871

34 I Hear Worse When I Wear Two Hearing Aids

Lauren Harvey and Wayne Wilson

34.1 Clinical History and Description

An 82-year-old female experienced hearing aid user was referred by her audiologist for further diagnostic assessment 1 year after receiving her third pair of bilateral behind-the-ear (BTE) hearing aids. JD had reported dissatisfaction with her hearing aids when listening in noisy environments.

JD is an 82-year-old woman returning to her audiologist 1 year after being fitted with bilateral BTE receiver-in-the-canal hearing aids with advanced signal processing technology and custom-made silicone earmolds. While JD remains a motivated hearing aid user, she reports increasingly limited benefit when wearing both of her hearing aids in noisy environments. The increasing stress and exhaustion from listening in noise is causing JD to withdraw from some social gatherings and events.

The audiologist had fitted JD's hearing aids to real ear insertion gain (REIG) targets (with correction for binaural summation) set by the National Acoustic Laboratories non-linear version 2 formula (NAL-NL2: NAL's prescriptive procedure for fitting non-linear hearing aids, version 2) real ear insertion gain (REIG) targets (with correction for binaural summation) before guiding JD through a 12-week trial period. The trial included several visits by the audiologist to JD's home in a retirement village where she worked with JD to manage the hearing aids and to communicate with family and friends during live social gatherings and events. The trial also included the use of a remote microphone coupled wirelessly to JD's hearing aids via a streamer and telecoil neck loop.

JD is an experienced hearing aid user having self-referred to her audiologist 8 years earlier for an audiologic examination and her first hearing aid trial. JD went on to wear two sets of bilateral BTE hearing aids to the end of their serviceable lifetimes, reporting moderate benefit from each set. While reporting benefit from previous trials of remote microphone technology, JD has always rejected this technology mostly on the grounds of cosmetics and a preference for fewer rather than more devices to assist her hearing. JD has no history of tinnitus, vertigo, noise exposure, or hearing loss in the family, and no significant medical history other than occasionally taking over-the-counter medication for headaches.

34.2 Audiologic Testing

▶ Fig. 34.1 reports the results of JD's audiologic examination performed by her audiologist on JD's return to the audiology clinic 1 year after receiving her most recent bilateral BTE hearing aids and communication training. No significant change was noted in JD's audiologic results over that 1-year period.

Pure-tone testing revealed bilateral symmetrical mild to moderately severe sensorineural hearing loss (SNHL) that is gradually falling in configuration. Speech audiometry testing showed JD's Speech Recognition Thresholds (SRT) and Word Recognition Scores (WRS) were consistent with the audiometric configuration bilaterally. JD's WRS improved with increased presentation level to a maximum of 100% bilaterally at an 80 dB

hearing level (HL) presentation level. No significant rollover was observed bilaterally at a 90 dB HL presentation level. The audiologist interpreted the lack of rollover as a negative finding for retrocochlear lesion (eighth cranial nerve and/or brainstem) although the poorer sensitivity of rollover to these lesions was noted. As the speech audiometry testing was completed in Australia, JD's WRS were obtained using the National Acoustics Laboratories Arthur Boothroyd (NAL AB) word lists and its recommended protocol.[1] The NAL AB word lists contain 15 lists of 10 monosyllabic words. The patient's response to each word is scored phonemically (giving 30 score-able items [phonemes] per list) such that correctly repeating 3, 2, 1, or 0 phonemes in each word elicits a score of 10, 7, 3, or 0% for that word, respectively. A performance-intensity (PI) function is obtained for each ear by presenting the first word list at the expected half-maximum level (HML: the level at which the patient is predicted to score 50%) and subsequent lists at levels 15 dB higher than the previous list until a maximum score is reached. If not already found for the first word list, a score is also obtained at a signal level 15 dB below HML. Speech noise masking is applied to the non–test ear according to the following formula: masking level in non–test ear = presentation level in test ear − 40 dB + air-bone gap in non–test ear + audiometer conversion factor (note: the audiometer conversion was clinically calibrated by placing speech and masking noise into the same headphone and determining the masker-to-signal ratio at which masking noise completely masks out a given intensity level of speech. It was determined to be 12 dB for the NAL AB word lists on the commercially available audiometers used, which was rounded to 10 dB for clinical application).[1] Once the PI functions are plotted, the SRT is estimated by extrapolating the presentation level required to reach the 50% score on the PI function.

On immittance testing, JD's results revealed ear canal volume, middle ear pressure, and static compliance to be within normal limits bilaterally. The audiologist used these results to rule out middle ear lesions that typically have a greater effect on tympanometry (such as middle ear effusion or Eustachian tube dysfunction), but not to rule out middle ear lesions that typically have lesser effects on tympanometry (such as early stage ossicular fixation or tympanosclerosis).

On Acoustic Reflex Threshold (ART) testing, JD's ARTs were absent to ipsilateral and contralateral stimuli using a maximum stimulus level of 100 dB HL. On analyzing JD's ART results, the audiologist considered four generalizations regarding ARTs to 500-, 1,000-, and 2,000-Hz stimuli in adults:

- The ART should occur at stimulus levels 70 to 100 dB above the person's hearing threshold at each frequency (i.e., at 70–100 dB sensation level [SL]).
- The ART typically cannot be elicited when recording the ART from an ear with a middle ear lesion (even if this lesion is not detected by pure-tone testing or tympanometry).
- The ART can be elicited at stimulus levels less than 70 dB SL when stimulating an ear that has cochlear recruitment.
- The ART is typically elicited at stimulus levels greater than 100 dB SL, or cannot be elicited at all, when stimulating an ear that has a retrocochlear lesion.

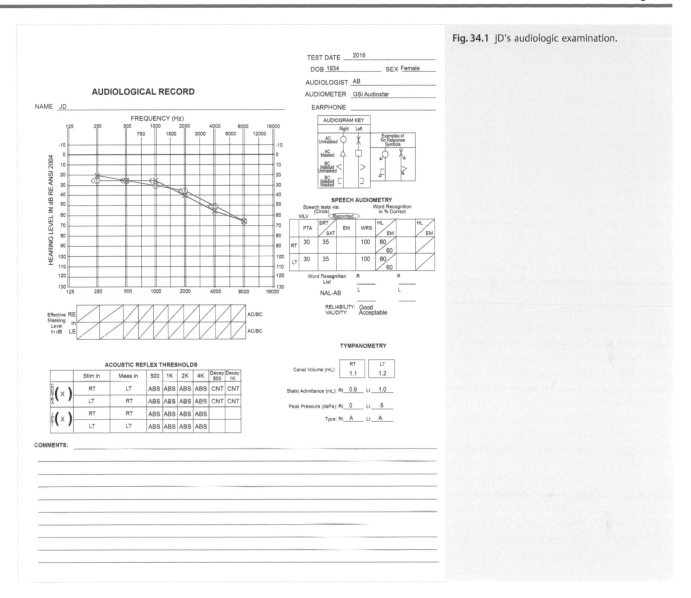

Fig. 34.1 JD's audiologic examination.

Using this approach, the audiologist was unable to isolate a specific site of lesion based on JD's ART results. JD's ART results could be explained by several possible sites of lesion. One possibility is bilateral mild middle ear dysfunction, which would cause all ARTs to be absent. A second possibility is bilateral cochlear sites of lesion without recruitment. As JD's best puretone threshold between 500 and 2,000 Hz is 25 dB HL, her best ARTs without recruitment would be expected at 70 to 100 dB SL. For JD, this equates to 95 to 125 dB HL, which is predominantly above the maximum stimulus level of 100 dB HL used by the audiologist. A third possibility is bilateral retrocochlear sites of lesion or a central (caudal brainstem) site of lesion. This could cause all ARTs to be present at greater than 100 dB SL, which for JD equates to greater than 125 dB HL, or all ARTs to be absent. Other possibilities include combinations of the above three possibilities.

After completing the testing described above, JD's audiologist assessed JD's hearing aids in a hearing aid analyzer. This assessment revealed JD's hearing aids were meeting the manufacturer's specifications for reference test gain (the amount of gain with a 50 dB sound pressure level (SPL) input and the volume control at normal position), full-on gain (FOG; the gain when the volume control is adjusted to maximum rotation), total harmonic distortion (THD [in %]: a measure of the total harmonics generated by the hearing aid when amplifying a standard reference input), and output sound pressure level 90 (OSPL90: the output saturation sound pressure level [SSPL] to a 90 dB SPL input measured over a frequency range, also called the saturation sound pressure level [SSPL]).

Finally, JD's audiologist also re-assessed JD's REIG results and revealed these results still met NAL-NL2 REIG targets and performed a listening check on JD's remote microphone device to confirm it was working properly.

34.3 Questions to the Reader

1. **Considering JD's reports regarding the performance of her hearing aids and the resulting assessments conducted by JD's audiologist to investigate these reports, what should JD's audiologist do next?**

34.4 Discussion of Questions

1. **Considering JD's reports regarding the performance of her hearing aids and the resulting assessments conducted by JD's audiologist to investigate these reports, what should JD's audiologist do next?**

An audiological reason for JD's increasingly limited benefit when wearing her hearing aids in noisy environments is not immediately obvious. JD is an experienced hearing aid user who has been using her current binaural BTE hearing aids for 1 year after a successful trial that included communication training in her home environment. No significant change was noted on JD's audiologic re-assessment and JD's hearing aids were shown to be working properly and meeting NAL-NL2 REIG targets. While JD reported some benefit when using her remote microphone, JD rejected this technology (as she had done in previous trials) on the grounds of cosmetics and a preference for fewer rather than more devices to assist her hearing.

The absence of an obvious audiological reason for JD's increasingly limited benefit when wearing her hearing aids in noisy environments led the audiologist to consider two other possibilities: (central) auditory processing ([C]AP) deficits and cognitive decline. To consider these reasons in more detail, the audiologist asked JD to elaborate on why she reported increasingly limited benefit when wearing both hearing aids in noisy environments. JD reported that when listening in a room with multiple speakers she felt the words of the speakers were becoming more and more "jumbled." This made it difficult for JD to follow the primary speaker. JD reported that while she used the communication strategies she had been taught during the hearing aid trial, these strategies only helped on some occasions. Interestingly, JD also reported that on some occasions, a more successful strategy was to remove her right hearing aid and only use her left hearing aid when listening in noisy situations. This sometimes helped JD to "unjumble" the words from the different talkers. JD's report of removing one hearing aid to improve her ability to listen in noise led the audiologist to decide to further investigate JD's (C)AP status prior to her cognitive status. To further investigate JD's (C)AP status, the audiologist referred JD to the Audiology Clinic at a nearby university for a comprehensive (C)AP assessment.

34.5 Additional Audiologic Testing

On arriving at the Audiology Clinic, JD's initial audiologic examination (conducted pure-tone testing only) revealed no significant change in hearing status. JD was then assessed using a behavioral (C)AP test battery based on the recommendations of the American Speech-Language-Hearing Association[2] and screened using a test of short-term and working memory. This assessment was conducted in the knowledge that some of the test results would be confounded by JD's SNHL. The (C)AP test battery included the competing sentences test, the two-pair dichotic digits (TPDD) test, the low-pass filtered speech (LPFS) test, and the frequency patterns (FP) test with a total test time of approximately 30 minutes (including rest breaks).

34.5.1 Competing Sentences (CS)

For each ear separately, JD was asked to repeat three blocks of 10 sentences presented at 80 dB HL (50 dB SL re: pure-tone average [PTA]) to the test ear while ignoring 10 equivalent competing sentences presented simultaneously at 80 dB HL (50 dB SL re: PTA, Block 1), 75 dB HL (45 dB SL re: PTA, Block 2), and 70 dB HL (40 dB SL re: PTA, Block 3) to the non–test ear. This sequence created three signal-to-noise ratios (SNR) for each ear: 0, +5, and +10 dB. The sentences were from the Auditec of St Louis (St Louis, MO) recordings of the Competing Sentences (CS) test that were six to seven words in length and had been recorded from a male talker.

34.5.2 Two-Pair Dichotic Digits (TPDD)

For both ears simultaneously, JD was asked to repeat 20 sets of four digits. Each set of four digits was presented sequentially as two digit pairs with one digit in each pair presented at 80 dB HL (50 dB SL re: PTA) to the right ear, while the other digit in that pair was simultaneously presented at 80 dB HL (50 dB SL re: PTA) to the left ear. The digits were from the U.S. Department of Veterans Affairs recording of the Two-pair Dichotic Digits (TPDD) test that included the numbers 1 through 10 (except 7) and had been recorded using a male talker.[3,4]

34.5.3 Low-Pass Filtered Speech (LPFS)

For each ear separately, JD was asked to repeat 25 monosyllabic words from equivalent word lists presented at 80 dB HL (50 dB SL re: PTA) to the test ear. The words were from the Auditec of St Louis recording of the Northwestern University Auditory Test No. 6 (NU-6) word lists 1C and 2C and had been recorded using a male talker.[5] These words had been low-pass filtered using a 1,000-Hz cutoff frequency.

34.5.4 Frequency Patterns (FP)

For each ear separately, JD was asked to describe in words (linguistic report) the FP contained in 25 sets of three tones presented monotonically at 80 dB HL (50 dB SL re: PTA). The FP were from the U.S. Department of Veterans Affairs recording of FP with each tone in each set of three tones being either 880 or 1,122 Hz.[3]

34.5.5 Memory

The tests of short-term and working memory were four subtests from the *Test of Auditory Processing Skills – Version 3* with a total test time of approximately 10 minutes.[6] The first subtest was auditory number memory forward (ANMF), which tested JD's ability to repeat increasing series of numbers in the order the numbers were spoken. The second subtest was auditory number memory backward (ANMB), which tested JD's ability to repeat increasing series of numbers in the reverse order the numbers were spoken. The third subtest was auditory word memory (AWM), which tested JD's ability to repeat increasing series of unrelated words not necessarily in the order they were spoken. The final subtest was auditory sentence memory (ASM), which tested JD's ability to repeat increasing length sentences exactly as they were spoken. The audiologist used monitored live voice to present these stimuli at a comfortable listening level.

34.6 Additional Question to the Reader

1. **What do the additional audiologic tests inform the audiologist about JD's hearing loss?**

34.7 Discussion of Additional Questions

1. **What do the additional audiologic tests inform the audiologist about JD's hearing loss?**

While JD's (C)AP test results were interpreted cautiously because of her SNHL, the results revealed the following main findings (▶ Table 34.1, column headed "Score [%] at baseline [pre-ARIA (auditory rehabilitation for interaural asymmetry) training]"). First, the CS test results showed JD found it almost impossible to repeat sentences presented to her right ear while ignoring equivalent competing sentences presented simultaneously to her left ear at all three SNR (0, +5, and +10 dB). In stark contrast, JD found it very easy to repeat sentences presented to the left ear while ignoring equivalent competing sentences presented simultaneously to the right ear at all three SNR (0, +5, and +10 dB). Second, the TPDD test results did not show the same significant difference between ears on this dichotic listening task. Instead, JD was generally able to repeat different digits played to each ear simultaneously. Third, the LPFS test results

showed JD found it difficult to repeat words played at an audible level when those words had been filtered to sound like the speaker was mumbling. Fourth, the FP test results showed JD was able to correctly describe auditory patterns. Finally, the tests of short-term and working memory showed JD had sufficient ability in these skill areas to complete the (C)AP testing.

From a functional perspective, these results provide some support for JD's reports of increased difficulty hearing in noisy listening environments and her strategy of occasionally removing the right hearing aid and using only the left hearing aid to listen better in noisy situations. From a (C)AP perspective, the strongest finding was the very asymmetrical performance in the competing CS test results (showing a much poorer performance on the signals sent to the left ear) despite JD's symmetrical SNHL. Interestingly, a much smaller asymmetrical performance was noted in the TPDD test results. While speculative, a possible reason for this smaller asymmetry could be related to the lower linguistic load of the digit stimuli in the TPDD test compared to the sentence stimuli in the CS test.

Asymmetrical performance between ears on dichotic testing has previously been reported in cases of unsuccessful binaural hearing aid fitting.[7,8,9] More recently, such asymmetries have been described as *amblyaudia*.[10]

Amblyaudia is a type of (C)APD characterized by deficits in the binaural integration of verbal information.[10] It is diagnosed by results from dichotic listening tests with the hallmark pattern being an abnormally large asymmetry between the ears. This suggests the presence of a "dominant ear." In JD's case, the processing of sentences presented to JD's left ear appeared to dominate the processing of equivalent sentences presented to her right ear on the CS test. This asymmetry was not observed on the presentation of the less complex and less linguistically loaded digit stimuli of the TPDD test. The underlying mechanisms of amblyaudia are unknown. Comparisons have been made to amblyopia, or "lazy eye," in the visual system where information from the dominant eye suppresses information from the nondominant eye.

34.8 Additional Questions to the Reader

1. **With amblyaudia being the dominant finding from the additional audiologic tests, what should the audiologist do next?**

34.9 Discussion of Additional Questions

1. **With amblyaudia being the dominant finding from the additional audiologic tests what should the audiologist do next?**

To address the amblyaudia, JD's audiologist suggested JD complete Auditory Rehabilitaion for Interaural Asymmetry (ARIA) training.[11] JD agreed and went on to complete four 1-hour sessions of ARIA training in the aided condition over a 3-week period. This training consisted of dichotic listening exercises in free field with digit, word, or sentence stimuli. These stimuli were played at a fixed level (80 dB HL) from the right loudspeaker (closer to JD's

Table 34.1 JD's (C)AP test scores at baseline (pre-ARIA training) and post-ARIA training

Test	Ear	SNR (dB)	Score (%) at baseline (pre-ARIA training)	Score (%) post-ARIA training
Competing sentences	R	0	*5*	*30*
	L	0	95	95
	R	+5	*5*	*70*
	L	+5	95	90
	R	+10	*0*	*90*
	L	+10	90	90
Two-pair dichotic digits	R		82.5	95
	L		100	98
Low-pass filtered speech	R		48	36
	L		44	56
Frequency patterns	R		80	86
	L		86	80

Note: Numbers in bold italics show the test scores that underwent the largest change pre- to post-ARIA training.

nondominant right ear) and at lower but adaptive levels from the left loudspeaker (closer to JD's dominant left ear) so that JD was always able to correctly repeat the stimuli from the right loudspeaker with approximately 80% accuracy. During each 60-minute training session, JD completed these exercises for the first 20 minutes, rested for the second 20 minutes, and completed more exercises for the last 20 minutes.

In the first of the four 1-hour sessions of ARIA training, JD was only able to accurately repeat the stimuli played on the side of her nondominant right ear at 80 dB HL when stimuli were played on the side of her dominant left ear at 40 to 50 dB HL. At the end of this first session of ARIA training, JD reported she was "exhausted" by the level of effort needed to listen for the target stimuli. JD's performance improved only slightly during the second session but improved dramatically in the third session of the ARIA training. By the end of the fourth session of ARIA training, JD was able to accurately repeat the stimuli played on the side of her nondominant right ear at 80 dB HL when the stimuli played on the side of her dominant left ear were from 70 to 80 dB HL. Furthermore, JD was able to do this without the levels of exhaustion experienced during the earlier ARIA training sessions.

34.10 Outcome

After the ARIA training, the audiologist reassessed JD using the same behavioral (C)AP test battery used to assess JD prior to the ARIA training. ▶ Table 34.1 shows JD's pre-ARIA and post-ARIA (C)APD test results. Post ARIA training, JD's CS test scores improved significantly for her nondominant right ear by 90% at + 10 SNR (right ear = 80 dB HL, left ear = 70 dB HL), 65% at + 5 SNR (right ear = 80 dB HL, left = 70 dB HL), and 25% at 0 SNR (right ear = 80 dB HL, left = 70 dB HL). This suggested the ARIA training significantly improved JD's dichotic processing skills for sentence stimuli. Post ARIA training, JD showed no significant changes for either ear on TPDD, LPFS, or FP testing. This was consistent with JD's already higher performances pre-ARIA training on the TPDD and FP tests. It also suggested the ARIA training did not affect the (C)AP skills required to complete the LPFS test.

After completing the ARIA training, JD's audiologist asked her to continue using her hearing aids and communication strategies in her home environment for 1 month. On returning to her audiologist, JD reported only mildly improved benefit when wearing both hearing aids in noisy environments. JD, however, also reported fewer occasions of taking one hearing aid out when listening in noisy situations and less stress and exhaustion from listening in noise. Unfortunately, JD also reported that she was still withdrawing from some social gatherings and events and continued to reject the option of using remote microphone technology to improve her listening in noise. As the next step, JD agreed to continue to work with her audiologist to manage her hearing aids and to monitor her amblyaudia. JD and her audiologist also agreed to investigate JD's cognitive status as another potential contributor to the increasingly limited benefit JD is receiving from her hearing aids. To do this, the audiologist referred JD to a psychologist for an initial cognitive assessment. The audiologist also sought to continue her efforts to finally convince JD of the benefits of remote microphone technology for listening in noise.

34.11 Summary

JD's audiologist identified amblyaudia as one possible reason for JD's increasingly limited benefit from her binaural hearing aids when listening in noisy environments. JD successfully completed the ARIA training program with her post-ARIA test scores showing evidence of greatly reduced amblyaudia. On returning to her audiologist 1 month after completing the ARIA training, JD reported mildly improved benefit when wearing both hearing aids in noisy environments and less stress and exhaustion from listening in noise, but continued withdrawal from some social gatherings and events. JD continues to work with her audiologist to manage her hearing aids and to monitor her amblyaudia, and JD has agreed to a cognitive assessment to further investigate the increasingly limited benefit she receives from her hearing aids.

34.12 Key Points

- While JD was an experienced hearing aid user, her reports of increasingly limited benefit when wearing both hearing aids in noisy environments contributed to a decision to conduct further audiologic assessments. These assessments led to a diagnosis of amblyaudia that may have otherwise gone undiagnosed.
- By having JD complete ARIA training, the audiologist was able to improve JD's dichotic listening abilities.
- JD reported only mild improvements post-ARIA training in the benefit she receives when wearing both hearing aids in noisy environments.
- JD and her audiologist continue to work together to further investigate the increasingly limited benefit JD receives from her hearing aids.

References

[1] Travers A. AB Word Lists: NAL Protocols. Sydney, Australia: National Acoustics Laboratories; 1990

[2] American Speech-Language-Hearing Association. (Central) auditory processing disorders. Available at: www.asha.org/policy/TR2005–00043.htm. Accessed December 22, 2016

[3] Wilson RH, Strouse A. Tonal and speech materials for auditory perceptual assessment, disc 2.0 [CD]. Mountain Home, TN: Department of Veterans Affairs; 1998

[4] Strouse A, Wilson RH. Stimulus length uncertainty with dichotic digit recognition. J Am Acad Audiol. 1999; 10(4):219–229

[5] Tillman TW, Carhart R. An expanded test for speech discrimination utilizing cnc monosyllabic words: Northwestern University Auditory Test No. 6. Technical Report no. SAM-TR-66–55. Brooks Air Force Base, TX: USAF School of Aerospace Medicine; 1966

[6] Martin N, Brownell R. Test of Auditory Processing Skills. 3rd ed. Novato, CA: Academic Therapy Publications; 2005

[7] Carter AS, Noe CM, Wilson RH. Listeners who prefer monaural to binaural hearing aids. J Am Acad Audiol. 2001; 12(5):261–272

[8] Chmiel R, Jerger J, Murphy E, Pirozzolo F, Tooley-Young C. Unsuccessful use of binaural amplification by an elderly person. J Am Acad Audiol. 1997; 8(1):1–10

[9] Jerger J, Silman S, Lew HL, Chmiel R. Case studies in binaural interference: converging evidence from behavioral and electrophysiologic measures. J Am Acad Audiol. 1993; 4(2):122–131

[10] Moncrieff D, Keith W, Abramson M, Swann A. Diagnosis of amblyaudia in children referred for auditory processing assessment. Int J Audiol. 2016; 55 (6):333–345

[11] Moncrieff DW, Wertz D. Auditory rehabilitation for interaural asymmetry: preliminary evidence of improved dichotic listening performance following intensive training. Int J Audiol. 2008; 47(2):84–97

35 You Need to Take Care of Your Front End!

Marshall Chasin

35.1 Clinical History and Description

MJ is a 70-year-old semiretired male rock musician. For some time he had been complaining of bilateral tinnitus and a gradual decrease in his ability to hear in noisier social environments. MJ has not reported any diplacusis or other pitch perception difficulties. He seems to be doing well when performing although he admits that he wishes the sound levels of his monitors were higher when he sings ballads. MJ had been seen twice for annual audiometric examinations at which time hearing aids were recommended. MJ now feels his problems in understanding speech in noise have increased and he is ready to try hearing aids.

MJ denied otalgia or vertigo. MJ's sound engineer always uses a sound level meter when setting up and testing the amplification equipment during rehearsal and performance. The reported sound levels typically ranged from 88 dBA to sustained periods in excess of 100 dBA. Other than his music, MJ reports no other sources of noise or music exposure.

35.2 Audiological Testing

▶ Fig. 35.1 reports the results of the most recent audiometric evaluation for MJ. Results revealed a bilateral symmetric slight to severe sensorineural hearing loss that is sharply falling in configuration beyond 500 Hz. This audiometric configuration is consistent with presbycusis and the impact of his exposure to music. Speech Recognition Thresholds (SRT) revealed a slight loss in the ability to receive speech in the right ear and a mild loss in the left ear. Word Recognition Scores (WRS) revealed normal ability bilaterally to recognize speech using full-list recorded versions of the NU-6 (Northwestern University Auditory Test Number 6) word list spoken by a male taker.

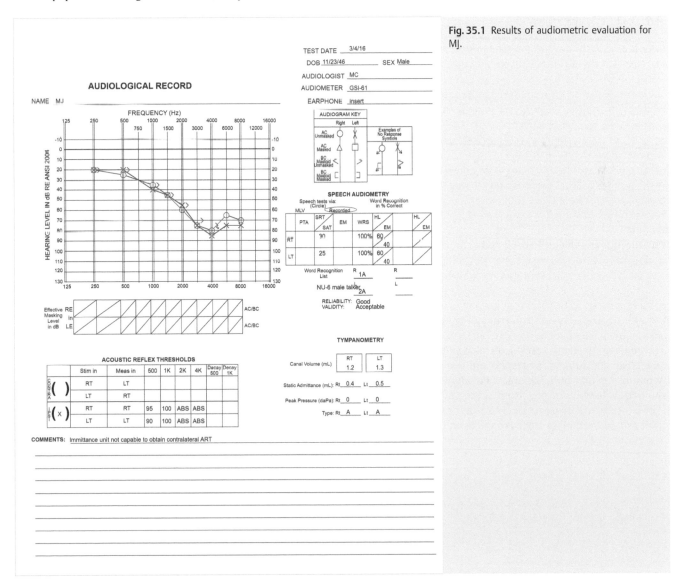

Fig. 35.1 Results of audiometric evaluation for MJ.

Tympanometry revealed normal middle ear function bilaterally and ipsilateral Acoustic Reflex Thresholds (ART) were consistent with MJ's audiometric thresholds. Contralateral ARTs could not be performed due to limitations of the equipment. Although not shown, Otoacoustic Emissions (OAE) revealed responses up to 1,000 Hz bilaterally with no responses above 1,000 Hz. This finding suggests relatively good outer hair cell function in the lower frequency region.

35.3 Hearing Aid Evaluation

After appropriate counseling, bilateral hearing aids were recommended for MJ. These nonoccluding receiver-in-the-canal (RIC) hearing aids had wireless capability and a large number of channels of signal processing. The custom RIC earmolds were ordered with a treble clef on the right earmold and a bass clef on the left earmold. Even before real ear measurements (REM) could be completed, however, while playing his tambourine, MJ removed the hearing aids and stated the hearing aids were "useless."

The clinician assured MJ that these hearing aids will probably match prescriptive real ear targets at 50 to 65 to 75 dB sound pressure level (SPL) providing significant benefit. MJ was encouraged to allow the clinician to proceed to measure the real ear gain of the hearing aids using REM.

Indeed, the measured real ear insertion gain (REIG) very closely matched the NAL-NL1 target bilaterally. MJ admitted that aided speech in the clinic sounded clearer and MJ felt his tinnitus had reduced slightly. Once again, however, MJs tambourine "informed" him of the poor sound quality of the hearing aids because the amplified sound of the tambourine sounded "distorted."

Assuming that MJs loudness discomfort levels (LDLs) had been exceeded, the clinician deduced that the output sound pressure level using a 90 dB SPL pure-tone sweep (OSPL90) of his hearing aids were programmed too high. After reducing the maximum output levels for his hearing aids, no improvement was reported and the tambourine was still considered to be of poor sound quality. MJ stated that the hearing aids were not excessively loud, but just sounded "fuzzy" and "distorted."

35.4 Questions to the Reader

1. **How is the spectrum (dB SPL) of speech different than the spectrum (dB SPL) of the tambourine?**
2. **Why wasn't MJ able to tolerate the amplified sound of his tambourine?**
3. **What other hardware or software changes could have been implemented to improve the sound quality of MJ's tambourine?**

35.5 Discussion of Questions

1. **How is the spectrum (dB SPL) of speech different than the spectrum (dB SPL) of the tambourine?**

The long-term speech spectrum has slight differences across languages, but most speech spectrums have most of its energy below 1,000 Hz with a 5 to 6 dB/octave roll-off above 500 Hz.

Table 35.1 Average and peak sound pressure levels (SPLs) of live music for the electric guitar, violin, and tambourine indicating peak input SPLs to a hearing aid in excess of 100 dB SPL. In contrast, peak speech SPL is typically less than 80 dB SPL.

Type of input to hearing aid	Average (RMS) dB SPL	Peak sound level (dB SPL)
Speech	65	77
Guitar	92	110
Violin	98	116
Tambourine	95	110

Abbreviation: RMS, root mean square.

The long-term average of speech is approximately 65 dB SPL at 1 m. In contrast, the tambourine has significant mid- and high-frequency sound energy with minimal sound energy below 500 Hz. This is not unlike the spectrum of a click stimulus for ABR (auditory brainstem response) that has broadband energy, but restricted to the higher frequency region. The other difference between the tambourine and speech is the peak input SPL. Whereas the peak SPL of conversational speech is approximately 80 dB SPL, the lowest SPL of the tambourine exceed 90 dB SPL with peak SPL approximately 110 dB SPL (see ▶ Table 35.1).

2. **Why wasn't MJ able to tolerate the amplified sound of his tambourine?**

Since reducing the OSPL90 did not improve the amplified sound quality of the tambourine or his acceptance of the amplified sound, this was not likely an issue related to the output of the hearing aids. With the higher input level to the hearing aids characteristic of the tambourine (and most other musical instruments), the input digitization of the amplified signal may be the cause of the problem. Specifically, the analog-to-digital (A/D) converter that all digital hearing aids have may have been overdriven. This is sometimes colloquially referred to as the "front-end" of the hearing aid. Most current A/D converters can only efficiently process input SPL around the mid-90 dB SPL range with many A/D converters only being able to manage significantly less than that. For speech, where the peak input SPL is approximately 80 dB SPL and therefore does not typically pose a problem. It can, however, become an issue with the higher peak input SPL of music. These higher peak input SPLs are above the optimal operating range of the A/D converter and no degree of software programming performed later can resolve this "front-end" problem.

Newer technologies have been introduced to more adequately address the higher peak input SPL. It needs to be stressed that these technologies are not beneficial only for musicians, but for anyone who enjoys listening to or plays music or listening to elevated speech levels in a noisy restaurant or bar (i.e., Lombard effect).

3. **What other hardware or software changes could have been implemented to improve the sound quality of MJ's tambourine?**

Once a high peak input SPL overdrives the A/D converter, there are no software changes that can be implemented to improve the sound quality. There can, however, be changes made to the hardware of the hearing aids. If the reader thinks of the A/D converter as a low-hanging bridge or doorway to the hearing aid, ducking under this bridge or increasing the height of the bridge could resolve this music sound quality issue. This may include using an assistive listening device with its own reduced volume control coupled to the hearing aids. Another option is reducing the sensitivity of the hearing aid microphones (i.e., "tricking" the A/D converter to "think" the peak input SPL is 10–12 dB SPL lower). Finally, there are a number of current hearing aid hardware technologies that increase or move the optimal operating range of the A/D converter to a region that is better suited to music to effectively process.

35.6 Current Hearing Aid Options for Improved Processing of Music

Since 2004 when this problem was initially identified,[1] the hearing aid industry has responded with four technologies designed to improve the sound quality of live music having higher peak input SPL. These advances would be beneficial to any patient who listens to or plays music (e.g., piano, violin, or singing) for self-enjoyment. These technologies can be explained by the bridge metaphor and relate to either ducking under the low-hanging bridge or increasing the height of the input digitization bridge. While the A/D converter, which digitizes the input signal, is always improving, there are a number of engineering design decisions typically based on issues related to power consumption and noise floor (i.e., internal noise generated by the components within the hearing aid) that limit the optimal operating range to input SPL below approximately 95 dB SPL. Some of the design decisions need to be made based on a broader set of engineering, cost, and marketing issues. Any input in excess of this *upper input limit* results in a distorted digitized signal. This becomes a hardware issue and cannot be corrected with clinical software programming changes.[2,3,4] Audio files are available that demonstrate this common phenomenon and can be found at www.chasin.ca/distorted_music.

35.7 Four Technical Innovations to Resolve the Front-End Problem

The hearing aid industry has responded with several innovative technologies to circumvent the "front-end" problem associated with the higher peak input SPL associated with listening and playing music as well as improve the sound quality of a hearing aid user's own voice (related to the close proximity of the hearing aid to the speaker's mouth). These technologies can be equally applied to nonmusicians who like to listen and perhaps play music or sing. Although some examples of hearing aid manufacturers that utilize a certain technology are mentioned, these approaches are constantly being redesigned and improved. The reader is encouraged to contact each hearing aid manufacturer to determine the current state of technology for improving aided sound quality of musicians.

There are four areas of technical innovation that are hardware based. These innovations can be implemented by software adjustments, but the hearing aid must have one or more of these technologies available:

- Less sensitive microphones can be used with hearing aids. Specifically, any hearing aid manufacturer can use a "–6 dB/octave" microphone. That is, one that is 6 dB less sensitive at 500 Hz and 12 dB less sensitive at 250 Hz. This has also been called a "low-cut microphone." With this technical innovation, the high-level, low-frequency components of the music (and a person's own voice, specifically the sonorants) would be reduced prior to the A/D converter in the front end. Depending on the magnitude and configuration of the hearing loss, there may be a requirement for low-frequency digital amplification to replace this low-frequency sound energy. Having a microphone that is less sensitive to low-frequency sounds occasionally mandates that this "missing" low-frequency sound energy needs to be replaced in the digital domain with gain that may exceed a prescriptive target. An example of a manufacturer using this approach is Unitron.

- A criticism of this approach is that the use of a "low-cut microphone" will increase the internal noise level in the hearing aid. This is true, but with expeditious use of expansion circuitry, the noise floor can be reduced to that of a wideband microphone that is typically used in the hearing aid industry. ▶ Fig. 35.2 reports this increase in noise level which is then reduced with expansion circuitry. With a "low-cut" microphone (i.e., less sensitive to low-frequency sounds), the internal noise level increases (upper violet curve), but with a judicious use of expansion, the noise level is reduced (black middle curve) to the level typically seen with broadband (red curve) microphones typically used in hearing aids.

- Increasing the typical input dynamic range that is typically from 0 to 95 dB to a dynamic range more suited to the acoustic features of music. Specifically, peak input SPL to 110 dB SPL can be transduced by such an A/D converter without appreciable distortion. The input dynamic range is typically stated in specification sheets without a suffix after the dB value. Like hearing aid gain, this is a difference measure between the quietest input SPL and the highest input SPL that can be digitized. With most 16-bit architecture found in hearing aids, the input dynamic range is typically 0 to 95 dB SPL (ranging from 0 to 95 dB SPL). While the upper limit of this range (95 dB SPL) is well suited for speech input, the upper range would fall short for most peak input SPL of music. The definition of "dynamic range" is, however, indeed only a range and not a set of absolute values. This "95 dB dynamic range" can also be from 15 to 111 dB SPL, a range that is more suited to the higher peak input SPL associated with music. Different manufacturers have accomplished this in different ways, but the effect is similar in that it raises the level of a low-hanging doorway or bridge. An example of a manufacturer that uses this approach is Bernafon.

- Yet another technical approach, albeit a throwback to the last generation of hearing aids, is using an analog compressor after the hearing aid microphone, but before the A/D converter. Then, digitally re-expand the amplified sound once digitized. This is analogous to ducking under a low-hanging doorway or bridge. An example of a manufacturer that uses this approach is ReSound.

- Recently, there have been a number of "post-16-bit architectures" that have entered the hearing aid marketplace.

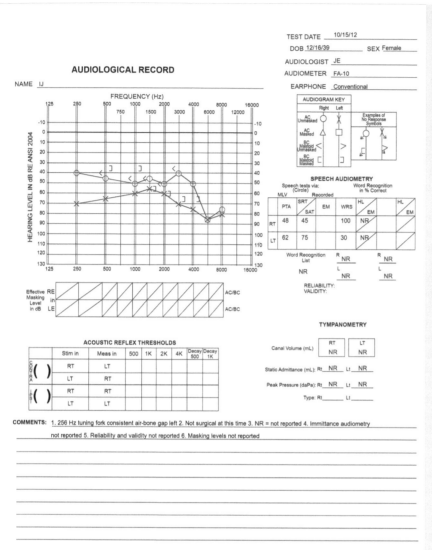

Fig. 36.1 Results for audiologic examination in 2012.

comprehensive audiologic evaluation was required to resolve the numerous discrepancies in the previous results.

IG agreed and the audiologist completed an audiologic examination including Olsen–Noffsinger tone decay test,[1] tympanograms, and contralateral and ipsilateral ART. Uncomfortable listening levels for pure tones were measured using the contour test instructions.[2] Results from the audiologic examination are reported in ▶ Fig. 36.3.

The audiologist did not feel there was a conductive component in the left ear although vibrotactile responses at 250 and 500 Hz suggest large air–bone gaps at those frequencies. IG was once again referred to a second large medical facility due to the asymmetry, dizziness/vertigo, tinnitus, and head pressure. The audiologist recommended a high-resolution contrast magnetic resonance imaging (MRI) with internal auditory canal (IAC) protocol (with and without Gadolinium contrast). The audiologist performed REM on IG's Costco hearing aids and found them to be well below an NAL-NL-2 target.[3] Finally, the audiologist measured bilateral aided Quick Speech in Noise (QUICKSIN) test[4] ability and found a signal-to-noise ratio hearing loss

(SNRHL) of 23.5 dB. This latter result indicated the patient's aided performance in noise was very poor.

36.3 Questions to the Reader

1. **At what point would an MRI with IAC protocol be appropriate in IG's management?**
2. **What factors might have contributed to the misdiagnosis of the mixed hearing loss in the left ear?**
3. **What battery of audiometric tests may have been more revealing for the correct diagnosis in the case of IG?**

36.4 Discussion of the Questions

1. **At what point would an MRI with IAC protocol be appropriate in IG's management?**

In cases of gradually progressive SNHL with one ear progressing more rapidly than the other, progressive diminution of vestibular

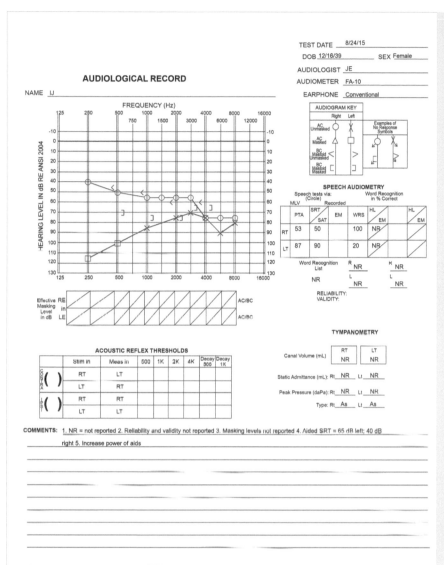

Fig. 36.2 Results for audiologic examination in 2015.

function, diplopia, ataxic gait, dysmetria, and nystagmus as reported by IG, an MRI with IAC protocol should be recommended to rule out the presence of a vestibular schwannoma (VS).[5] While the cost of an MRI is an appropriate consideration, it is the opinion of the author that it is better to err on the side of caution when these symptoms are presented. This is particularly true because the incidence of VS was 1.74% in postmortem examinations of patients with nonoperated VS.[6]

While there is considerable discussion as to what constitutes asymmetrical hearing loss, it has been recently noted[5] that the best criterion is the average difference in bone conduction thresholds at two to three high frequencies with 2,000 Hz being the most important.

2. What factors might have contributed to the misdiagnosis of the mixed hearing loss in the left ear?

Without recording of appropriate masking levels, it is conceivable that insufficient masking may have produced an artefactual air–bone gap on the left ear. Specifically, if there were insufficient masking into the right ear when testing the left ear bone conduction, it is possible the better right ear bone conduction thresholds are being tested. Thus, documenting the mask-ing levels used when measuring air and bone conduction thresholds, SRT, tone decay (when appropriate) and word recognition is highly recommended. Further, it is apparent that use of the Rinne test would not offer accurate information in a patient with a significant sensorineural asymmetry because the bone conduction threshold of the better ear could produce a positive Rinne on the poorer ear even if both ears had SNHL.

3. What battery of audiometric tests may have been more revealing for the correct diagnosis in the case of IG?

Clinicians[7] have reported that combining the contralateral ARTs, tone decay, and WRS with auditory brainstem response (ABR) can improve the prediction of identifying VS.

36.5 Additional Testing

36.5.1 Vestibular Results

As noted above, IG had been referred to a vestibular clinic for testing. The results from this clinic showed generally normal responses for eye movements, vertebral artery and cervical vertigo tests, standard Romberg with eyes open and closed, gaze,

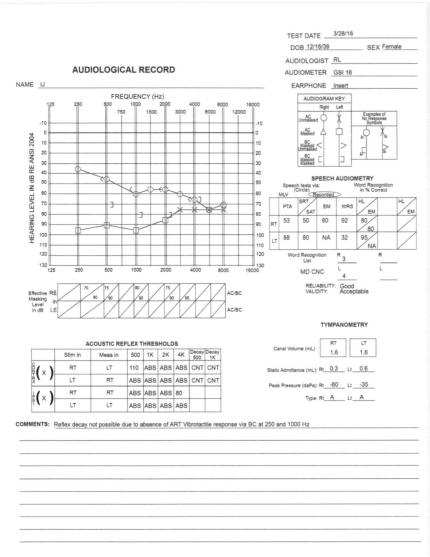

Fig. 36.3 Results for audiologic examination in 2016.

smooth pursuit/oscillating tracking and random saccades, positional, caloric, Hallpike, optokinetic reflex, rotational tests of the horizontal vestibular ocular reflex (VOR) including single signs and step test, visual enhancement of the VOR, visual suppression of the VOR, and subjective visual vertical.

Conversely, caloric testing showed normal response on the right ear and decreased amplitude on the left. The caloric weakness was 78% in the left ear. Horizontal semicircular canal responses to whole body rotation revealed an abnormally large phase lead, short VOR time constants, and a bias to the right.

36.5.2 Magnetic Resonance Imaging Results

An MRI with IAC protocol revealed a predominantly T1 and T2 hypointense enhancing lesion of approximately 1.5 cm along the left cerebellopontine angle, which extended along the left eighth cranial nerve into the porus acusticus and IAC. The cochlea, vestibule, semicircular canals, and endolymphatic sac were found to be normal.

36.6 Additional Questions to the Reader

1. **Why were the results from the vestibular evaluation not more revealing of IG's VS?**
2. **Once a VS is identified, do audiologists play a further role in the care of the patient?**
3. **Can cochlear symptoms be present in a disorder thought to be primarily neural?**
4. **To what extent might an audiologist disagree with other professionals and recommend the patient pursue another opinion?**
5. **Would over-the-counter (OTC) hearing aids as recommended[8] and the current OTC bill[9] result in appropriate management of this patient?**
6. **An often repeated business adage is "The customer is always right." Does this adage apply to IG?**

36.7 Discussion of Additional Questions

1. Why were the results from the vestibular evaluation not more revealing of IG's VS?

The vestibular test battery pointed to a left ear weakness, but no subtest accurately identified the presence of a VS. This finding is not surprising based on comprehensive literature review of the differential diagnostic capabilities of many vestibular tests at identifying VS discussed elsewhere.[10] IG did exhibit a significant and time-accelerating left ear weakness during caloric testing, but caloric testing did not specifically point to a VS.

2. Once a VS is identified, do audiologists play a further role in the care of the patient?

It has been noted[11] interventions for treating a VS can result in additional hearing problems ranging from minor changes in hearing sensitivity to an inability to recognize speech in quiet or noise. Hearing degradation can change the patient from a binaural listener to a monaural listener along with changes in spatial hearing. The patient may also experience clinically significant age-related hearing loss complicated by additional hearing loss from the VS. This may require hearing aid reprogramming or dispensing a more powerful receiver or hearing aids.

If subsequent MRIs and audiologic examinations reveal no changes over 2 to 5 years, the frequency of these examinations can be decreased or ended.[11] Patients with a severe or profound unilateral hearing loss (UHL) following VS removal are significantly disabled in a number of situations such as hearing sounds from the impaired side, and hearing in the presence of background noise and localizing sounds.

It is further noted that patients need to be counseled about communication difficulties created by UHL and about implanted bone conduction devices, Contralateral Routing of Signals (CROS) hearing aid, and/or use of external microphones.

If fall risk is apparent from screening as described elsewhere,[12] vestibular therapy should be recommended. While audiologists cannot bill Medicare for such therapy, the success of the American Institute of Balance (http://dizzy.com/) and other facilities show that many patients are willing to pay privately for such services from audiologists.[12] In all cases, accurate measures of hearing sensitivity and balance function are important for making these decisions. It behooves audiologists to assist physicians in the proper diagnosis, treatment, and recommendations of balance disorders to show the diversity and value of the audiologist's expertise.

3. Can cochlear symptoms be present in a disorder thought to be primarily neural?

VS is often considered a purely retrocochlear lesion. However, in recent years, otoacoustic emission data have shown significant secondary labyrinthine pathology in patients with VS.[13] Some symptoms associated with VS may arise from labyrinthine factors rather than neural factors. Since the inner ear is more accessible to therapeutic interventions by intratympanic injection of drugs, new therapeutic possibilities for symptom control in VS patients may arise in cases where the tumor is stable and does not require invasive intervention. In IG's case, the tumor was growing and symptom control was not recommended. Rather surgical or radiological intervention was ultimately recommended as noted below.

4. To what extent might an audiologist disagree with other professionals and recommend the patient pursue another opinion?

Audiologists strive to establish working relationships with physicians and other hearing health care providers. In this instance, the health implications for the patient outweighed the potential problems related to suggesting more information from other professionals. The "second-opinion" decision must be made on a case-by-case basis. All members of the hearing health care team should be apprised of the rationale for additional referral.

5. Would over-the-counter (OTC) hearing aids as recommended[8] and the current OTC bill[9] result in appropriate management of this patient?

OTC hearing aid provision assumes that patients with mild to moderate hearing loss do not often have other significant health problems that warrant comprehensive evaluation.[14,15] This was not true for IG who initially presented with moderate hearing loss as seen in ▶ Fig. 36.1. This "rare-occurrence assumption" is the basis of several recommendations[8] "for improving acquisition and affordability of hearing health care." The "insufficient medical need" assumption also underlies a pending regulation that seeks to legalize sale of OTC hearing aids.[9]

While VS is rare in the general population, there are a large number of auditory-vestibular–related disorders that do require additional and ongoing audiological attention. Since these recommendations[8] were published, the author has documented the number of patients in his clinic with mild to moderate hearing loss presenting with additional medical issues. These data show nearly 50% of patients have medical issues contraindicating purchase of hearing aids without further attention. In short, these recommendations[8,9] appear to run counter to best audiological practice. Had IG purchased OTC hearing aids, the identification of her VS and treatment options would not have been addressed. In addition, in all probability, the amount of amplification she would have received in all likelihood would have been less than sufficient to overcome her magnitude of hearing loss.

6. An often repeated business adage is "The customer is always right." Does this adage apply to IG?

IG made it very clear during her initial visit that she was there only to obtain "better" hearing aids. She was displeased that the audiologist continued medical questioning. After all, in her mind, she had already obtained four audiometric exams and had visited an otolaryngologist on two occasions. IG's initial intention was to use our clinic as a retail hearing aid dispensary. In this case, the "customer" was incorrect. The audiologist refused to provide hearing aids without first addressing medical concerns. Over time, IG's view changed. The diagnostic outcome could have gone in a different direction had she not returned for a second, third, and fourth visit. Audiologists must apply best practices even when such application runs counter to the patient's wishes.

36.8 Diagnosis and Recommended Treatment

The vestibular laboratory noted IG may benefit from another round of vestibular rehabilitation/balance therapy. In view, however, of the progressive loss of vestibular function and hearing on the left side and the persistent and debilitating symptoms she was experiencing, IG was encouraged to seek the advice of a neurotologist to discuss the advantages and disadvantages of various medical options such as surgical intervention, medication options, or possibly gentamicin therapy to chemically destroy the remaining vestibular function in the left ear.

In a subsequent follow-up conference, IG was counseled that her imbalance was likely secondary to her left VS. She was cautioned that the surgery was not minor and recovery time was substantial. While radiation therapy was discussed, it was not strongly recommended. Vestibular rehabilitation was again suggested.

At our request, IG returned to the clinic to discuss her options. At this visit, IG once again discussed the numerous life-limiting symptoms produced by the VS. Based on these reports, an additional consult at another out-of-state medical center was recommended. Also at this visit, IG was fitted with new hearing aids that were programmed using REM to the NAL-NL2 (National Acoustics Laboratories prescriptive procedure for fitting non-linear hearing aids, version 2) target.

In conversation with this last medical facility, the audiologist was informed that when a VS greater than 1 cm is detected, the physicians recommend surgical or radiation options to IG.

36.9 Outcome

IG is currently considering her treatment options and has currently taken no steps to schedule surgical or radiation intervention. She is effectively using her new hearing aids with streaming capabilities on her cell phone, television, and other media, and using the wireless remote microphone provided with the hearing aids.

36.10 Key Points

- Hearing aid dispensing must not be the focus of patient care. Comprehensive, best-practice diagnostics and rehabilitation need to be the primary focus. When serious audiological diagnostic/treatment errors occur, the perpetuating error often occurs early in the process. Everything completed thereafter magnifies the initial error. Even though IG insisted that she be allowed to purchase hearing aids during the first visit, the audiologist refused because prior audiometric results showed best-practice diagnostics had not been performed. This refusal to dispense hearing aids until medical issues were addressed initially resulted in IG being dissatisfied with the audiologist. It is not uncommon to encounter patients who request specific services not in agreement with best practices. In all instances, these requests are refused.

○ Recently, the Food and Drug Administration (FDA) ruled they will not enforce the requirement that individuals 18 years and older receive a medical evaluation or sign a waiver prior to purchasing most hearing aids.[16] In addition, the FDA, acting upon the recommendations of the President's Council of Advisors on Science and Technology (PCAST) announced its commitment to consider creating a category of OTC hearing aids without medical oversight. At a time when hearing aid provision is viewed as a retail transaction, it is more important than ever that audiologists provide medically defensible diagnostics and rehabilitation despite patient insistence to the contrary. IG now disagrees with this assessment of "no benefit" to medical evaluation and "rare occurrence of medical need."

- The belief that patients will self-diagnose their hearing and balance problems based on information provided in the hearing aid user instructional brochure, as suggested by PCAST, is not supported in the literature. Many experienced hearing aid users armed with such information present at our clinic with significant cognitive problems, fall risk, history of recurrent recent falls, precancerous lesions of the pinna, otitis externa, otitis media, fungal infections of the ear canal and impacted cerumen, and a host of other medical problems recognized by the audiologist.

- The "customer is not always right." Best audiological practices are always appropriate and second, third, and fourth opinions may be needed for appropriate diagnosis and treatment.

- None of the audiometric or vestibular test results, in isolation, pointed to a VS. Any patient, however, with unexplained symptoms, asymmetric hearing loss, or unilateral tinnitus should raise "red flags." Even if VS is not shown as the cause, there are therapeutic needs that should be addressed as discussed earlier.

References

[1] Olsen WO, Noffsinger D. Comparison of one new and three old tests of auditory adaptation. Arch Otolaryngol. 1974; 99(2):94–99

[2] Cox RM, Alexander GC, Taylor IM, Gray GA. The contour test of loudness perception. Ear Hear. 1997; 18(5):388–400

[3] Keidser G, Dillon H, Carter L, O'Brien A. NAL-NL2 empirical adjustments. Trends Amplif. 2012; 16(4):211–223

[4] Killion MC, Niquette PA, Gudmundsen GI, Revit LJ, Banerjee S. Development of a quick speech-in-noise test for measuring signal-to-noise ratio loss in normal-hearing and hearing-impaired listeners. J Acoust Soc Am. 2004; 116(4, Pt 1):2395–2405

[5] Metselaar M, Demirtas G, van Immerzeel T, van der Schroeff M. Evaluation of magnetic resonance imaging diagnostic approaches for vestibular schwannoma based on hearing threshold differences between ears:added value of auditory brainstem responses. Otol Neurotol. 2015; 36(10):1610–1615

[6] Eckermeier L, Pirsig W, Mueller D. Histopathology of 30 non-operated acoustic schwannomas. Arch Otorhinolaryngol. 1979; 222(1):1–9

[7] Callan DE, Lasky RE, Fowler CG. Neural networks applied to retrocochlear diagnosis. J Speech Lang Hear Res. 1999; 42(2):287–299

[8] Blazer DG, Domnitz S, Liverman CT, eds. Hearing Health Care for adults: Priorities for improving access and affordability committee on accessible and affordable hearing Health Care for Adults. Washington, DC: National Academies Press; 20001

[9] Grassley C, Warren E. The over-the-counter hearing aid act of 2016. Hear Rev. http://www.warren.senate.gov/files/documents/2016-11-07_Hearing_Aid_-Bill_Text.pdf. Published November 8, 2016. Accessed November 8, 2016

[10] von Kirschbaum C, Gürkov R. Audiovestibular function deficits in vestibular schwannoma. BioMed Res Int. 2016; 2016:4980562

[11] Popelka G. Vestibular schwannoma. In: Valente M, Valente LM, eds. The Adult Audiology Casebook. New York, NY: Thieme Medical Publishers; 2015:44–50

[12] Jagger S. How to incorporate VHIT into your practice. Paper presented at Annual Academy of Doctors of Audiology Conference. 2016. San Diego, CA

[13] Telischi F. An objective method of analyzing cochlear versus noncochlear patterns of distortion-product otoacoustic emissions in patients with acoustic neuromas. Laryngoscope. 2000; 110(4):553–562

[14] Lin FR. Hearing loss and aging: consequences, implications, and creating better outcomes through alternative models of care. Paper presented at Annual Academy of Doctors of Audiology Conference. November 2014

[15] Lin F. Hearing loss and healthy aging: a public health perspective. ASHA. http://cred.pubs.asha.org/article.aspx?articleid=2494934. Accessed November 2015

[16] FDA takes steps to improve hearing aid accessibility. http://www.fda.gov/NewsEvents/Newsroom/PressAnnouncements/ucm532005.htm. Accessed January 7, 2017

37 Innovative Hearing Device for the Treatment of Mild to Severe Sensorineural Hearing Loss

Laura Street

37.1 Clinical History and Description

This case reviews test procedures and treatment options for a patient with bilateral symmetrical high-frequency sensorineural hearing loss (SNHL). Challenges that may interfere with the effective restoration of high-frequency speech cues are also discussed.

FY is a 77-year-old male who volunteered to participate in a pilot study conducted by a privately held company. The study's protocol was approved by the Western Institutional Review Board and informed consent was obtained prior to participation. At his initial visit, FY reported bilateral hearing loss for at least 20 years due to the cumulative effects of aging and noise exposure. He stated he is a retired hardware engineer with previous exposure to greater than 10 years of low- to moderate-level machine noise without the use of hearing protection. He denied otalgia, aural fullness, tinnitus, and vertigo. His medical history was negative for known familial hearing loss, rapidly progressive and/or fluctuating hearing loss, ototoxic drug exposure, frequent middle ear infections, ear surgery, head trauma, and stroke.

37.2 Audiological Testing

After taking a case history, audiometric and immittance data were obtained (▶ Fig. 37.1) to determine if FY met the inclusion criteria for the study. Pure-tone testing revealed normal hearing at 125 Hz to 500 Hz sloping to a moderate SNHL at 750 to 1,000 Hz and then sloping to a severe SNHL at 1,500 to 8,000 Hz. Speech Reception Thresholds (SRTs) revealed a bilateral mild loss in the ability to receive speech and agreed with the two-frequency pure-tone average (PTA). Word Recognition Scores (WRS) indicated slight difficulty to recognize speech in the right ear and moderate difficulty in the left ear. Tympanometry was consistent with normal middle ear function bilaterally. The absent ipsilateral Acoustic Reflex Threshold (ART) at 2,000 and 4,000 Hz agreed with the patient's magnitude of hearing loss. Neither contralateral ARTs nor acoustic reflex decay could be assessed due to limitations with the equipment.

In terms of amplification history, FY reported bilateral hearing aid use for the past four years with his current devices being a pair of basic open-fit, Receiver-In-the-Canal (RIC) hearing aids. Although FY reported overall satisfaction with his hearing aids, he wished he could follow conversations with his wife and daughter better without having to ask them to repeat themselves so often. He also reported that the clarity of soft speech was degraded. When asked about his device coupling, FY reported that his audiologist originally recommended a closed fitting, but an open-fit device was selected because he responded negatively to the occlusion associated with a closed fitting.

37.3 Questions to the Reader

1. **What type of pathophysiology is generally associated with severe-to-profound SNHL and how might one better diagnose its presence in the cochlea?**
2. **Since the most common complaint associated with SNHL is difficulty hearing in noise, what additional testing might further improve the treatment selection process?**

37.4 Discussion of Questions

1. **What type of pathophysiology is generally associated with severe-to-profound SNHL and how might one better diagnose its presence in the cochlea?**

Severe-to-profound SNHL is generally associated with dead regions or clusters of sensory cells that are no longer functional within the cochlea. This means that the absolute thresholds obtained for patients with one or more dead regions may not reflect the true degree of hearing loss if off-place listening is not suppressed. To review, a pure-tone elicits a response at a normal or characteristic place along the basilar membrane in a normal-hearing ear. This characteristic place then corresponds to a specific frequency response in the brain. In a severely hearing-impaired ear, a tone's place of maximal stimulation may not be situated at its normal place, but at a different place due to the presence of a dead region. Off-place listening occurs whenever the normal place for a specific tone falls within a dead region, and the tone, when made sufficiently loud, elicits a response from functional sensory cells at a different yet nearby place along the basilar membrane. By presenting a broadband masker, the responses of functional sensory cells outside of a dead region can be masked and off-place listening suppressed.[1] Thus, the audiogram—in combination with a test that utilizes a broadband masker—can be used to help predict which regions of the cochlea are the most amenable to amplification. The Threshold Equalization Noise (TEN) test is one test that was specifically developed for this purpose.[2]

The TEN test prevents off-place listening through the presentation of broadband noise that produces nearly equal masked thresholds between 250 and 10,000 Hz in listeners that, based on the findings of psychophysical tuning curves, lack dead regions. If a patient presents with a dead region, the TEN masked threshold(s) corresponding to the affected frequency range will be significantly higher than expected. As such, clinicians should consider the TEN test whenever patients present with audiometric thresholds ≥ 40 to 50 dB hearing level (HL) as this population will have dead regions at least 29% of the time, particularly if the patients exhibit a rising configuration or severe-to-profound hearing thresholds.[1,3] For patients with hearing thresholds better than 40 to 50 dB HL, performing the

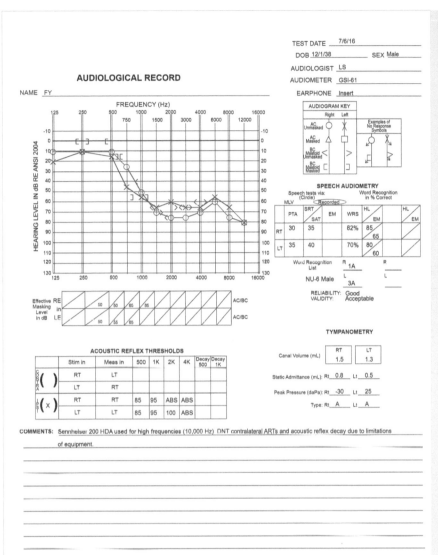

Fig. 37.1 Audiometric results. Sennheiser 200 HDA circumaural headphones were used to assess thresholds at 10,000 Hz and the thresholds at 12,000 Hz were actually thresholds obtained at 10,000 Hz.

TEN test is likely superfluous as there is generally minimal to no inner hair cell dysfunction associated with lesser degrees of SNHL. Notable exceptions to this trend include neural and central hearing losses where thresholds may be normal to profound despite the existence of healthy, functional inner hair cells.

2. **Since the most common complaint associated with SNHL is difficulty hearing in noise, what additional testing might further improve the treatment selection process?**

Speech-in-noise (SIN) testing addresses the most common complaint among patients with SNHL. As such, SIN testing can be used to verify difficulty hearing in noise as well as to better inform the treatment selection process. Clinically, there are several SIN tests to choose from. Some of these tests include the Bamford–Kowal–Bench (BKB) SIN test,[4] the Connected Speech Test (CST),[5] the Hearing In Noise Test (HINT),[6] and the QuickSIN test.[7] When selecting a SIN test, the clinician must consider the overall speed and ease of administering the test given few reimbursement options, the representativeness of the test compared to real-world listening situations, and the perceived difficulty of

the test in relation to possible floor and ceiling effects.[8] In other words, the test should be sensitive enough to separate the performance of individuals with normal hearing ability in noise from those with varying degrees of hearing difficulty in noise. The difficulty of the test should also be such that individuals cannot frequently respond with all correct or all incorrect responses. Depending on a patient's performance, the clinician may choose to give priority to devices equipped with remote microphone and/or Frequency Modulation (FM) system compatibility.

37.5 Additional Testing

As part of the study protocol, the clinician completed the TEN test and results suggested high-frequency dead regions at 8,000 and 10,000 Hz for each ear. These results were of interest as FY was participating in a sound-quality pilot study where he would compare the performance of two pairs of devices—his current open-fit hearing aids and a new set of extended bandwidth hearing aids. If pervasive dead regions were present, FY might not have been able to effectively utilize the additional frequency components supplied by a wider bandwidth.

Next, the clinician completed real-ear measures with FY's open-fit hearing aids. ► Fig. 37.2 represents the Real-Ear Aided Responses (REARs) for soft (55 dB sound pressure level [SPL]), average (65 dB SPL), and loud (75 dB SPL) speech inputs displayed as pink, green, and blue lines, respectively, with a clear roll-off in the frequency response observed beyond 4,000 Hz. When compared to NAL-NL2 (National Acoustics Laboratories' Nonlinear Fitting Procedure, version 2) targets for soft speech (pink crosses), average speech (green crosses), and loud speech (blue crosses), the targets are undershot and mostly inaudible between 2,000 and 8,000 Hz for the right ear and between 1,500 and 8,000 Hz for the left ear. Even when NAL-NL2 targets are corrected for binaural summation effects,[9,10] these findings are not altogether unexpected as moderately severe to severe

high-frequency SNHL cannot be optimally treated with open domes. Since FY's low-frequency thresholds are essentially normal through 500 Hz, FY's open-fit hearing aids are likely providing benefit only at 750 and 1,000 Hz. The poor speech intelligibility index (SII) values reported in ► Fig. 37.2 represented by the numbers in the pink, green, and blue bars further support this conclusion. Although not displayed in ► Fig. 37.2, the Maximum Power Output (MPO) of the hearing aids was also measured and found to be below the patient's predicted Uncomfortable Loudness Levels (UCLs). SIN results will be discussed later.

Following completion of real-ear measures, FY's user settings were not adjusted or "optimized" for three reasons. First, the obtained measures seemed consistent with open-fit devices being used to treat moderately severe to severe high-frequency SNHL. As most hearing aid manufacturers report, the fitting

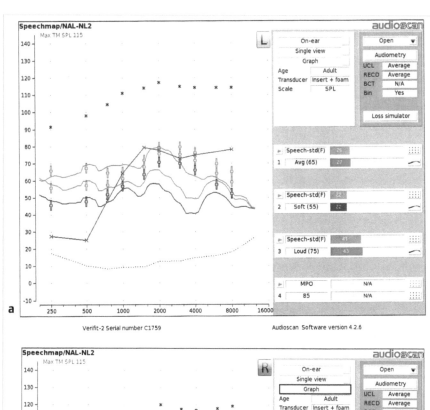

Fig. 37.2 Real-ear aided response (REAR) measures for soft (pink; 55 dB SPL), average (green; 65 dB SPL), and loud (blue; 75 dB SPL) speech using the patient's (a) left and (b) right open-fit hearing aids.

range for open domes typically bottoms out between 60 and 70 dB HL. Second, patients with steeply sloping SNHL are generally considered a difficult population to fit given the need for significant high-frequency amplification without the bothersome occlusion introduced by a closed fitting. Thus, how one defines an "optimized" fitting for this patient population is likely controversial even with additional patient counseling and changes to the hearing aid programming. Third, one goal of this pilot study was to identify which audiometric configurations and patient populations might be most well suited to receive benefit from the proposed intervention. A repeat study will likely take place in the future including a fitting optimization period with the patients' own acoustic hearing aids prior to treatment.

37.6 Additional Questions to the Reader

1. **What are some potential reasons why the TEN test has not been more widely adopted in the clinic?**
2. **How are the test stimuli used for many current SIN tests spectrally limited, and are there any new SIN tests that can assess the benefit of extended high-frequency hearing aids in noise?**

37.7 Discussion of Additional Questions

1. **What are some potential reasons why the TEN test has not been more widely adopted in the clinic?**

Given the potential utility of the TEN test to diagnose dead regions, one might ask why its use has not been more widely adopted in the clinic. Some of the arguments presented against using the TEN test include the following[1,11]:

- The original TEN test—called the TEN(SPL) test—is difficult and time consuming to administer because the test stimuli were calibrated in dB SPL rather than dB HL. This means that the clinician must first measure the patient's audiometric thresholds in dB SPL and then administer the TEN test knowing that the presentation levels listed on the audiometer require a correction factor.
- The more recent TEN(HL) test eliminates many of the calibration issues associated with the original, but uses a broadband noise that is limited between 354 and 6,000 Hz. This is useful for reducing distortion and maintaining patient comfort at elevated test levels, but limiting for identifying dead regions beyond 4,000 Hz. Given that high-frequency SNHL is the most common audiometric configuration, this change is a little counterintuitive unless one believes that providing amplification beyond 4,000 Hz is not overly beneficial (as one might argue using one or more frequency importance functions) or even realistically possible (as is generally the case with open-fit hearing aids).
- A dead region cannot be confirmed diagnostically if an absolute or masked threshold is unobtainable due to the severity of the hearing loss or patient sound tolerance issues. Fortunately, if patient thresholds cannot be measured due to

the former reason, the likelihood of a dead region is high given the degree of SNHL.
- The validity of the TEN test has been questioned by some researchers who have assessed the agreement between the findings of psychophysical tuning curves (PTCs) and the TEN test.[12] Although PTCs are the current "gold standard" for diagnosing dead regions in humans, they are not without error, and false negatives resulting from beats or combination tones may account for the reported discrepancy.[1]
- As is the case for many audiological services, reimbursement for completing the TEN test is lacking.
- Finally, although the TEN test can be used to better understand the pathophysiology of high-frequency SNHL, its administration is not necessarily required to treat or counsel patients with high-frequency SNHL. Research has shown that patients with suspected dead regions have elevated pure-tone thresholds and poorer than predicted performance on speech measures in quiet and noise.[3] This confirms that the presence of a dead region does not alter a clinician's decision to treat patients with high-frequency SNHL but rather perhaps how to treat patients with high-frequency SNHL.

2. **How are the test stimuli used for many current SIN tests spectrally limited, and are there any new SIN tests that can assess the benefit of extended high-frequency hearing aids in noise?**

One limitation of many current SIN tests is that spectral energy above 8,000 Hz is not available to the listener. This means that clinicians and researchers are restricted in their ability to verify manufacturer claims regarding extended-bandwidth hearing aid benefit in noise. Although not yet commercially available, a new version of the HINT, the hearing in speech test (HIST),[13] was recently developed to include high-frequency information through 20,000 Hz. Professionals interested in obtaining a copy of the HIST should contact Earlens Corporation for additional details.

The HIST employs the same adaptive test protocol as the HINT, but with re-recorded test tokens, novel masking signals, and two spatial test configurations. Rather than presenting target sentences and speech-shaped noise from 0 degrees azimuth, the HIST assesses performance either in diffuse noise (i.e., target sentences presented from 0 degrees azimuth and four maskers presented from ± 45 and ± 135 degrees azimuth) or while utilizing the head shadow effect (i.e., target sentences presented from − 45 degrees azimuth and two collocated maskers presented from + 45 degrees azimuth). Each masking signal is a recording of a different male speaker reading the Rainbow passage[14,15] and the Television passage.[16] These protocol changes to the HINT were designed to make the HIST more representative of a real-world listening environment.

The diffuse noise condition of the HIST shares some similarities with the HINT when combined with the R-SPACE simulation.[17,18] For those unfamiliar with the R-SPACE simulation, uncorrelated restaurant noise is produced via eight loudspeakers set 45 degrees apart in a circular array. The HINT stimuli are then presented from the front at 0 degrees azimuth with the patient seated in the middle of the array. As such, the HIST and the R-SPACE simulations are similar because they both utilize a complex array of loudspeakers as well as real speech maskers. They are different, however, because the HIST neither presents a masker from 0 degrees azimuth nor utilizes stimuli spectrally limited above 8,000 Hz. This latter characteristic is what makes the HIST especially suited to testing hearing aids with advertised bandwidths beyond 4,000 or 6,000 Hz.

The HIST is completed in approximately 10 to 15 minutes and then a reception threshold for sentences (RTS in dB) is calculated for each spatial condition. These values represent the speech-in-noise ratios (SNRs) required to repeat 50% of the target sentences correctly in noise. More negative RTS values represent better performance in noise; more positive RTS values represent poorer performance in noise. To assist the clinician to interpret the test data, normative values have been developed and the test has been validated against the HINT using 24 normal-hearing listeners. When the HIST was completed on 25 participants with mild-to-severe SNHL, the participants' average RTS value improved significantly by 1.3 dB when a simulated hearing aid bandwidth was extended to 10,000 Hz and the participants were permitted to utilize the head shadow effect. This finding suggested that the participants could experience as much as an 11.6% (1.3 dB × 8.9% per dB[19]) improvement in sentence recognition under these conditions. A nonsignificant SNR improvement of 0.5 dB was then observed for the diffuse condition when extending the simulated hearing aid bandwidth.

37.8 Additional Testing

The clinician performed HIST testing after verifying that FY's hearing aids had a directional response in the Audioscan Verifit 2. Upon completing the HIST, the computer produced an RTS value of + 3.0 dB for FY. This finding indicated that FY needed the speech signal to be 3.0 dB louder than the noise for FY to correctly repeat 50% of the sentences while wearing his directional hearing aids and utilizing the head shadow effect. Under the same conditions, 24 normal-hearing listeners without hearing aids achieved a mean RTS value and standard deviation of - 4.9 ± 1.26 dB. As such, FY's performance with open-fit hearing aids was significantly poorer than that of normal-hearing listeners. Lack of audibility above 1,000 Hz, a reduced directional response with open-fit hearing aids,[20] and an impaired ability to differentiate between speech and noise due to hearing loss likely contributed to FY's performance.

While somewhat unconventional for verifying hearing aid fittings today, functional gain (FG) was assessed by measuring FY's unaided and aided sound-field thresholds. These data are presented in ▶ Fig. 37.3, with "O" symbols representing the unaided responses and "X" symbols representing the aided responses for each ear. Sound-field threshold testing was completed with the non-test ear plugged and a loudspeaker

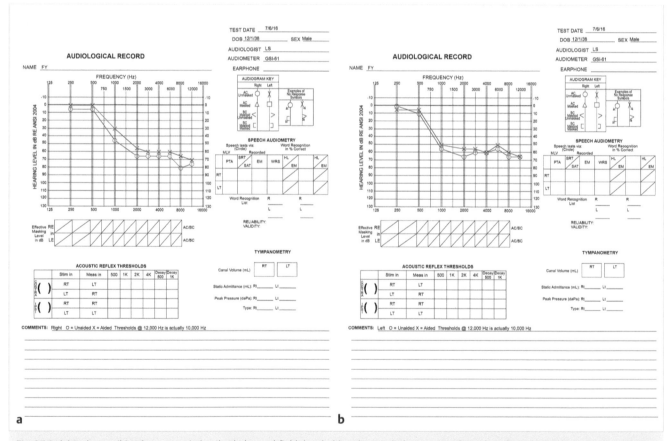

Fig. 37.3 (a) Right ear. **(b)** Left ear. Unaided and aided sound-field thresholds indicating little to no significant benefit in the high frequencies with FY's acoustic hearing aids. Thresholds at 750 and 1,500 Hz were not measured because testing at these frequencies was not part of the study protocol despite the patient's sloping configuration. A standing wave may have affected the right unaided threshold at 8,000 Hz. The 12,000 Hz thresholds were actually thresholds measured at 10,000 Hz. O, unaided sound-field threshold; X, aided sound-field threshold.

positioned at 0 degrees azimuth 1 m from the patient at ear level in a sound booth. When comparing unaided and aided sound-field thresholds, an improvement of ≥ 15 dB HL was noted for FY at 1,000 Hz for the right ear only. This finding agreed with the real-ear measures obtained earlier.

FG is the difference between a patient's unaided and aided sound-field thresholds. Many clinicians use FG measures to help verify cochlear implants, middle ear implants, and bone-anchored hearing aids (i.e., devices that cannot be verified via real-ear measures). FG measures are less likely to be used today to verify hearing aid performance because the validity and reliability of FG measures can be compromised more easily than real-ear measures. Some of the ways in which the data from sound-field threshold testing, and therefore FG measures, can be contaminated include the following[21,22,23,24,25]:

- Incorrectly assuming that unaided thresholds obtained under headphones are equivalent to those obtained by various loudspeaker arrays in the sound field.
- Conducting testing in a sound booth that has not been acoustically treated in the proper manner (i.e., not all sound booth surfaces were acoustically treated with sound absorbing tile, foam, and/or carpeting, and unnecessary equipment was kept in the test booth).
- Using test stimuli more susceptible to standing waves particularly in the reverberant field where both direct and reflected sound sources exist (e.g., using pure tones instead of frequency-modulated (FM) tones or warble tones).
- Presenting test stimuli at high intensity levels without proper ipsilateral or contralateral masking can cause
  - The test loudspeaker or hearing aid transducer to saturate and produce distortion.
  - The plugged non-test ear to respond in patients with asymmetrical hearing loss.
  - Off-place listening to occur in patients with dead regions.
- Using a test loudspeaker other than the one utilized for calibration via the substitution method (e.g., using of the 90 degree azimuth loudspeaker rather than 0 degree azimuth loudspeaker as was previously calibrated).
- Allowing the patient to adjust the hearing aid settings or move away from the precalibrated test position in the reverberant field (i.e., changing the distance, height, or angle of the patient's ear in relation to the designated test position).
- Failing to eliminate the presence of low-level noise from the hearing aid circuit or in the test environment that can mask the stimuli for listeners with normal hearing or mild low-frequency hearing loss.
- Ignoring the effects that hearing aid compression characteristics can have on stimulus presentation levels (e.g., nonlinear hearing aids generally provide more gain to soft-level inputs and less gain to high-level inputs albeit differently across manufacturers relative to their time constants and compression thresholds).

Although issues related to calibration and data contamination are potentially significant, careful measures can yield useful results. For example, in FY's case, FG measures supported conclusions drawn from real-ear measures.

37.9 Diagnosis and Treatment

Pure-tone testing and immittance findings for FY were consistent with bilateral symmetrical high-frequency SNHL likely related to the cumulative effects of aging and noise exposure. Real-ear measures and HIST results further suggested that FY could receive additional benefit from hearing aids if he could tolerate the high-frequency amplification. The TEN test indicated that FY could likely use high-frequency speech cues at least through 6,000 Hz. Since FY was previously unsuccessful with closed-fit air conduction hearing aids and since he met the inclusion criteria for a paired-comparison pilot study, FY was fitted with Earlens hearing aids bilaterally.

37.10 Additional Questions to the Reader

1. **What treatment options are available for patients with high-frequency SNHL and what are some of the advantages and disadvantages of each option?**
2. **What are the major components and features of the Earlens hearing aid?**
3. **What are the advantages and disadvantages of the Earlens?**
4. **How does a clinician verify the performance of the Earlens without using real-ear probe tube microphone measures?**

37.11 Discussion of Additional Questions

1. **What treatment options are available for patients with high-frequency SNHL and what are some of the advantages and disadvantages of each option?**

Closed-fit hearing aids, open-fit hearing aids, frequency-lowering technology, hybrid cochlear implants, and hearing assistive technology (HAT) have all been proposed as possible treatment options for high-frequency SNHL. The advantages and disadvantages of each of these options are briefly summarized below:

- Hearing aids with a custom earmold or custom shell are closed-fit devices if the vent is sufficiently narrow. RIC and slim-tube hearing aids with closed or double domes can also be viewed as closed-fit devices, but domes are generally more comfortable, less capable of providing retention in the ear canal, less suitable for providing high-frequency gain, and less successful at preventing feedback oscillation compared to custom earmolds. Regardless of the coupling, the greatest disadvantage of a closed fitting is the potential for patient discomfort. For example, custom earmolds and shells can cause discomfort particularly if they are seated deeply in the ear canal. Also, closed-fit hearing aids can result in bothersome occlusion particularly if the patient has normal or near-normal low-frequency thresholds. While custom earmolds or shells can be modified or remade until a comfortable fit is achieved, occlusion can only be "solved" by counseling the patient or compromising the fit by resorting to a more open vent or ordering a new earmold or shell that resides deeper in the ear canal.

- Open-fit devices are those employing an earmold, a custom shell, or a dome with the maximum vent size possible. The advantages and disadvantages of an open fitting are essentially the reverse of those for a closed fitting. Open-fit devices generally are more comfortable and provide less occlusion at the cost of significant gain and acoustic feedback prevention. As such, digital feedback cancellation will likely need to be enabled for almost any open-fit acoustic hearing aid. Additional drawbacks to open-fit devices include a reduced directional response[20] and poorer streaming performance due to increased leakage of amplified low-frequency signals out of the ear canal.

- Hearing aids with frequency-lowering technology are sometimes recommended for patients when high-frequency information is unavailable due to the existence of cochlear dead regions, a hearing aid's inability to restore high-frequency audibility, or a patient's intolerance of high-frequency amplification. To overcome one or more of these issues, frequency-lowering technology alters the spectral content of the input signal so that all or part of the output signal is presented to a lower frequency region in the cochlea. In short, the potential advantage of frequency lowering is the ability to "extend" a patient's usable bandwidth by exploiting his or her residual low-frequency hearing. Hearing aids with frequency-lowering technology typically use one of two approaches: frequency transposition or frequency compression. Devices with frequency transposition present high-frequency information as though it is lower in frequency by a fixed amount. For example, if frequencies above 3,000 Hz are shifted down by 1,000 Hz, a 4,000 Hz signal would be presented as a 3,000 Hz signal, a 6,000 Hz signal would be presented as a 5,000 Hz signal, etc. While this is one way to ensure that patients have access to high-frequency speech cues, sound quality and speech clarity are negatively affected when the high frequencies are transposed into mid-frequency bands that are already occupied by other frequencies. For instance, vowel formants and nasal antiformants may be masked by transposed high-frequency information. In the above example, overlapping frequency components could theoretically occur between 2,000 and 3,000 Hz. Frequency compression is related to frequency transposition in that frequencies are transposed not by a fixed amount, but by a fixed ratio. For instance, if frequencies above 3,000 Hz are compressed at a ratio of 2:1, a 4,000 Hz signal would be presented as a 3,500 Hz signal, a 6,000 Hz signal would be presented as a 4,500 Hz signal, etc. Frequency compression is advantageous in that high-frequency information is made accessible without the need to overlap frequency bands. Undesirable effects can occur, however, if a large frequency compression ratio is selected or if frequency compression is applied below 1,500 Hz where pitch cues reside. At present, evidence-based recommendations for how and when to utilize frequency-lowering technology (if at all) are lacking as each manufacturer uses its own method, and research examining the effects of various frequency-lowering parameters (e.g., the frequency at which frequency lowering should start, the compression ratio, etc.) is sparse. Of the studies that have been conducted thus far, frequency lowering appears to be advantageous for some patients in quiet so long as frequency lowering is not applied below 1,500 Hz, the transposition shift or compression ratio is not overly large, and/or the hearing loss is not steeply sloping. While many clinicians verify that the phonemes /s/ and /ʃ/ are audible with frequency lowering, it is important to ensure that other phonemes are not negatively impacted at the same time.[26,27]

- The term *hybrid cochlear implant* is used to describe a configuration where a cochlear implant (CI, hereafter) and a hearing aid are worn on the same ear. The CI provides high-frequency information via electrical stimulation, and the hearing aid provides low-frequency information via acoustic stimulation. At present, the crossover frequency (or frequencies) where it is best to transition from acoustic to electrical stimulation has not been well defined, but it may be worthwhile to begin providing electrical stimulation to frequencies presenting with dead regions. Given the method of signal transmission, a hybrid fitting is generally recommended for patients with steeply sloping high-frequency SNHL (i.e., patients with several "unaidable" high-frequency thresholds). The benefit of utilizing a hybrid system is that the CI and the hearing aid can provide more information together than would be possible with each device alone. For instance, studies evaluating speech perception in quiet and noise have found that a patient will oftentimes perform significantly better with a hybrid system than a CI or a hearing aid individually. In this way, a hybrid system can be thought of as a device providing the "best of both worlds" for patients with steeply sloping hearing loss—the CI provides the "unaidable" high-frequency information and a hearing aid provides the aidable low-frequency information.

- As one might expect, the drawback to utilizing a hybrid system is that it requires an invasive surgery that carries its own risks. For example, low-frequency hearing may not be preserved postoperatively due to cochlear trauma. Low-frequency hearing may also degrade gradually or even spontaneously years later. According to a recent review article, 24 dB HL was the mean low-frequency PTA shift for 26 patients 6 months after implantation with a short electrode array.[28] When low-frequency hearing is reduced following cochlear implantation, it can have important implications for the hearing aid benefit achieved in the implanted ear. Once again, as is the case for many audiological services, insurance coverage and payment options for fitting hybrid devices and providing aural rehabilitation are limited.

- Finally, since patients with high-frequency SNHL oftentimes present with difficulties hearing in noise, FM systems or remote microphones using the 2.4-GHz wireless band may prove helpful. FM systems and remote microphones are advantageous in that they improve the SNR by effectively reducing the distance that exists between the speaker and the hearing aid user. Although an FM system can improve the SNR by as much as 25 dB,[29] patients may find hearing aid accessories aesthetically unappealing and/or cumbersome to use in addition to their hearing aids.

2. **What are the major components and features of the Earlens?**

The Earlens hearing aid[30] is a new device for treating mild-to-severe SNHL and has received approval from the FDA (Food and Drug Administration) in 2015 and experienced a limited commercial release in 2016. It is priced competitively with high-end acoustic hearing aids and is composed of a peritympanic transducer, a behind-the-ear (BTE) hearing aid, a laser diode, and a battery charging station. The Earlens is a novel device that mechanically drives the tympanic membrane via a transducer placed deeply in the ear canal by an otologist or otolaryngologist.

The *tympanic lens* or the *tympanic membrane transducer (TMT)* consists of a tiny circular surface that contacts the umbo of the tympanic membrane, a microactuator that drives the system, and a photodetector that collects light to power the system. ▶ Fig. 37.4 illustrates the major components of the lens. To prevent lens extrusion with long-term wear, a parylene-coated perimeter platform and a small chassis with compression springs are customized to fit each patient's anatomy and to allow the tympanic membrane to move normally with breathing, swallowing, coughing, etc. Epithelial migration is also permitted through the maintenance of a thin layer of mineral oil between the lens' surfaces and the external auditory meatus.

The BTE component of the Earlens, called the *photon processor*, functions similarly to other devices on the market. It includes a digital signal processor (DSP) with 20 channels; a rechargeable battery providing at least 16 hours of battery life per 4-hour charging session; two configurable buttons that can be programmed to turn the devices on and off, change programs, or make volume adjustments; and automatic adaptive directional microphones that produce omnidirectional, bidirectional, hypercardioid, and cardioid patterns. While the Earlens processor does not presently include a telecoil, it does have a Bluetooth antenna that can be enabled for made-for-iPhone (MFi) compatibility. Since the company's value proposition is to make a broader bandwidth audible to the patient, the Earlens processor does not presently make use of frequency-lowering technology. Finally, the Earlens fitting (ELF) software permits the creation of as many as four programs and the adjustment of as many as nine gain handles. The noise reduction, feedback cancellation, and acclimatization features can all be modified in ELF as well. For instance, the clinician can choose to acclimatize the high frequencies above 4,000 Hz for an experienced hearing aid user or the full bandwidth between 125 and 10,000 Hz for new users.

An additional way in which Earlens is unique is that it does not utilize a receiver in the ear canal such as an RIC hearing aid. Instead, the Earlens employs a laser diode embedded in an open earmold called a *Light Tip* to convey information. The frequency response of the hearing aid is, thus, presented by an invisible laser light in two ways: (1) the frequency components of the signal are represented by the on/off pattern of the emitted light and (2) the intensity of the signal is represented by the power of the emitted light. Upon leaving the Light Tip, the infrared light is converted back into mechanical energy at the level of the tympanic membrane by the peritympanic transducer vibrating the umbo. Videos that depict how the Earlens works and how a lens is nonsurgically placed into the ear canal are included with the electronic version of the Adult Audiology Casebook (2nd edition) at https://ecomsci.thieme.com./. These videos can also be accessed online at https://youtu.be/O554HdSZhKk and https://youtu.be/2BqXM G2wDBl.

3. What are the advantages and disadvantages of the Earlens?

By driving the tympanic membrane via a peritympanic transducer and by presenting a light stimulus rather than an auditory stimulus, the Earlens can provide more stable gain over a wider frequency bandwidth than is presently possible with an open-fit acoustic hearing aid. According to a study by the manufacturer, the Earlens can produce an average of 40 dB of stable gain between 670 and 10,000 Hz using an open earmold and no active feedback suppression.[31] Although the Earlens can occasionally be driven to feedback at high intensities, feedback is far less likely to occur and far easier to manage given the device's unique method of sound transmission. Other benefits of the

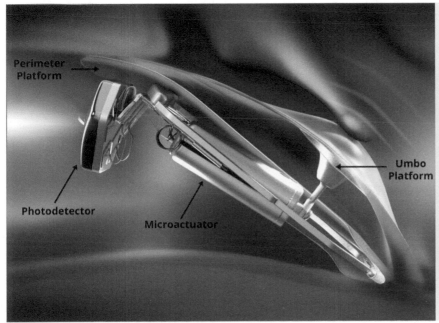

Fig. 37.4 *Lens* component of the Earlens. Refer to the text for additional details.

Perimeter Platform

Photodetector

Microactuator

Umbo Platform

Earlens include improved performance in noise compared to an unaided condition on the HINT and the HIST as well as an ability to nonsurgically remove the lens at the patient's request, at the physician's discretion, or prior to magnetic resonance imaging (MRI). Statistically significant data from the manufacturer also indicate that no change in residual hearing occurs following removal of the lens.[32]

One potential disadvantage for patients wearing the Earlens is an increased likelihood of experiencing generally mild perceptual effects (e.g., autophony and/or damped hearing) caused by mass loading the tympanic membrane with the lens. According to the manufacturer, approximately 62% of participants ($N = 13$) reported a noticeable damping effect (measured as 0–7 dB on average across all frequencies) to which they acclimatized following a few weeks of lens wear.[31] Another potential disadvantage of the Earlens is the need for a deeply seated, yet still open, earmold to ensure proper alignment of the laser light and the photodetector. Although occlusion is not an issue, earmold modifications and/or remakes may be required to achieve a more comfortable fit.

4. **How does a clinician verify the performance of the Earlens without using real-ear probe tube microphone measures?**

For clinicians who routinely perform hearing aid verification measures, another possible disadvantage to Earlens is that it is not compatible with probe tube microphone measures due to the lack of acoustic output. Instead, the clinician must calibrate the device using an in situ test called *Light Calibration*. During light calibration, the clinician measures patient thresholds between 125 and 10,000 Hz using tones generated by the hearing aid on the ear. The hearing aid software then uses the data to generate transfer functions characterizing the amount of light energy required to produce each in situ threshold. These transfer functions—combined with the patient's audiometric thresholds and the Cambridge Method for Loudness Equalization 2 - High-Frequency (CAM2) fitting formula[33]—are used to generate the input–output characteristics of the Earlens hearing aid.

In addition to the required in situ calibration step, the clinician may measure the patient's unaided and aided sound-field thresholds to determine the FG provided by the Earlens. During testing, aided sound-field thresholds can be measured either with the patient's user settings or with a special test mode called *FG mode*. When the device is set to FG mode, the hearing aid provides linear insertion gain and all advanced features are disabled except for feedback cancellation. The gain prescribed during FG mode is equal to the user's prescribed insertion gain at the compression threshold and is, thus, comparable to the CAM2 prescribed gain for soft speech.[34]

FG mode allows for assessment of the insertion gain provided for soft, average, and loud inputs as long as the MPO is not reached. In this way, testing with FG mode can serve as verification that the device is meeting some target (e.g., aided sound-field thresholds of ~20 dB HL for hearing losses ≤ 40 dB HL or at least 50% improvement in aided sound-field thresholds for hearing losses ≥ 45 dB HL)[24,35] and that the Light Calibration data were recorded accurately.

Although sound-field threshold testing cannot measure the response of nonlinear hearing aids to different input levels, unaided and aided sound-field thresholds are useful because they can account for middle ear impedance variability across patients as well as verify that the prescribed gain levels are adequate for reaching threshold.[36] In a study conducted by the manufacturer, mean FG for 39 subjects fitted with the Earlens was 31 dB between 2,000 and 10,000 Hz and 39 dB between 9,000 and 10,000 Hz.[32] This is significant as current acoustic hearing aids can neither provide broadband amplification of this magnitude nor restore high-frequency audibility above 4,000 and 6,000 Hz where hearing is most commonly impacted by SNHL.

While the Earlens is designed to be a light-driven device, the processor can be coupled to an RIC for some device verification purposes. For instance, some investigators at Earlens can verify the functionality of the directional microphones and/or the noise reduction feature using a coupler. Gain and output characteristics, however, are not assessed using an RIC because coupler measures would not reflect the true performance of the Earlens when coupled to a Light Tip. At present, Earlens RICs are unavailable, but may be offered in the future for ear canal and tympanic membranes that cannot accommodate the Lens.

37.12 Outcome

FY completed a 2-month fitting optimization period that provided him the opportunity to adjust to the increased high-frequency amplification he was receiving from his Earlens. At FY's initial fitting, gain was provided over the full bandwidth between 125 and 10,000 Hz, but with the acclimatization feature active for frequencies above 4,000 Hz. The acclimatization period was then completed in 1 month's time. Gain was provided over the full range of frequencies despite the possibility that high-frequency dead regions could negatively impact FY's word recognition performance and/or sound quality ratings. This decision was made as recent research has suggested that patients typically perform better (or at least not poorer) on speech perception tasks when high-frequency amplification is provided even in the presence of dead regions.[1,3,37,38] FY's experience was consistent with these findings as he reported significant benefit and a general appreciation for the extended bandwidth and additional high-frequency gain provided by his Earlens. He also denied autophony and a noticeable damping effect on his hearing following Lens placement.

At the end of FY's fitting optimization period, aided sound-field threshold testing and the HIST were repeated with the Earlens. ▶ Fig. 37.5 displays FY's hearing aids and Earlens aided sound-field thresholds. When the results for FY's original open-fit devices were compared to those for his Earlens, improvements of 25 to 40 dB HL were noted between 2,000 and 10,000 Hz for the right ear and 20 to 35 dB HL were noted between 1,000 and 10,000 Hz for the left ear. These findings suggest significant improvement in terms of FY's access to high-frequency speech information. The slightly reduced low-frequency sound-field thresholds obtained with the Earlens were likely due to the noise floor of the hearing aids at that time.

FY's HIST results indicated that the signal needed to be −2.8 dB softer than the noise for FY to correctly repeat 50% of the target sentences. When compared to the HIST result for FY's open-fit hearing aids, the SNR improvement achieved with Earlens was 5.8 dB, suggesting up to 51.62% (5.8 dB × 8.9% per dB) improvement in sentence recognition in noise when listening

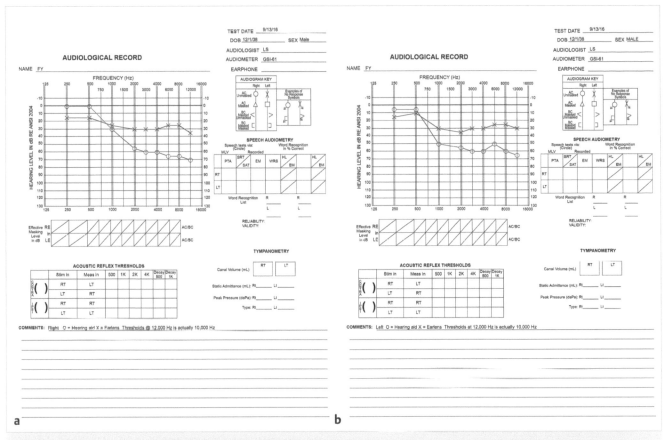

Fig. 37.5 **(a)** Right ear. **(b)** Left ear. Aided sound-field thresholds indicating significant benefit in the high frequencies with Earlens. There was no significant difference between the Earlens-aided sound-field thresholds obtained with the patient's user settings versus the *Functional Gain Mode* settings. Thresholds at 750 and 1,500 Hz were not measured because testing at these frequencies was not part of the study protocol. The 12,000-Hz thresholds were actually measured at 10,000 Hz. O, hearing aid–aided sound-field threshold; X, Earlens-aided sound-field threshold.

with Earlens and taking advantage of the head shadow effect. Collectively, the aided sound-field threshold and HIST data suggested that the audible extended bandwidth delivered by Earlens was providing FY with significant objective benefit in both quiet and noisy listening situations under laboratory conditions.

After completing his Earlens trial, FY agreed to have the lenses removed so he could return to wearing his acoustic hearing aids for a period of 2 weeks. After wearing his acoustic hearing aids for 2 weeks, FY returned and completed a manufacturer-developed questionnaire whereby he indicated that speech and music sounded clearer and more natural with his Earlens when compared to his acoustical devices. At the end of the pilot study, FY had the opportunity to either continue with his acoustic hearing aids or return to his Earlens devices at no cost. FY elected to return to his Earlens devices and he has continued to volunteer for additional studies at Earlens, having acquired an appreciation for hearing aid research and the quality of life improvements his new devices have afforded him.

37.13 Key Points

- When testing patients with high-frequency SNHL, clinicians should be conscientious of the possibility of cochlear dead regions.

- Although confirming the existence of cochlear dead regions with the TEN test does not alter the clinician's decision to treat patients with high-frequency SNHL, it may impact how the clinician chooses to treat patients with high-frequency SNHL.
- Unlike other SIN tests, the HIST can be used to assess the benefit of extended bandwidth hearing aids in noise.
- Closed-fit hearing aids, open-fit hearing aids, frequency-lowering technology, hybrid CI, HAT, and the new Earlens are all options for treating patients with SNHL.
- The Earlens provides gain between 125 and 10,000 Hz because it directly drives the tympanic membrane via a transducer placed deeply in the ear canal. It can only be verified with sound-field threshold testing as it utilizes a laser diode rather than a receiver to present the signal.

37.14 Acknowledgments

The author would like to thank Suzanne Levy, PhD, Director of Clinical Research at Earlens Corporation, for providing constructive comments on earlier versions of this case study. Her feedback, along with those of the editors, significantly improved the depth and quality of the information discussed. Sincere appreciation is also given to FY who has continued to exhibit curiosity and enthusiasm for hearing aid research.

References

[1] Moore BC. Dead regions in the cochlea: diagnosis, perceptual consequences, and implications for the fitting of hearing AIDS. Trends Amplif. 2001; 5(1):1–34

[2] Moore BC, Huss M, Vickers DA, Glasberg BR, Alcántara JI. A test for the diagnosis of dead regions in the cochlea. Br J Audiol. 2000; 34(4):205–224

[3] Preminger JE, Carpenter R, Ziegler CH. A clinical perspective on cochlear dead regions: intelligibility of speech and subjective hearing aid benefit. J Am Acad Audiol. 2005; 16(8):600–613, quiz 631–632

[4] Bench J, Kowal A, Bamford J. The BKB (Bamford-Kowal-Bench) sentence lists for partially-hearing children. Br J Audiol. 1979; 13(3):108–112

[5] Cox RM, Alexander GC, Gilmore C. Development of the connected speech test (CST). Ear Hear. 1987; 8(5) Suppl:119S–126S

[6] Nilsson M, Soli SD, Sullivan JA. Development of the hearing in noise test for the measurement of speech reception thresholds in quiet and in noise. J Acoust Soc Am. 1994; 95(2):1085–1099

[7] Killion MC, Niquette PA, Gudmundsen GI, Revit LJ, Banerjee S. Development of a quick speech-in-noise test for measuring signal-to-noise ratio loss in normal-hearing and hearing-impaired listeners. J Acoust Soc Am. 2004; 116(4, Pt 1):2395–2405

[8] Wilson RH, McArdle RA, Smith SL. An evaluation of the BKB-SIN, HINT, Quick-SIN, and WIN materials on listeners with normal hearing and listeners with hearing loss. J Speech Lang Hear Res. 2007; 50(4):844–856

[9] Audioscan Verifit® User's Guide (Version 3.16). Ontario, Canada: Etymonic Design Inc.; 2016:105

[10] Audioscan Verifit® User's Guide (Version 4.8). Ontario, Canada: Etymonic Design Inc.; 2016:56

[11] Moore BC, Glasberg BR, Stone MA. New version of the TEN test with calibrations in dB HL. Ear Hear. 2004; 25(5):478–487

[12] Summers V, Molis MR, Müsch H, Walden BE, Surr RK, Cord MT. Identifying dead regions in the cochlea: psychophysical tuning curves and tone detection in threshold-equalizing noise. Ear Hear. 2003; 24(2):133–142

[13] Levy SC, Freed DJ, Nilsson M, Moore BC, Puria S. Extended high-frequency bandwidth improves speech reception in the presence of spatially separated masking speech. Ear Hear. 2015; 36(5):e214–e224

[14] Fairbanks G. Voice and Articulation Drillbook. 2nd ed. New York, NY: Harper & Row; 1960:124–139

[15] Cox RM, Moore JN. Composite speech spectrum for hearing and gain prescriptions. J Speech Hear Res. 1988; 31(1):102–107

[16] Nilsson M, Ghent RM, Bray V, Harris R. Development of a test environment to evaluate performance of modern hearing aid features. J Am Acad Audiol. 2005; 16(1):27–41

[17] Compton-Conley CL, Neuman AC, Killion MC, Levitt H. Performance of directional microphones for hearing aids: real-world versus simulation. J Am Acad Audiol. 2004; 15(6):440–455

[18] Valente M, Mispagel KM, Tchorz J, Fabry D. Effect of type of noise and loudspeaker array on the performance of omnidirectional and directional microphones. J Am Acad Audiol. 2006; 17(6):398–412

[19] Soli SD, Nilsson MJ. Predicting speech intelligibility in noise: the role of factors other than pure tone sensitivity. J Acoust Soc Am. 1998; 101(5):3201

[20] Klemp EJ, Dhar S. Speech perception in noise using directional microphones in open-canal hearing aids. J Am Acad Audiol. 2008; 19(7):571–578

[21] Morgan DE, Dirks DD, Bower DR. Suggested threshold sound pressure levels for frequency-modulated (warble) tones in the sound field. J Speech Hear Disord. 1979; 44(1):37–54

[22] Walker G, Dillon H, Byrne D. Sound field audiometry: recommended stimuli and procedures. Ear Hear. 1984; 5(1):13–21

[23] Kuk FK. Considerations in modern multichannel nonlinear hearing aids. In: Valante M, ed. Hearing Aids: Standards, Options, and Limitations. 2nd ed. New York, NY: Thieme Medical Publishers; 2002:178–213

[24] Kuk F, Ludvigsen C. Reconsidering the concept of the aided threshold for nonlinear hearing AIDS. Trends Amplif. 2003; 7(3):77–97

[25] Hawkins DB. Limitations and uses of the aided audiogram. Semin Hear. 2004; 25(1):51–62

[26] Simpson A. Frequency-lowering devices for managing high-frequency hearing loss: a review. Trends Amplif. 2009; 13(2):87–106

[27] Dillon H. Advanced signal processing schemes. In: Dillon H, ed. Hearing Aids. 2nd ed. New York, NY: Thieme Publishers; 2012:225–255

[28] Incerti PV, Ching TY, Cowan R. A systematic review of electric-acoustic stimulation: device fitting ranges, outcomes, and clinical fitting practices. Trends Amplif. 2013; 17(1):3–26

[29] Crandell C, Smaldino J. Room acoustics and amplification. In: Valente M, Roeser R, Hosford-Dunn H, eds. Audiology: Treatment Strategies. New York, NY: Thieme Medical Publishers; 2000:601–637

[30] Perkins R, Fay JP, Rucker P, Rosen M, Olson L, Puria S. The EarLens system: new sound transduction methods. Hear Res. 2010; 263(1–2):104–113

[31] Fay JP, Perkins R, Levy SC, Nilsson M, Puria S. Preliminary evaluation of a light-based contact hearing device for the hearing impaired. Otol Neurotol. 2013; 34(5):912–921

[32] Gantz BJ, Perkins R, Murray M, Levy SC, Puria S. Light-driven contact hearing aid for broad-spectrum amplification: safety and effectiveness pivotal study. Otol Neurotol. 2017; 38(3):352–359

[33] Moore BCJ, Glasberg BR, Stone MA. Development of a new method for deriving initial fittings for hearing aids with multi-channel compression: CAMEQ2-HF. Int J Audiol. 2010; 49(3):216–227

[34] Arbogast T, Moore BCJ, Puria S, Edwards B, Levy SC. Real-world experience with CAM2 high frequency gain prescriptions provided with the light-driven contact hearing aid. Poster presented at IHCON; Tahoe City, CA; August 2016

[35] Bray V, Nilsson M. Assessing hearing aid fittings: an outcome measures battery approach. In: Valante M, ed. Strategies for Selecting and Verifying Hearing Aid Fittings. 2nd ed. New York, NY: Thieme Medical Publishers; 2002:151–175

[36] Dillon H. Electroacoustic performance and measurement. In: Dillon H, ed. Hearing Aids. 2nd ed. New York, NY: Thieme Publishers; 2012:81–127

[37] Cox RM, Alexander GC, Johnson J, Rivera I. Cochlear dead regions in typical hearing aid candidates: prevalence and implications for use of high-frequency speech cues. Ear Hear. 2011; 32(3):339–348

[38] Cox RM, Johnson JA, Alexander GC. Implications of high-frequency cochlear dead regions for fitting hearing aids to adults with mild to moderately severe hearing loss. Ear Hear. 2012; 33(5):573–587

38 It Is Never Too Late

Therese C. Walden

38.1 Clinical History and Description

This case study illustrates the need for providers to try alternatives with each patient until the correct balance of treatment outcomes is reached.

Treatment of hearing loss is a process. There are multiple steps in the process that help ensure the patient's hearing needs are addressed properly. Sometimes, however, the initial solution selected for the patient is not the solution that will bring about the greatest benefit. This case study illustrates the need for providers to try alternatives with each patient until the correct balance of treatment outcomes is reached.

SE is an 87-year-old female with a long-standing history of hearing loss and bothersome tinnitus. Within the past several years, SE developed intermittent dizziness and had a feeling of being off-balance without any symptoms of vertigo. SE was seen 2 years ago in the practice on referral from an otolaryngologist because of the above symptoms. At that first visit, SE was diagnosed with a bilateral moderate to severe sensorineural hearing loss, and it was recommended she be fitted with hearing aids. It was decided that custom half-shell In-The-Ear (ITE) hearing aids would be best in terms of ease of insertion and overall use. SE returned for the hearing aid fitting and the new hearing aids were programmed to 70% of the prescribed NAL-NL1 target[1] (corrected for binaural summation and multiple channel summation). This 70% to target fitting seemed loud to SE, but she was willing to try amplification to help her hearing loss as well as possibly her tinnitus. In addition, at this initial hearing aid fitting appointment, a Dix–Hallpike test was performed as SE's cardiologist recommended the procedure to rule out Benign Paroxysmal Positional Vertigo (BPPV). The test was negative for positional nystagmus; however, SE reported slight dizziness on the left-sided movement. At this point, the Epley maneuver was completed and that seemed to alleviate the dizziness. One month later, SE's daughter returned the hearing aids. She said SE did not acclimatize to the hearing aids and with all her other medical issues, the daughter felt it best to wait before adding any more medical interventions to SE's list.

Two years later, SE returned to have her hearing reevaluated and determine if hearing aids would help. The patient's current medical status was reviewed. SE is treated for chronic obstructive pulmonary disease (COPD). COPD is a progressive lung disease that may include emphysema, bronchitis, and asthma. Symptoms include increased breathlessness, frequent coughing, and wheezing. COPD may have a genetic component as well as environmental (pollutants) and behavioral (smoking and exposure to second-hand smoke) contributions.[2] SE uses three inhalers to help reduce the acute symptoms of her COPD (coughing, wheezing, etc.) and SE takes Zyrtec, an antihistamine, to help reduce her asthma and other allergic symptoms. SE's chronic coughing became an issue for the treatment of her hearing loss, as will be discussed.

In addition to the medications for the COPD, SE is taking vitamin D supplements and Synthroid, which are both common prescriptions for an older patient. SE is being treated for hypothyroidism or an underactive thyroid. Symptoms of hypothyroidism are nonspecific and may be missed. For example, as many as 25% of nursing home residents have undiagnosed hypothyroidism.[3] Hypothyroidism may manifest as cognitive decline, memory loss, sleepiness, weight gain, or constipation. These symptoms can also be associated with "normal aging." Diagnosis of hypothyroidism then is a combination of presenting symptoms, the patient's past medical conditions, family history, and laboratory tests. Finally, SE has recently been evaluated by a neurologist for memory loss and cognitive decline. SE's daughter reported that there was no imaging testing completed nor is she aware of any laboratory tests to determine if the memory loss and cognitive decline are the result of dementia. Because of SE's hearing loss, however, the neurologist referred SE to an otolaryngologist for evaluation of hearing loss, which eventually led SE to our practice.

In addition to the medications and treatments listed above, SE is taking Lyrica and Elavil, as prescribed by a pain specialist for peripheral neuropathy in her feet that is caused by spinal stenosis. SE's daughter reports that the prescription for Ambien was given to help SE sleep. SE has had difficulty sleeping in part because of the bothersome tinnitus. All of SE's current medications are listed in ▶ Table 38.1. Clearly, SE has several comorbidity conditions having similar symptomology.

SE is relatively active, moving well under her own power, and does not use a cane for walking assistance. She has maintained a healthy weight into her older years as well. The dizziness she reports is not vertiginous, (i.e., she is not reporting spinning sensations nor nausea or vomiting). Although dizziness can occur due to aging, a review of the list of medications in ▶ Table 38.1 clearly indicates that many of the medications SE is taking cite dizziness as a possible side effect. Additionally, endocrine system imbalances (i.e., hypothyroidism) can cause dizziness. Since SE did not report positional dizziness, but rather an intermittent sensation of lightheadedness, the audiologist did not perform the Dix–Hallpike test again to determine if BPPV was the cause of the dizziness.[4]

To address her tinnitus, the audiologist had SE rate how aware she was of the tinnitus throughout the day and how bothered she was by the tinnitus. An internal 10-point rating scale is used such that, in terms of awareness, 1 = "mildly aware" and 10 = "aware all the time." In terms of bothersomeness, a similar scale is use whereby 1 = "mildly bothered" and 10 = "severely bothered." SE rated both awareness and bothersomeness as 7/10. The audiologist counseled SE that the conditions for which she is being treated and the medications used to treat her symptoms can readily cause dizziness and tinnitus. In addition, hearing loss, certainly to the degree of loss SE has, can contribute to the presence of tinnitus.

38.2 Audiologic Testing and Diagnosis

Audiologic testing was performed after completing the extensive medical history review. Again, with the use of an internal

Table 38.1 List of medications for SE

Medication	Purpose	Dose	Side effect(s)
Vitamin D	Support absorption of calcium to prevent bone loss, prevent cognitive issues	2,000 mg/daily (older adult dose)	None unless taking excessive amounts
Synthroid	Replacement hormone to help regulate the body's metabolic processes	50 mcg/morning	Sensitivity to heat, headache, irritability
Zyrtec	Antihistamine to treat asthma, allergy symptoms	Each morning	Drowsiness, dry mouth
Anoro inhaler	Prevents wheezing; treatment for COPD	Once daily	Nervousness, dizziness
Albuterol inhaler	Bronchodilator; relaxes airway muscles	Twice daily	Shakiness, dizziness, insomnia
QVAR inhaler	Treats wheezing, shortness of breath	Twice daily	Dry mouth, headache
Lyrica	Seizures, nerve pain	100 mg/bedtime	Dizziness
Elavil	Depression, anxiety	25 mg/bedtime	Dizziness
Ambien	Sedative, insomnia	5 mg/bedtime	Dizziness, memory problems

Abbreviation: COPD, chronic obstructive pulmonary disease.

subjective rating scale, SE rates her overall hearing ability as 3/10 on a 10-point scale where 1 = "I can hear everything" and 10 = "I can't hear at all." SE denied ear infections, ear surgeries, a history of hazardous noise exposure, no head trauma, and no adult-onset hearing loss in the family.

Audiometric test results are shown in ▶ Fig. 38.1. Results indicated a slight overall decrease in hearing thresholds compared to the audiologic examination completed 2 years earlier. This magnitude of hearing loss can clearly compromise SE to hear and participate in most, if not all, everyday listening situations. These thresholds are also in agreement with SE's overall hearing ability rating of 3/10 as well as the report by SE's daughter that the family is struggling to keep SE included in their conversations. Loudness Discomfort Levels (LDL) were assessed at 500 and 3,000 Hz and resulted in uncomfortable levels at 85 and 90 dB hearing level (HL) in each ear. These results are consistent with a significantly reduced dynamic range.

Speech Recognition Threshold (SRT) and Word Recognition Score (WRS) testing were not completed at this visit. The results from 2 years ago indicated 60% WRS in each ear. Therefore, repeating WRS testing would not have resulted in any additional information concerning SE's ability to hear in the presence of background noise that SE reported was most problematic.

▶ Table 38.2 reports the results of the Quick Speech-in-Noise (QuickSIN) testing.[5] The QuickSIN is a speech recognition–in-noise test that evaluates one's ability to hear in noise. The test uses sentences recorded in a four-talker babble at various (favorable to unfavorable) Signal-to-Noise Ratios (SNR). There are five keys words in each sentence that are scored as correct or incorrect. The resultant score represents SNR loss, that is, the increased SNR necessary for an individual to understand speech in noise compared to a person with normal hearing. All Quick-SIN testing was completed binaurally. The QuickSIN was initially completed at SE's preferred listening level (PLL) in an auditory-only condition. The PLL is simply a comfortable loudness level that allowed SE to hear the audiologist via insert earphones. At SE's PLL (65 dB HL), her SNR ability was severely compromised (i.e., + 19.5 dB SNR HL). SE could only repeat the complete sentence at the most favorable SNR (+ 25 dB). At more unfavorable SNR conditions, SE struggled. With an increase of 10 dB (75 dB HL), SE could extract a greater number of keywords at a less favorable SNR (i.e., + 14.5 dB SNR HL), but still her overall performance was poor.

Because of SE's memory loss and severe SNR HL, the audiologist administered the QuickSIN sentences via insert earphones with and without visual cues (and no background noise) to determine if the memory loss impacted performance. As indicated in ▶ Table 38.2, when the background noise was removed, SE could repeat the keywords in the QuickSIN sentences with and without visual cues at the + 10 dB S/N level (i.e., SNR HL improved from + 14.5 to + 5.5 dB) increasing. Although this cannot be reported as an SNR HL (as there was no background noise), SE's ability to hear and repeat back the QuickSIN sentences is prognostically encouraging. It allows SE to understand she can comprehend sentences in quiet and it illustrates to her the highly adverse effects of background noise.

At the completion of testing, the results were discussed with SE and her daughter and they were convinced, especially because of the quantitative QuickSIN results, that treatment of the hearing loss was necessary. They also stated they were encouraged by the comprehensive medical review, testing, and discussion that the treatment of the hearing loss this time will be effective.

38.3 Recommended Treatment

Since SE had used custom half-shell ITE hearing aids previously, it was suggested that ITEs be tried again. Slim-tube Behind-The-Ear (BTE) hearing aids, however, were also discussed and SE decided to try the BTE aids this time. The audiologist counseled SE and her daughter on how the slim-tube hearing aids work, how they should be used, and how hearing aids may help reduce/relieve the awareness and bothersomeness of tinnitus.

SE returned for a hearing aid fitting to program the hearing aids and verify the fitting using the NAL-NL1 prescriptive target. Power domes were used with the slim-tube BTE aids, but Real Ear Measurements (REM) indicated that the slim-tube/power dome fitting was ineffective in providing appropriate gain to meet NAL-NL1 targets as well as control feedback. A pair of Receiver-In-the-Canal (RIC) hearing aids was selected from stock (again, using power domes) and REM indicated sufficient gain for input levels of 50, 65, and 80 dB SPL. Also, minimal feedback was present once feedback management was adjusted

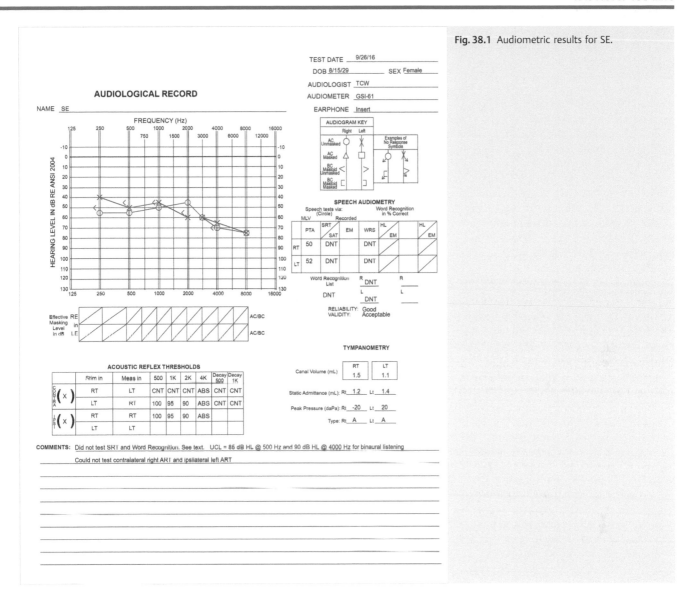

Fig. 38.1 Audiometric results for SE.

Table 38.2 QuickSIN results for SE

Presentation level	SNR HL	Test condition
65 dB HL (preferred loudness)	19.5 dB SNR HL	Auditory only/insert phones
75 dB HL (increased loudness)	14.5 dB SNR HL	Auditory only/insert phones
75 dB HL	5.5 dB (S/N 10 level)	Auditory and visual/no babble
75 dB HL	5.5 dB (S/N 10 level)	Auditory only/no babble

Abbreviations: HL, hearing level; QuickSIN, Quick Speech-in-Noise test; SNR, signal-to-noise ratio.

in the programming software. Because SE was effectively a "new" hearing aid user, the overall gain profile was reduced to 70% of target in the default listening program. A second speech-in-noise program with adaptive directionality and slightly reduced overall gain was selected. This second program allowed SE (or her daughter) to reduce the overall loudness as SE began the acclimatization period with the hearing aids. Although SE felt the overall gain was still "too loud," she agreed to try the hearing aids in the current settings for several hours each day. SE added more listening time as she adapted to the hearing aids. The Real Ear Saturation Response (RESR) with a 90 dB SPL swept tone (RESR$_{90}$) was measured to ensure the patient's severely reduced dynamic range was addressed.

After the verification and fitting procedures were completed, the care and use of the hearing aids was discussed. SE could only partially insert the hearing aids on her own, but her daughter could easily insert the hearing aids for SE and she intended to practice with SE at home. During the counseling session, SE kept asking why she was wearing something in her ears and why she needed something in her ear *and* behind her ear if the hearing loss was *in* the ear. SE also made the comment that the ears "just pick up sound" and that "the brain does all the understanding." SE is a retired nurse and her knowledge of the human body and how it works was still embedded in her memory. This would prove useful throughout the treatment process. The introduction of the hearing aids was completed slowly to allow SE to determine the pace at which she could absorb the information she was receiving. Although SE's daughter was handling most of the technical issues of the hearing aid usage (i.e., changing batteries, cleaning the aids, etc.), it still was SE who had to acclimate to her new world of sound and this process would simply take time.

Engaging SE as a patient as well as SE being an educated professional immensely expedited the entire process. The audiologist discussed the use of the hearing aids as "medicine" for the brain and instantly this resonated with SE. SE proclaimed, "Medicine has to be taken every day!" SE was correct about the need for consistency in the use of hearing aids for the brain to acclimatize and enliven the auditory processing centers in the central auditory system. In addition, consistency of use is necessary to help SE realize reduction of her tinnitus. The session concluded with her daughter taking the responsibility for the care of the hearing aids. SE was scheduled for a follow-up appointment in 2 weeks. During the 2 weeks, SE's son called to report that SE was using the aids and enjoying how the hearing aids reconnected her to the family. He reported that the hearing aids had made "quite a bit of difference in her life so far."

At the 2-week follow-up appointment, the family said that one of the new hearing aids had been lost. They were not sure how it happened and they looked extensively for the aid. It is possible SE removed the aid or it fell off because the dome was not inserted into the ear canal sufficiently. Although the audiologist fitted a new aid to replace the lost one, SE's daughter was not sure the RIC style was best for SE. The family asked if the hearing aids could be worn when SE was sleeping. It was explained that there was no reason to remove the aids if SE preferred to wear them at night, but it was suggested that a lower gain setting be used. It was also suggested they would need to check for the aids each morning to ensure that one or the other had not come dislodged in the bedding overnight. Another 2-week follow-up appointment was scheduled.

At the next appointment, there was a clear change in SE's demeanor. Whereas previously SE had been quite loud when she spoke, her voice had now softened. Previously, she had laughed at inappropriate times and repeated things, but now she made appropriate humorous statements about herself and others. When asked about the tinnitus, SE responded, "What tinnitus?" The ear noises had significantly subsided. SE's daughter reported that when the family goes for dinner, SE is part of the conversation and that she is reconnecting with them. Her overall personality has steadied and SE is more likely to start a conversation than she has in many years and she clearly is hearing others in the environment because her questions are appropriate and timely. The effort, however, to insert and remove the RIC hearing aids is a bit tiresome for SE and her daughter, and SE sometimes forgets that she has the aids in her ears. Also, when brushing her hair, the hearing aids get caught in the brush or comb and this could result in the loss of one or both hearing aids.

38.4 Questions to the Reader

1. **What options are available that would provide SE with the benefits of amplification and address the ease of and consistency of her issues with use?**

38.5 Discussion of Questions

What options are available that would provide SE with the benefits of amplification and address the ease of and consistency of her issues with use?

Although SE was receiving benefit from the current RIC hearing aids, the ease of use was problematic. The discussion about using ITE hearing aids was revisited. ITEs had been tried previously and it was possible that a half-shell or In-The-Canal (ITC) hearing aid could be easier for SE and her family. Additionally, "extended-wear" hearing aids were discussed. One of the benefits of extended-wear hearing aids is the ability to insert the hearing aid once and leave it in the ear canal, undisturbed, until the battery in the device needs to be replaced or the device is removed proactively toward the end of the expected battery life. Also, this style of hearing aid allows the patient to bathe or shower normally, sleep with the device in the ear, and adjust the volume setting with the use of a magnet. After considering the advantages and disadvantages of custom hearing aids versus extended-wear hearing aids, it was decided to try the extended-wear devices. SE was an appropriate candidate for the device in terms of physical fit in the ear canal. The extended-wear hearing aids were programmed and subjectively verified based on the patient's report and aided sound-field measurements. Real ear measurements could not be completed due to collapsing of the probe tube with insertion of the extended-wear hearing aids. SE reported that her own voice sounded "echoic" with the extended-wear hearing aids. As a result of this report, reprogramming was completed to reduce low-frequency gain. This had not occurred with the RIC hearing aids. SE reported no adverse effects from the insertion and seating of the hearing aids and she was pleased to not have to be concerned with insertion/removal of the new hearing aids.

At the first follow-up visit, 1 week later, the hearing aids were in place and SE and her family were delighted with the ease of use. No programming changes were made. One week later, SE returned with the left device removed by her daughter because it was causing pain. The ear canal was inspected and found to have some redness midway down the ear canal. The daughter reported that SE complained of the ear pain following a persistent coughing episode several days before the device had been removed. Recall that SE is being treated for COPD and a hallmark symptom of COPD is excessive coughing. Knowing that the coughing could have dislodged the device, the audiologist decided to wait 1 week to have the ear canal heal completely.

At the next visit, the audiologist inserted the next larger size device using a small amount of lubrication liquid. The thought was that the larger size might reduce the chance of slippage from coughing episodes. SE reported that the larger device felt tighter, but not uncomfortable. SE wore the hearing aids another week and had no problems with ear pain even though she had coughed. The audiologist discussed with the family about adjusting the volume of the extended-wear device, but overall, SE was acclimatizing well and she did not request any adjustments. SE left the hearing aids in the default volume setting and they did not interfere with her sleep. Recall also that SE has been prescribed Ambien for sleep.

At this last appointment, SE's other daughter accompanied SE and to ensure all family members knew how to inspect the ear and use the magnetic volume wand. She videotaped the session with her smartphone to share the information with her siblings. The audiologist also took several photographs with the smartphone to show how the ear looked in terms of positioning of the hearing aids in the ear canal as well as how the ear canal should look when there is no redness or other abnormalities. The use of smartphones to counsel patients and their family members has been effective in reducing "information overload" that can occur at these long visits when significant information is provided.

SE is currently doing very well. She is scheduled for programmed replacement of the extended-wear hearing aids *before* their expected battery lifespan every 7 to 8 weeks and SE seems to understand that she is in control of her hearing. SE reports her tinnitus is controlled and her dizziness has subsided. Follow-up visits with the family indicate that SE's other health care providers are impressed with how treatment of SE's hearing loss and tinnitus has not only improved communications with SE, but also that her overall quality of life has improved. SE's daughter reports that SE is more optimistic and more confident and the family believes SE's cognitive abilities are improved. SE routinely hugs the clinicians in the practice who work with her and she and her family cannot express how grateful they are for all the efforts expended on her behalf.

38.6 Key Points

- Although SE and her family waited many years to address the significantly compromising hearing loss and although the hearing loss may have contributed to or exacerbated some of her other medical conditions, it is never too late to start treating hearing loss. In fact, as Robert N. Butler of the International Longevity Center in New York has stated about health promotion, "It's never too late to start and always too soon to stop."[6]
- Treatment of hearing loss is a process of which the selected device(s) is only a component. Since there are myriad choices available, knowing the advantages and disadvantages of each device option ensures that patients are well educated in their decisions about hearing aids that best suit their lifestyle and hearing needs.
- Co-morbid medical and disease conditions can complicate a patient's life so much so as to delay treatment for hearing loss

as it is deemed "the least of their problems." In fact, untreated hearing loss can exacerbate many medical symptoms and conditions. Early diagnosis and treatment of hearing loss could help the patient. Recent research has determined that dementia and cognitive decline are inextricably linked to untreated hearing loss with the resultant loss of societal contact and connections.[7]

- REM as a method/procedure to verify hearing aid fittings is a requirement for those who use hearing aids as part of the treatment process. Without REM, there is no way to know the amount of gain/output that is generated in the ear canal for the various input levels. REM ensures that the settings are not so soft as to not allow a long-term difference or so loud that the patient will reject the hearing aids. Without the use of REM to verify the fitting is completed correctly, the audiologist is simply guessing and that is unethical.
- Smartphones can be very helpful in the hearing aid counseling process.

References

[1] Byrne D, Dillon H, Ching T, Katsch R, Keidser G. NAL-NL1 procedure for fitting nonlinear hearing aids: characteristics and comparisons with other procedures. J Am Acad Audiol. 2001; 12(1):37–51

[2] The COPD Foundation. What is COPD? Available at: http://www.copdfoundation.org/What-is-COPD/Understanding-COPD/What-is-COPD.aspx. Accessed January 17, 2017

[3] American Thyroid Association. Thyroid disease in the older patient. Available at: http://www.thyroid.org/thyroid-disease-older-patient/. Accessed January 17, 2017

[4] MedicineNet.com. Dizziness (Dizzy). Available at: http://www.medicinenet.com/dizziness_dizzy/article.htm. Medically reviewed by a doctor 8/4/2016. Accessed January 10, 2017

[5] Etymōtic Research, Inc. QuickSIN Test. Elk Grove Village, IL: Etymōtic Research, Inc.; 2001

[6] Butler RN. Strategies for Health Promotion. Grand Challenges of Our Aging Society: Workshop Summary. National Research Council of the National Academies. Washington, DC: The National Academies Press; 2010

[7] Lin FR, Metter EJ, O'Brien RJ, Resnick SM, Zonderman AB, Ferrucci L. Hearing loss and incident dementia. Arch Neurol. 2011; 68(2):214–220

Suggested Reading

[1] Mueller HG. 20Q: real-ear probe microphone measurements—30 years of progress? Audiol Online. Available at: http://www.audiologyonline.com/articles/20q-probe-mic-measures-12410. Published January 13, 2014. Accessed January 8, 2017

39 Hearing Aid Prescriptive Methods in an Adult Patient

Jacqueline Busen

39.1 Clinical History and Description

AZ is a long-term hearing aid user who self-referred to the audiology clinic for hearing aid reprogramming. AZ reported difficulty understanding speech, hearing in the presence of background noise, and hearing while using the telephone. Due to concerns of hearing becoming progressively poorer, a comprehensive audiologic evaluation was recommended and performed. AZ was counseled on a hierarchy of treatment options. Ultimately, he requested that his current hearing aids be reprogrammed. Initially, electroacoustic analysis was completed on his current hearing aids to determine if both hearing aids met the American National Standards Institution (ANSI S3.22–2009) specification.[1] Then, AZ's hearing aids were reprogrammed using Real-Ear Measures (REM) to NAL-NL2 (National Acoustics Laboratories' nonlinear fitting procedure, version 2)[2] and Desired Sensation Level v5.0 (DSL v5.0) for adult and child.[3] Upon completion of reprogramming to NAL-NL2 and DSL v5.0 for adults and then children, AZ indicated a preference for the fitting using the DSL v5.0 for child target.

39.2 Audiological Testing

▶ Fig. 39.1 reports the results of AZ's audiologic examination. The audiological examination was obtained with good reliability and validity and revealed a bilateral symmetrical mild to profound sensorineural hearing loss at 250 to 8,000 Hz with no measureable hearing at 6,000 to 8,000 Hz. The speech recognition thresholds revealed a moderate loss in the ability to receive speech in each ear and were in agreement with the pure-tone averages. Word Recognition Scores (WRS) were assessed using the **computer-assisted speech perception assessment**. An averaged WRS was obtained using three lists at each presentation level in each ear. Results revealed very poor ability to recognize speech at two input levels in each ear. Compared to an audiologic examination 3 years earlier, the results from the current evaluation revealed a significant decrease in hearing sensitivity at 2,000 Hz in the right ear and at 6,000 to 8,000 Hz in both ears. Immittance audiometry revealed normal middle ear pressure, ear canal volume, and static admittance in each ear. The ipsilateral and contralateral Acoustic Reflex Thresholds (ARTs) were present at 500 to 2,000 Hz at reduced Sensation Levels (SL), suggesting the hearing loss to be cochlear in origin. ARTs were absent at 4,000 Hz, which is related to the magnitude of hearing loss at that frequency. Acoustic reflex decay was negative at 500 and 1,000 Hz in each ear.

Because AZ reported hearing difficulties in background noise, the Quick Speech-in-Noise (QuickSIN)[4] was administered during this same appointment. AZ's QuickSIN Signal-to-Noise Ratio Hearing Loss (SNRHL) was 20 dB. This result suggests that maximum improvement in the SNR is required,[4] which included directional microphones plus Hearing Assistive Technology (HAT) because hearing aids alone would not sufficiently improve his performance in a noisy listening environment.

39.3 Questions for the Reader

1. **Based on AZ's significant decrease in hearing sensitivity over the course of 3 years, what recommendation should be made prior to any further audiologic treatment?**
2. **Based on AZ's current hearing loss and his reports of specific hearing difficulties while taking the case history, what treatment options should the audiologist counsel AZ to consider?**
3. **Based on AZ's decreased hearing, what changes could an audiologist make to AZ's hearing aids?**
4. **Should an audiologist complete any additional testing of the hearing aids?**

39.4 Discussion of Questions

1. **Based on AZ's significant decrease in hearing sensitivity over the course of 3 years, what recommendation should be made prior to any further audiologic treatment?**

Due to the significant change in AZ's hearing at 2,000 Hz in the right ear and 6,000 to 8,000 Hz in each ear over 3 years, it was recommended that AZ be referred to an otologist for a medical evaluation prior to reprogramming his hearing aids. The otologist examined AZ and referred him for a magnetic resonance image (MRI). Based on the report from AZ's otologist, no abnormalities were noted on the examination or MRI. AZ was referred back to the audiologist to counsel on treatment options.

2. **Based on AZ's current hearing loss and his reports of specific hearing difficulties while taking the case history, what treatment options should the audiologist counsel AZ to consider?**

At the follow-up hearing aid evaluation, AZ was counseled on the following potential treatment options:

- Reprogramming his hearing aids to meet a valid prescriptive target.
- Purchasing new hearing aids with improved signal processing, availability of a wireless remote microphone without the need of an intermediary streamer. Also, with some current smartphone applications, it is possible to stream the signal from his phone directly to his hearing aids, allowing for bilateral listening during telephone communication. Recall that one of AZ's reports was difficulty when communicating on the phone.
- Cochlear implant evaluation.
- Additional options of HAT.

At the author's clinic, the most cost-effective option for AZ was to have his current hearing aids reprogrammed based on his change in hearing. Due to the age of his hearing aids, as described earlier, AZ was also counseled on updated technology that would be available to him if he were to purchase new hearing aids. Further, based on AZ's poor word recognition ability

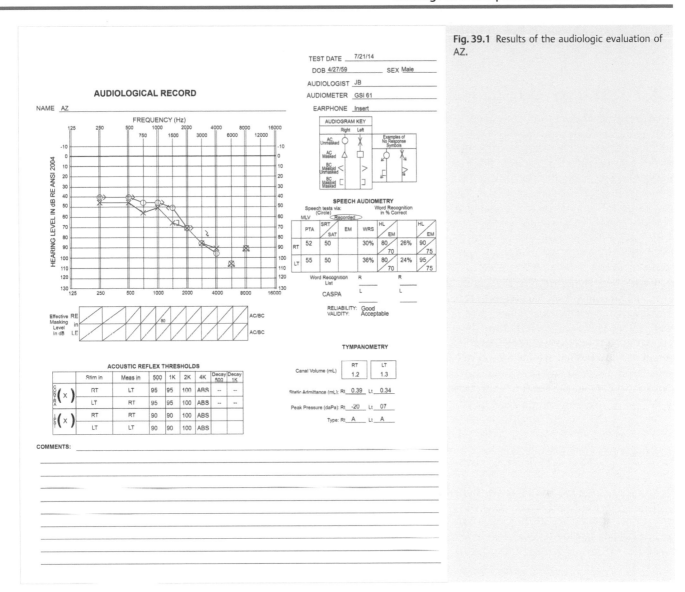

Fig. 39.1 Results of the audiologic evaluation of AZ.

and his audiologic thresholds, AZ should be counseled about potential cochlear implant candidacy. While cochlear implant candidacy requirements differ for each manufacturer, AZ may be a candidate for a cochlear implant in one or both ears. To assess his candidacy, aided speech testing using a sentence measure, such as the AZBio, must be completed.[5,6] This testing should take place after his hearing aids are reprogrammed based on his hearing changes to ensure that AZ is evaluated using his best aided performance. After the hearing aid reprogramming, it was recommended that AZ schedule a cochlear implant evaluation; however, this has not taken place at the time of preparing this case report.

HAT technology was also discussed with AZ due to his reported difficulties hearing in background noise and his Quick-SIN results. Currently, when AZ is in background noise, he manually changes to a "noise" program with directional microphones and the noise reduction algorithm is activated. AZ was counseled on the potential benefit that a wireless remote microphone or an FM (frequency modulated) system could provide. AZ was interested in this technology, but preferred to proceed with reprogramming his hearing aids and possibly a cochlear implant evaluation prior to pursuing these other options.

3. **Based on AZ's decreased hearing, what changes could an audiologist make to AZ's hearing aids?**

AZ's hearing aids should be reprogrammed using REM to meet a prescriptive target using his most recent hearing thresholds. While it is known that AZ may need greater gain at the frequencies where his hearing decreased, the most appropriate procedure is to reprogram his hearing aids to a prescriptive target based on his most recent audiometric results.[7] Prescriptive methods are algorithms that consider the patient's hearing loss and other demographic information to provide target gain or output settings for the "average" patient. Prescriptive targets are an excellent starting point, after which fine-tuning can be utilized to appropriately reprogram AZ's hearing aids.[8]

4. **Should an audiologist complete any additional testing of the hearing aids?**

Since AZ has not been seen for a hearing aid appointment in several years, electroacoustic analysis of each hearing aid was recommended and completed to ensure that the hearing aids were meeting manufacturer specifications and performing how they performed at previous visits.[7] To reprogram the hearing aids to a target-based prescriptive method, REM using speech-mapping measurements was completed.[7]

39.5 Hearing Aid Programming

Electroacoustic analysis was completed to determine if AZ's hearing aids were meeting the ANSI S3.22–2009 specifications.[1] All measurements were within the ANSI specifications provided by the hearing aid manufacturer. The maximum output, the high-frequency maximum output, the high-frequency full-on gain, and the total harmonic distortion were all within manufacturer specifications. This indicated that AZ's hearing aids were working properly and did not require any service or repair at the time of the appointment.

Real-ear-to-coupler difference measurements were completed in each ear and AZ's hearing aids were then reprogrammed to meet the NAL-NL2 targets for input levels of 50, 65, and 75 dB sound pressure level (SPL; ▶ Fig. 39.2).[2] After reprogramming to NAL-NL2, AZ indicated that his hearing aids were "too quiet." AZ reported that the loud presentation level (i.e., 75 dB SPL) was "most comfortable" when his response should have been "loud, but OK," while the average (65 dB SPL) and soft (50 dB SPL) input levels were both judged as "too soft." After a brief discussion of other prescriptive formulas, AZ agreed to try being reprogrammed using the DSL v5.0 for child target (▶ Fig. 39.3).[3] DSL v5.0 for child target was selected because this provides greater output than the DSL v5.0 for adult

target. After reprogramming to the DSL V5.0 for child targets, AZ indicated that the sound quality and loudness were significantly better NAL-NL2.

39.6 Additional Questions for the Reader

1. **When should electroacoustic analysis measurements be completed?**
2. **What are the primary differences between NAL-NL2 and DSL v5.0 targets?**

39.7 Discussion of Additional Questions

1. **When should electroacoustic analysis measurements be completed?**

Electroacoustic analysis should be completed before fitting new hearing aids as a means of quality control.[7] Initial measures can serve as a benchmark for future visits. Electroacoustic analysis should also be completed after patients decide they will keep their hearing aid(s) and any time the audiologist suspects there may be a problem with the hearing aid(s). If a patient complains that their hearing aids sound weak or require adjustment, an audiologist should first complete an electroacoustic analysis to determine if the

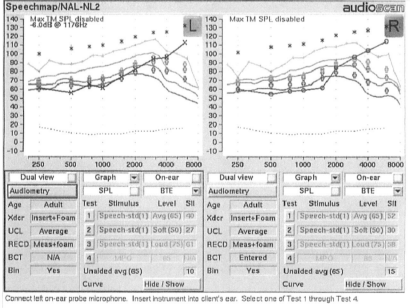

Fig. 39.2 Speechmap obtained for NSL-NL2 (National Acoustics Laboratory's nonlinear fitting procedure, version 2) prescriptive method. Real-ear measures at input levels of 50, 65, and 75 dB SPL for AZ for his left and right hearing aids for NAL-NL2.

		250	500	750	1K	1K5	2K	3K	4K	6K	8K	10K	12K5
HL	L	45	45	55	50	65	70	85	90	105			
	R	40	40	45	45	50	70	85	95	105			
UCL	L												
	R												
BCT	L												
	R	40	40	45	45	50	70	85	95	105			
RECD (HA-1)	L	2	4	4	5	7	10	12	12	15			
	R	6	7	7	8	10	13	14	15	16			
WRECD	L												
	R												
Hz		250	500	750	1K	1K5	2K	3K	4K	6K	8K	10K	12K5

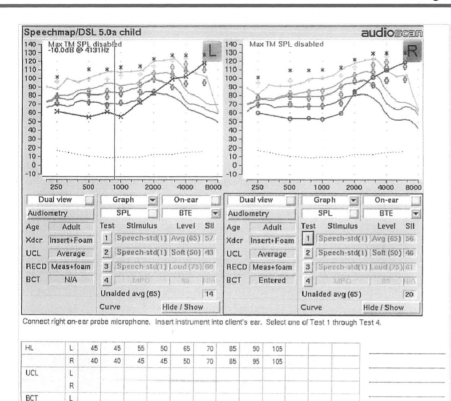

Fig. 39.3 Speechmap obtained foe DSL v5.0 (Desired Sensation Level v5.0) child prescriptive method. Real-ear measures at input levels of 50, 65, and 75 dB SPL for AZ for his left and right hearing aids for DSL v5.0 for child target.

		250	500	750	1K	1K5	2K	3K	4K	6K	8K	10K	12K5
HL	L	45	45	55	50	65	70	85	90	105			
	R	40	40	45	45	50	70	85	95	105			
UCL	L												
	R												
BCT	L												
	R	40	40	45	45	50	70	85	95	105			
RECD (HA-1)	L	2	4	4	5	7	10	12	12	15			
	R	6	7	7	8	10	13	14	15	16			
WRECD	L												
	R												
Hz		250	500	750	1K	1K5	2K	3K	4K	6K	8K	10K	12K5

Table 39.1 Comparison of DSL v5.0 and NAL-NL2 prescriptive methods[1]

	DSL v5.0	NAL-NL2
Patient's previous hearing aid experience	No changes	Increase in gain for experienced users Decrease in gain for new users
Patient's gender	No changes	1-dB increase in gain for males 1-dB decrease in gain for females
Bilateral fittings	3-dB decrease in gain for bilateral fittings	Bilateral gain correction that increases with input level
Listening in noise	Targets for speech are reduced by 3–5 dB for low importance frequencies for noise program	No changes
Corrections for conductive hearing loss	Raises the predicted uncomfortable levels (UCL) by 25% of the average air–bone gap, which raises the upper limit of the target input/output curve, resulting in small corrections for gain for most audiograms	First applies prescribed gain for the sensorineural component and then adds 75% of the air–bone gap to this value
Loudness discomfort levels (LDLs)	Will accept patient-specific LDLs; will alter its prescription of gain and output for not only high input levels that approximate the loudness discomfort measure, but also the desired output for average and soft output levels	Does not alter its prescription of gain and output at any input level based on LDLs

Abbreviations: DSL v5.0, Desired Sensation Level v5.0; NAL-NL2, National Acoustics Laboratories' nonlinear fitting procedure, version 2.

complaint is due to an issue with the hearing aids or with the programming of the aids.

2. What are the primary differences between NAL-NL2 and DSL v5.0 targets?

NAL-NL2 and DSL v5.0 are the two primary prescriptive approaches used to program hearing aids.[2,3] Each prescriptive approach represent revisions of previous versions. A brief outline of the primary differences between the two approaches is provided in ▶ Table 39.1. A comparison of the fitting targets for soft (55 dB SPL), average (65 dB SPL), and loud (75 dB SPL) input levels for NAL-NL2 and DSL v5.0 for AZ's left hearing aid are shown in ▶ Fig. 39.4. In addition, a comparison of the fitting targets for soft, average, and loud input levels for DSL v.50 for child

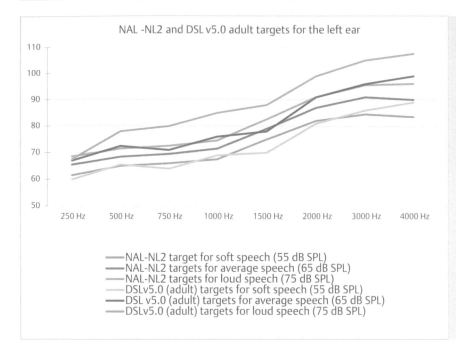

Fig. 39.4 Real ear aided response (REAR) for 50, 65, and 75 dB SPL for AZ for his left hearing aid for NAL-NL2 and DSL v5.0 for adult target.

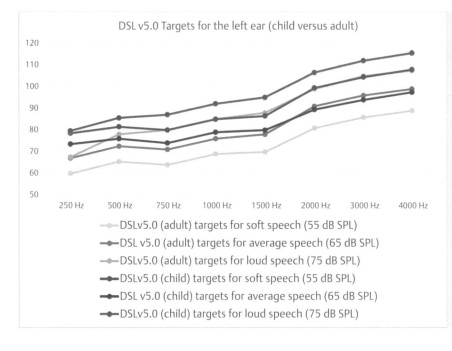

Fig. 39.5 Real ear aided response (REAR) for 50, 65, and 75 dB SPL for AZ for his left hearing aid for DSL v5.0 adult and child targets.

and adult targets for AZ left hearing aid is reported in ▶ Fig. 39.5. These figures clearly illustrate the greater output provided by the DSL v5.0 for child targets in comparison to the DSL v50 for adult and NAL-NL2 targets.

39.8 Outcome

AZ was pleased with the loudness and sound quality after being programmed to DSL v50 for child target. To minimize the impact of ambient noise, AZ required a decrease in output for the soft low-frequency input level. AZ is currently scheduled for a cochlear implant evaluation. He has been provided with literature to review before that appointment in order to familiarize AZ with the advantages and disadvantage of the available technologies.

39.9 Key Points

- This case illustrates the importance of annual audiologic examinations and medical referrals as part of the hearing aid–fitting process.
- It is important to fit to a prescriptive method when fitting hearing aids; however, individualizing fitting targets for each patient is beneficial. When AZ indicated that his reprogrammed hearing aids were still "too quiet" when reprogrammed to the NAL-NL2, reprogramming to DSL v5.0 for child target resulted in a more satisfactory outcome because of the increased output.
- The importance of keeping current with the most recent advancements in hearing aid technology and candidacy for

cochlear implants so that the highest level of care can be provided to patients.

- It is important to understand the differences between prescriptive targets in order to select the most appropriate target based on patient's preferences.

References

[1] American National Standards Institute. Specification of Hearing Aid Characteristics. New York, NY: American National Standards Institute; 2009

[2] Keidser G, Dillon H, Flax M, Ching T, Brewer S. The NAL-NL2 prescription procedure. Audiology Res. 2011; 1(1):e24

[3] Scollie S, Seewald R, Cornelisse L, et al. The desired sensation level multistage input/output algorithm. Trends Amplif. 2005; 9(4):159–197

[4] Killion MC, Niquette PA, Gudmundsen GI, Revit LJ, Banerjee S. Development of a quick speech-in-noise test for measuring signal-to-noise ratio loss in normal-hearing and hearing-impaired listeners. J Acoust Soc Am. 2004; 116(4, Pt 1):2395–2405

[5] Spahr AJ, Dorman MF, Litvak LM, et al. Development and validation of the AzBio sentence lists. Ear Hear. 2012; 33(1):112–117

[6] New Minimum Speech Test Battery (MSTB) for Adult Cochlear Implant Users. 2011

[7] Valente M, Abram H, Benson D, et al. Guidelines for the audiologic management of adult hearing impairment. AudiolToday. 2006; 18(5):1–44

[8] Bentler R, Mueller G, Ricketts T. Modern Hearing Aids: Verification, Outcome Measures, and Follow-Up. San Diego, CA: Plural Publishing, Inc.; 2016

Suggested Readings

[1] Keidser G, Dillon H, Carter L, O'Brien A. NAL-NL2 empirical adjustments. Trends Amplif. 2012; 16(4):211–223

[2] Polonenko MJ, Scollie SD, Moodie S, et al. Fit to targets, preferred listening levels, and self-reported outcomes for the DSL v5.0 a hearing aid prescription for adults. Int J Audiol. 2010; 49(8):550–560

[3] Dillon H. Hearing Aids. 2nd ed. New York, NY: Thieme Publishers; 2012:286–335

40 Quick Fit versus Programming Hearing Aid Fittings: Acoustic and Perceptual Differences

Amyn M. Amlani

40.1 Clinical History and Description

This case demonstrates acoustic and perceptual differences between the Quick-Fit and programmed real-ear protocols in a hearing aid fitting.

AQ is a 56-year-old man seeking an audiologist to assess his hearing sensitivity. AQ, a social worker, reported a gradual decline over the past few years in his ability to communicate, especially in environments with competing background noise as well as when using the telephone. He further reported a history of noise exposure from previously serving in the military, regular firearm use, the occasional use of power tools, and daily use of earbuds while listening to streamed music. The patient reported that previous audiologic testing performed 30 years prior while he served in the military revealed hearing sensitivity to be within normal limits. All other audiologic, medical, and family history was unremarkable.

40.2 Audiologic Testing

▶ Fig. 40.1 reports the results of AQ's most recent audiologic assessment. Pure-tone testing revealed a bilateral symmetrical mild to moderate severe gradually sloping sensorineural hearing loss. Speech recognition thresholds indicated a mild loss in the ability to receive speech and were consistent with the pure-tone average. AQ's word recognition scores indicated normal ability to recognize speech in the right and left ears. Immittance audiometry revealed normal ear canal volume, static admittance, and middle ear pressure for the right and left ears. Acoustic Reflex Thresholds (ARTs) were within normal limits bilaterally, with the exception of slightly elevated ARTs at 2,000 and 4,000 Hz for left ipsilateral stimulation and 4,000 Hz for left contralateral stimulation.

At the audiometric evaluation, the audiologist calculated AQ's audibility using the $A_o(6)$ method.[1] Using this method, audibility is quantified from 0.00 to 1.00 with values closer to 0.00 representing no availability of speech cues and 1.00 representing the availability of all the speech cues. Audibility can also be reported as a percentage and derived by simply multiplying the audibility value by 100 (e.g., audibility = 0.61 or 61% [0.61 × 100]). The $A_o(6)$ method quantifies audibility based on the audiometric thresholds at octave and mid-octave frequencies between 250 and 6,000 Hz under the premise that speech cues important to speech recognition range are between 20 and 50 dB HL (i.e., 30 dB dynamic range of speech). The speech cues are premised on speech stimuli presented in quiet, spoken with normal vocal effort, and at a distance of 1 m from the listener. Together, the overall presentation level of speech is presumed to be 65 dB Sound Pressure Level (SPL), as measured in sound field.

To illustrate the clinical application of $A_o(6)$, the audiologist noted that the unaided earphone threshold of the right ear in ▶ Fig. 40.1 at 500 Hz is 20 dB HL. At this frequency, all 30 dB of audibility (i.e., 50 – 20 dB HL) is available to the listener. On the other hand, at 1,000, 2,000, 3,000, 4,000, and 6,000 Hz, audibility is 15, 5, 0, 0, and 10 dB, respectively. The amount of available speech information to AQ is 0.44, or 44% (▶ Table 40.1). The amount of audibility available to AQ in the unaided condition was derived by summing the amount of audibility at the three lower frequencies (i.e., 30 + 15 + 5 = 50) and adding it to the average audibility in the three higher frequencies (i.e., [0 + 0 + 10]/3 = 3.3). Together, these values equal 53.3 (i.e., 50 + 3.3), which is then divided by 120, or the maximum number of audible decibels (see Box 24.1 (p. 206) for details), yielding 0.44 (i.e., 53.3/120) or 44% (i.e., [53.3/120] × 100). For additional assistance with this calculation, the reader is referred to Amlani et al.[2]

> **Box 24.1**
>
> The precursor to the Ao(6) procedure was the Ao(4) procedure, which weighted speech using octave bands at the frequencies between 500 and 4,000 Hz. Because the Ao(6) procedure maintains the octave band speech weightings, thresholds from the mid-octaves of 3,000 and 6,000 Hz are averaged together with thresholds from the octave band at 4,000 Hz.

AQ was counseled on the results of his audiologic evaluation and agreed to a trial period with a pair of smartphone-enabled receiver-in-the-canal hearing aids with open domes, as well as a wireless remote microphone. The inclusion of the remote microphone was to improve AQ's ability to hear speech in environments with competing noise. Also, by using the smartphone application, telephone calls via his cellphone are now wirelessly streamed to each hearing aid to address the concern raised by AQ that he noticed increased difficulty communicating on the telephone.

Prior to the initial hearing aid fitting, the audiologist measured the performance of the hearing aids in a HA1 2-mL coupler to confirm that the electroacoustic properties of the hearing aids met the manufacturer American National Standards Institution (ANSI-2009) specifications. Memory 1 of the hearing aids was then programmed to the NAL-NL2 (National Acoustics Laboratories' nonlinear fitting procedure, version 2) prescriptive target[3] by selecting the "target" icon (i.e., Quick-Fit) in the manufacturer's software and all features (e.g., directional microphones, noise reduction, and spectral enhancement) and any additional memories were disabled. At the time of the fitting, AQ was counseled on the use and maintenance of the devices and provided communication strategies. AQ was then fitted with the devices with no additional testing and was scheduled to return in 1 week for a follow-up appointment. At the follow-up appointment, AQ informed the audiologist that the devices did not improve his ability to understand speech and that he wished to terminate the trial period.

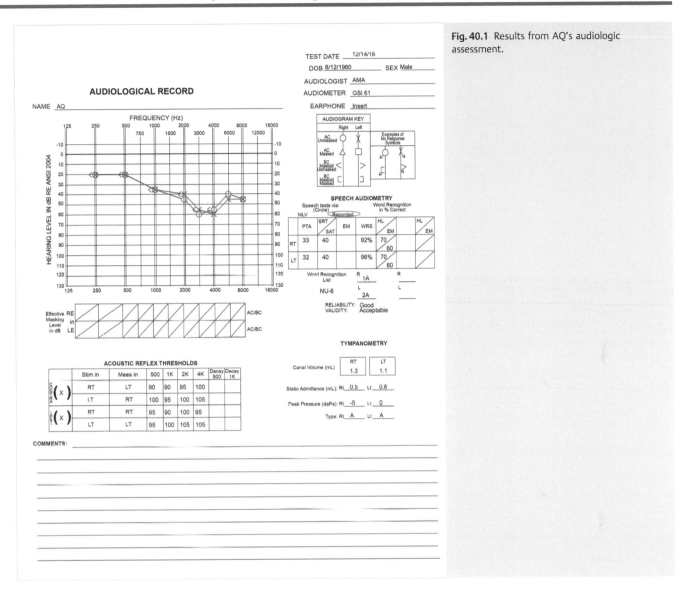

Fig. 40.1 Results from AQ's audiologic assessment.

Table 40.1 Audibility calculation unaided and for a hearing aid programmed using the Quick-Fit approach for a 65 dB SPL input signal

		Frequency (Hz)					
		500	1,000	2,000	3,000	4,000	6,000
A. Audibility calculation	Unaided threshold	20	35	45	60	55	40
		30	15	5	0	0	10
		0.44					
B. Convert dB HL to dB SPL	Thresholds (dB HL)	20	35	45	60	55	40
	MAP corrections	+10	+9	+13	+13	+15	+16
	Thresholds (dB SPL)	30	44	58	73	70	56
C. REAR and REIG (65-dB-SPL input)	REAR: measured	31.7	51.7	74.6	86.3	85.9	68.7
	REIG: measured	0	0.9	4.3	5.7	6.7	2.2
D. Calculate aided threshold	Thresholds (dB HL)	20	35	45	60	55	40
	REIG	0	−0.9	−4.3	−5.7	−6.7	−2.2
	Aided threshold	20	34.1	40.7	54.3	48.3	37.8
E. Audibility calculation	Aided threshold	20	34.1	40.7	54.3	48.3	37.8
	Audibility	30	15.9	9.3	0	1.7	12.2
	$A_0(6)$ method: aided	0.60					

Abbreviations: MAP, minimum audible pressure; REAR, real-ear aided response; REIG, real-ear insertion gain.

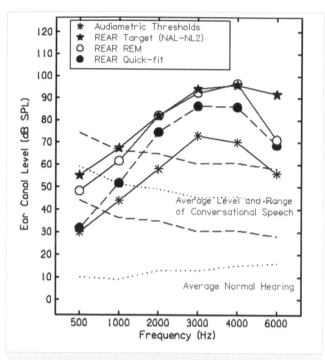

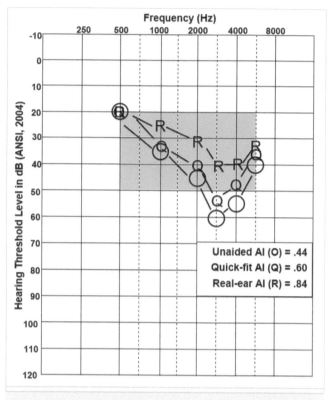

Fig. 40.2 Audiometric thresholds, converted to dB SPL (decibel sound pressure level) at the ear canal (*asterisks*), along with real-ear aided responses (REAR) for the NAL-NL2 (National Acoustics Laboratories' nonlinear fitting procedure, version 2) target (*filled stars*), REAR obtained using the REM (real-ear measurement) approach (*open circles*), and REAR obtained using the Quick-Fit approach (*filled circles*). Also represented is the average normal hearing curve (*square dotted line*), and the average level (*round-dotted line*) and range of conversational speech (*dashed lines*).

Fig. 40.3 Audiogram representation of audibility in the right ear, calculated using the $A_o(6)$ method, unaided (*O*), real-ear measurement (REM) obtained for the Quick-Fit approach (*Q*), and REM obtained for the programming approach (*R*).

40.3 Questions for the Reader

1. **Why did AQ report the hearing aids hindered his ability to understand speech?**
2. **How would employing Real-Ear Measurement (REM) have aided the audiologist in overcoming the limitations provided by Quick-Fit?**
3. **How could programming using REM improve the likelihood of AQ adopting amplification?**

40.4 Discussion of Questions

1. **Why did AQ report the hearing aids hindered his ability to understand speech?**

▶ Fig. 40.2 illustrates the amplification received at AQ's eardrum of his right ear. Note that the asterisks in the middle of ▶ Fig. 40.2 report AQ's audiometric thresholds converted to dB SPL using minimum audible pressure transformation values[4] (denoted by the asterisks and calculated in ▶ Table 40.1). Also reported in ▶ Fig. 40.2 is the target for the NAL-NL2 Real-Ear Aided Response (REAR) for a 65-dB-SPL input level (represented by the filled stars) for a binaural fitting. The measured REAR provided by the manufacturer's Quick-Fit formula is characterized by the closed circles in ▶ Fig. 40.2. Note that the manufacturer REAR significantly under-amplified the prescribed NAL-

NL2 target at every test frequency. Research indicates that using the Quick-Fit approach can deviate from the prescribed target by greater than 10 dB.[5] When aided audibility was calculated using the Quick-Fit approach, results revealed that the Quick-Fit approach resulted in a value of 0.60 (▶ Table 40.1), or a 0.16 increase in audibility compared to the unaided condition (i.e., 0.44).

Audibility was derived by subtracting the real-ear insertion gain (REIG; see Box 24.2 (p.208] for converting REAR to REIG) provided by the real-ear analyzer (section C in ▶ Table 40.1) and, had REM been performed, from AQ's earphone thresholds (▶ Fig. 40.1; first row in ▶ Table 40.1).

> ### Box 24.2
>
> Real-ear insertion gain (REIG) is derived by transforming real-ear aided response (REAR) data to REAG (minus input signal [obtained at 65 dB in this example]) and subtracting the patient's real-ear unaided gain [REUG]). This transformation results in REIG (i.e., REIG = REAG – REUG), which is then subtracted, when REIG is positive, from unaided thresholds.

These data are replotted on an audiogram and labeled as **Q** in ▶ Fig. 40.3. This represents the predicted aided sound-field thresholds at 250 to 6,000 Hz using the Quick-Fit formula.

Table 40.2 Audibility calculation unaided and for a hearing aid programmed using the real-ear approach

		Frequency (Hz)					
		500	1,000	2,000	3,000	4,000	6,000
A. Audibility calculation	Unaided threshold	20	35	45	60	55	40
	Audibility	30	15	5	0	0	10
	$A_o(6)$ method: unaided	0.44					
B. Convert dB HL to dB SPL	Thresholds (dB HL)	20	35	45	60	55	40
	MAP corrections	+10	+9	+13	+13	+15	+16
	Thresholds (dB SPL)	30	44	58	73	70	56
C. REAR and REIG (65-dB-SPL input)	REAR: measured	48.2	61.6	82.1	92.3	96.5	71.1
	REIG: measured	0	8.7	14.6	18.8	13.9	4.7
D. Calculate aided threshold	Thresholds (dB HL)	20	35	45	60	55	40
	REIG	0	−8.7	−14.6	−18.8	−13.9	−4.7
	Aided threshold	20	26.3	30.4	41.2	41.1	35.3
E. Audibility calculation	Aided threshold	20	26.3	30.4	41.2	41.1	35.3
	Audibility	30	23.7	19.6	8.8	8.9	14.7
	$A_o(6)$ method: aided	0.84					

Abbreviations: MAP, minimum audible pressure; REAR, real-ear aided response; REIG, real-ear insertion gain.

2. **How would employing REM have aided the audiologist in overcoming the limitations provided by Quick-Fit?**

Performing REM would have resulted in increased audibility because REM would have afforded the audiologist the information needed to program the hearing aid's REAR to meet the prescribed NAL-NL2 target. The open circles in ▶ Fig. 40.2 represent the measured REAR programmed by the audiologist. Note that the programmed REAR matched target between 2,000 and 4,000 Hz. Because of the open fit, the frequencies ≤ 1,000 Hz do not meet the NAL-NL2 target because the amplified sound is exiting the ear canal through the open dome. A recalculation of aided audibility for the programmed REAR indicates a value of 0.84 (▶ Table 40.2), or an increase in audibility of 0.40 compared to the unaided condition (i.e., 0.44). In addition, the aided audibility for the programmed condition yielded an increase of 0.24 relative to the Quick-Fit approach (i.e., 0.60). Audibility (i.e., $A_o(6)$ method) for the real-ear approach is shown in ▶ Table 40.2, and represented on an audiogram as predicted aided sound-filed threshold as **R** in ▶ Fig. 40.3.

3. **How could programming using REM improve the likelihood of AQ adopting amplification?**

Recall that AQ terminated the trial period with amplification primarily because the audiologist failed to provide adequate aided audibility using the Quick-Fit approach. Had the audiologist initially programmed the hearing aids to the NAL-NL2 target using REM, AQ would have received increased aided audibility and increased the likelihood of adopting the hearing aids.

Often overlooked is that the protocol for fitting hearing aids goes beyond audibility. A recent study[6] assessed patient psychological perception in three groups of listeners (experienced users of hearing aids; patients owning hearing aids, but do not use them; and no experience with hearing aids) toward audiologic service for hearing aids fit using the Quick-Fit versus programmed approaches. Findings revealed that the programmed protocol, compared to the Quick-Fit protocol, improved the perception and confidence of the patient toward the provider and the quality of service received, as well as self-perception toward success with amplification. In short, programming hearing aids to a valid prescriptive target using REM enhanced the value of the experience of obtaining amplification. This potentially can lead to greater patient benefit with amplification, as well as increased satisfaction and loyalty to the provider and, ultimately, increase in the practice's revenue.

40.5 Key Points

- AQ experienced hearing difficulties and sought the assistance of an audiologist to provide treatment to overcome his communication difficulties.
- The audiologist provided hearing aids that could lessen AQ's communication difficulties, but used the Quick-Fit approach that provided less than adequate (1) aided audibility and (2) confidence in the audiologist's clinical skills to treat his hearing loss. As a result of this experience, AQ had a negative reaction toward his audiologist and possible benefit provided by hearing aids.
- This scenario could have been mitigated had the audiologist simply used REM to program the hearing aids to a valid prescriptive target, which would not only have probably yielded a satisfied patient, but could have also increased patient loyalty and referrals.

References

[1] Pavlovic CV. Articulation index predictions of speech intelligibility in hearing aid selection. ASHA. 1988; 30(6–7):63–65

[2] Amlani AM, Punch JL, Ching TY. Methods and applications of the audibility index in hearing aid selection and fitting. Trends Amplif. 2002; 6(3): 81–129

[3] Keidser G, Dillon H, Flax M, Ching T, Brewer S. The NAL-NL2 prescription procedure. Audiology Res. 2011; 1(1):e24

[4] Bentler RA, Pavlovic CV. Transfer functions and correction factors used in hearing aid evaluation and research. Ear Hear. 1989; 10(1):58–63

[5] Sanders J, Stoody T, Weber J, Mueller HG. Manufacturers' NAL-NL2 fittings fail real-ear verification. Hear Rev.. 2015; 21(3):24–32

[6] Amlani AM, Pumford J, Gessling E. Improving patient perception of clinical services through real-ear measurements. Hear Rev.. 2016; 23(12):12–16

Suggested Readings

[1] Aazh H, Moore BC, Prasher D. The accuracy of matching target insertion gains with open-fit hearing aids. Am J Audiol. 2012; 21(2):175–180

[2] Abrams HB, Chisolm TH, McManus M, McArdle R. Initial-fit approach versus verified prescription: comparing self-perceived hearing aid benefit. J Am Acad Audiol. 2012; 23(10):768–778

[3] Mueller HG. 20Q: real-ear probe-microphone measures-30 years of progress? AudiologyOnline, Article 12410. Available at: http://www.audiologyonline.com

41 Fitting Hearing Aids to a Patient with Mild Hearing Loss

Steven Smith and Brianna Schmitt

41.1 Clinical History and Description

NH is a 67-year-old woman who returned for an annual audiometric evaluation. In the previous audiometric evaluation, NH stated difficulty understanding speech in noise; however, she did not feel she experienced sufficient difficulty to warrant intervention. Upon returning for her annual evaluation, NH noticed greater difficulty with hearing, especially in noise. NH stated she is asking people to repeat more often and thinks it might be time to consider hearing aids. She reported tinnitus bilaterally that is more noticeable in her right ear. NH reported occasional dizziness and vertigo, but feels this may be related to the medication, which was previously discussed with her primary care physician. NH denied otalgia or aural fullness as well as noise exposure.

41.2 Audiologic Testing

NH underwent a comprehensive audiometric examination (▶ Fig. 41.1). Testing in the right ear revealed a slight Sensori-Neural Hearing Loss (SNHL) from 250 to 3,000 Hz, sloping to mild SNHL at 4,000 Hz, rising to slight SNHL at 6,000 Hz, and then sloping to a mild SNHL at 8,000 Hz. Results for the left ear revealed normal to slight SNHL from 250 to 2,000 Hz, sloping to mild SNHL from 3,000 to 4,000 Hz, sloping to moderate SNHL at 6,000 Hz, and then rising to a mild SNHL at 8,000 Hz. Speech recognition thresholds revealed a slight loss in the ability to receive speech in each ear. Word recognition scores revealed normal ability to recognize speech bilaterally. Tympanograms revealed normal ear canal volume, static compliance, and middle ear pressure bilaterally. Acoustic reflex thresholds were present and normal for ipsilateral and contralateral stimulation at 500 to 4,000 Hz bilaterally. Acoustic reflex decay was negative from 500 Hz and 1,000 Hz for each ear. A slight decrease in hearing thresholds of 15 dB HL were noted in the right ear at 4,000 and 6,000 Hz from the previous evaluation.

41.3 Questions for the Reader

1. **How much hearing loss should be present before hearing aids can be expected to provide benefit?**
2. **How important is verification for a successful hearing aid fitting?**
3. **How can one measure the successful use of hearing aids?**

41.4 Discussion of Questions

1. **How much hearing loss should be present before hearing aids can be expected to provide benefit?**

A clinician may review the audiometric results in ▶ Fig. 41.1 and conclude there is insufficient hearing loss for NH to notice or achieve benefit from hearing aids. Some clinicians may view

NH as a patient who may return the hearing aids for credit due to lack of sufficient benefit. The magnitude of hearing loss required for successful use with hearing aids is very subjective. Many clinicians who dispense hearing aids and care for adult patients use 25 dB HL as the "cutoff" for normal hearing. Using those criteria, NH has very minimal hearing loss. No prior data, however, are available for the past 5 or 10 years. It is possible that hearing thresholds were normal at that time. Therefore, NH could be noticing threshold changes of approximately 20 dB HL in the lower frequencies and 30 dB HL in the higher frequencies since she had her hearing initially evaluated. In this case, NH reported she is experiencing sufficient difficulty that she is interested in how hearing aids may assist her with her hearing concerns. As long as realistic expectations are maintained throughout the process of the hearing aid counseling and fitting, the patient may notice benefit and increased quality of life from using hearing aid technology. When fitting individuals with minimal hearing loss, the clinician must strongly consider patient motivation. If the patient is highly motivated, a higher rate of success will be obtained. If there is minimal motivation, there may be an increased probability of dissatisfaction. When this occurs, the patient may wait many years before trying amplification again. In addition to this, a patient may perpetuate the idea that hearing aids do not function well and share this opinion with those around him or her, thus affecting how others may perceive the benefits of hearing aids. As a clinician, it is important to recognize when a patient is motivated or not motivated to pursue amplification.

2. **How important is verification for a successful hearing aid fitting?**

The selection of appropriate hearing aid technology is part of the overall solution when fitting hearing aids. Just as important, however, is the use of Real-Ear Measurements (REM). The typical procedure that is followed when fitting hearing aids is to enter the patient's audiometric results into the manufacturer's Noah module. The manufacturer Noah module applies prescribed gain or output to the hearing aids dependent on the severity of the entered hearing loss at each frequency. How much gain or output that is applied may be different for each manufacturer and will depend on the manufacturer's proprietary formula (i.e., manufacturer first-fit). Many audiologists take these formulas at face value when programming hearing aids and are not using REM.[1] In essence, the audiologist assumes that the fitting formula is providing sufficient gain or output for the patient. It has been demonstrated in numerous studies that this method of fitting hearing aids is not providing sufficient gain/output in the high frequencies that are important for speech understanding.[2,3] REM must be performed for all patients to verify the amount of gain/output provided by hearing aids.

Verification measures are performed through the use of a real-ear analyzer having a reference microphone and probe tube connected to a probe microphone on the ear to be tested. A probe microphone assembly is placed above the aided ear and includes a reference microphone and a probe tube from a probe microphone placed in the ear canal 4 to 6 mm from the

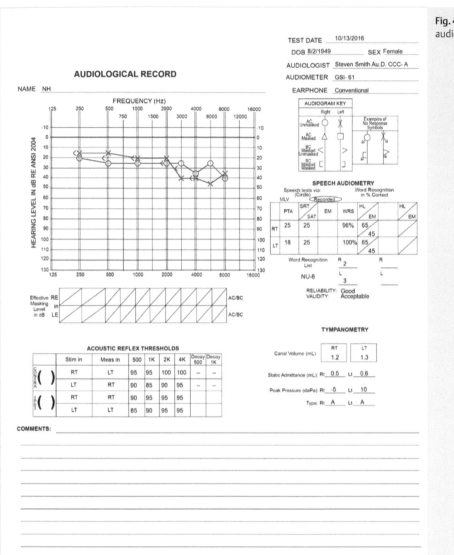

Fig. 41.1 Results from NH's comprehensive audiometric examination.

eardrum. At this point, the reference and probe microphone are calibrated. Once this is completed, the unaided ear canal resonance may be measured. The ear canal resonance is used to assist in calculating the real-ear insertion gain (REIG) once the hearing aid is placed in the ear canal. The hearing aid is then inserted into the ear canal and measurements are obtained of hearing aid performance in real time and the REIG or real-ear aided response is measured. Through this method, the gain/output can be programmed to increase or decrease at any frequency region depending upon the number of frequency bands available for programming to better "fit" the hearing aid to the prescriptive target. Both American Academy of Audiology (AAA)[4] and the American Speech-Language-Hearing Association (ASHA)[5] have endorsed using REM as components for best practice. When REM is not performed, optimal results may not be obtained, leading to unnecessary adjustments as well as frustration to the patient and clinician.

3. How can one measure the successful use of hearing aids?

Determining if hearing aid use is successful is best performed through the utilization of objective and subjective measures.

Prior to the fitting of hearing aids, questionnaires can be administered to the patient regarding subjective judgments of the impact of hearing loss. Many validated questionnaires such as the COSI[6] (Client Oriented Scale of Improvement) and COAT[7] (Characteristics of Amplification Tool) can assist the clinician to obtain a greater understanding of hearing needs and wishes of the patient. These questionnaires can provide meaningful information from the patient in terms of hearing difficulties. After fitting the hearing aids and allowing a period of time to adjust to amplification, these questionnaires can be repeated to determine subjective benefit or satisfaction with the hearing aids (i.e., aided – unaided = benefit). This provides helpful subjective data to the patient as well as to the clinician regarding hearing aid benefit/satisfaction and if the hearing aids achieved the stated goals as expressed by the patient. Independent surveys such as EARTrack[8] have been proven effective in measuring patient satisfaction. Patients are provided with the independent survey either on paper or online. Once performed by the patient, these data can be analyzed for satisfaction with amplification and used to improve quality of care.

Objective benefit can also be measured through the use of speech in noise testing. One method of obtaining this information is through using the Quick Speech-in-Noise (QuickSIN).[9] This test can be performed relatively quickly. The QuickSIN presents sentences to the patient either through headphones or in the sound field along with a four-talker babble. When each sentence is presented, the level of the noise is increased by 5 dB HL until a 0-dB Signal-to-Noise Ratio Hearing Loss (SNRHL) is achieved. Keywords are used to score each sentence (i.e., number of underlined words correctly identified). The score for each of the six sentences in each list is summed and subtracted from 25.5 dB to obtain the SNRHL for the patient (▶ Fig. 41.2). An SNRHL of 0 to 2 dB is considered normal or near normal, 2 to 7 dB a mild SNRHL, 7 to 15 dB a moderate SNRHL, and greater than 15 dB a severe SNRHL. One of the goals is to determine the deficit in hearing in noise for a patient and provide useful information in the intervention for that patient. For example, if a patient has a 9.5-dB SNRHL, this would suggest the need of hearing aids plus the addition of a Hearing Assistive Technology (HAT) such as a remote microphone to improve the SNRHL to as close to 0 dB as possible. In our clinic, when performing the QuickSIN in sound field, the patient is placed in the sound field with sentences presented at 0 degrees and the noise presented at 180 degrees. The QuickSIN can be performed prior to the fitting of hearing aids (i.e., unaided) and after an adjustment period (i.e., aided), where the difference can determine improvement in aided hearing in noise. Depending on the magnitude of improvement, appropriate counseling can be provided regarding realistic expectations in noise as well as additional intervention in the form of a remote microphone or HAT.

QUICKSIN – Unaided

List 1 – Track 24   Score

1. A white silk-jacket goes with any shoes. — S/N 25 — 0
2. The child crawled into the dense grass. — S/N 20 — 0
3. Footprints showed the path he took up the beach. — S/N 15 — 4
4. A vent near the edge brought in fresh air. — S/N 10 — 0
5. It is a band of steel three inches wide. — S/N 5 — 1
6. The weight of the package was seen on the high scale. — S/N 0 — 3
   25.5 – TOTAL = 17.5 dB SNR Loss

List 2 – Track 25

1. Tear a thin sheet from the yellow pad. — S/N 25 — 0
2. A cruise in warm waters in a sleek yacht is fun. — S/N 20 — 5
3. A streak of color ran down the left edge. — S/N 15 — 3
4. It was done before the boy could see it. — S/N 10 — 0
5. Crouch before you jump or miss the mark. — S/N 5 — 0
6. The square peg will settle in the round hole. — S/N 0 — 0
   25.5 – TOTAL = 17.5 dB SNR Loss

List 6 – Track 29

1. The leaf drifts along with a slow spin. — S/N 25 — 3
2. The pencil was cut to be sharp at both ends. — S/N 20 — 0
3. Down that road is the way to the grain farmer. — S/N 15 — 0
4. The best method is to fix it in place with clips. — S/N 10 — 0
5. If you mumble your speech will be lost. — S/N 5 — 0
6. A toad and a frog are hard to tell apart. — S/N 0 — 3
   25.5 – TOTAL = 19.5 dB SNR Loss

Average: 18.17 dB

QUICKSIN Aided

List 8 – Track 31

1. The sun came up to light the eastern sky. — S/N 25 — 5
2. The stale smell of old beer lingers. — S/N 20 — 4
3. The desk was firm on the shaky floor. — S/N 15 — 5
4. A list of names is carved around the base. — S/N 10 — 5
5. The news struck doubt into restless minds. — S/N 5 — 1
6. The sand drifts over the sill of the old house. — S/N 0 — 0
   25.5 – TOTAL = 5.5 dB SNR Loss

List 10 – Track 33

1. Dots of light betrayed the black cat. — S/N 25 — 5
2. Put the chart on the mantel and tack it down. — S/N 20 — 5
3. The steady drip is worse than a drenching rain. — S/N 15 — 4
4. A flat pack takes less luggage space. — S/N 10 — 5
5. The gloss on top made it unfit to read. — S/N 5 — 4
6. Seven seals were stamped on great sheets. — S/N 0 — 3
   25.5 – TOTAL = -0.5 dB SNR Loss

List 11 – Track 34

1. The marsh will freeze when cold enough. — S/N 25 — 0
2. A gray mare walked before the colt. — S/N 20 — 5
3. Bottles hold four kinds of rum. — S/N 15 — 4
4. He wheeled the bike past the winding road. — S/N 10 — 5
5. Throw out the used paper cup and plate. — S/N 5 — 4
6. The wall phone rang loud and often. — S/N 0 — 4
   25.5 – TOTAL = 3.5 dB SNR Loss

Average: 2.98 dB

Fig. 41.2 SNRHL (Signal-to-Noise Ratio Hearing Loss) in dB for NH's unaided (upper) and aided (lower) QuickSIN (Quick Speech-in-Noise).

41.5 Outcome

NH was counseled regarding her hearing loss and the difficulty she has been experiencing hearing in noise. Recommendations were provided, which included annual audiologic testing, hearing protection in noise to prevent further hearing loss, amplification, and HAT such as amplified phones and TV ears. Due to the difficulty NH was experiencing daily, NH decided to pursue bilateral amplification. A recommendation was provided for the use of bilateral open-fit receiver-in-the-canal hearing aids with open domes. NH reported difficulty hearing when using her cell phone and therefore made-for-iPhone hearing aids were ordered.

NH returned for her hearing aid fitting. Prior to her arrival, the hearing aids were verified in a 2-mL coupler to ANSI S3.72–2009 on test setting and were compared to the manufacturer's specification. Also, the performance of the directional microphones was verified. The hearing aids were fitted using REM. The hearing aids were programmed to the NAL-NL1 (National Acoustic Laboratories' nonlinear fitting procedure, version 1) fitting formula[10] corrected for binaural and channel summation at input levels of 50, 65, and 80 dB SPL (sound pressure level) using a speech-weighted modulated digital signal. Slight adjustments were made for comfort and sound quality preferences after programming to NAL-NL1 (▶ Fig. 41.3; **upper is for the left ear; lower is for the right ear**). Loudness judgment levels

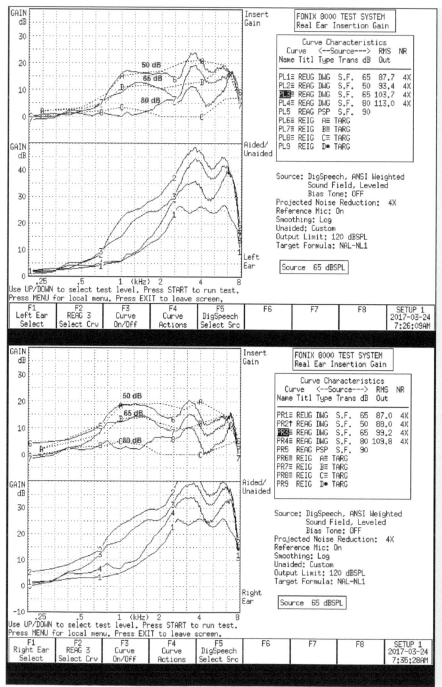

Fig. 41.3 REIG (Real-Ear Insertion Gain) measures to NAL-NL1 (National Acoustics Laboratories' nonlinear fitting procedure, version 1) for the left (upper) and right (lower) hearing aids in response to input levels of 50, 65, and 80 dB SPL (sound pressure level) using a speech-weight digital speech signal.

Hearing Aid Self-Assessment Scale

Patient Name: <u>NH</u>   Age:<u>67</u>   Date of Birth:<u>08/02/49</u>

Date:<u>11/10/16</u>   Key: Unaided **(U)** Aided **(A)**

Fig. 41.4 Unaided (U) and aided (A) responses to the Washington University Self-Assessment Questionnaire where when aided response to the right of the unaided response indicate improved aided performance.

HEARING DIFFICULTY

Single Talker Situations	Always	Often	Sometimes	Rarely	Never
At home, one-on-one			U		A
Riding in a car with a friend			U		A
Sports, such as playing golf			N/A		N/A
Talking to someone in a social setting			U	A	
Doctor appointment/Pharmacist			U		A
At work, conversation with co-worker			U	A	
Walking on a noisy street			U	A	
Shopping/Guided tours			U	A	

HEARING DIFFICULTY

Telephone Situations	Always	Often	Sometimes	Rarely	Never
Using mobile phone			U	A	
Using cordless home phone			U		A
Using landline phone			U		A

HEARING DIFFICULTY

Multi-Talker Situations	Always	Often	Sometimes	Rarely	Never
Noisy restaurant, courtroom, shopping mall		U	A		
Places of worship, theaters, movies, auditoriums		U	A		
Business meetings, social functions		U	A		

HEARING DIFFICULTY

Entertainment Device Situations	Always	Often	Sometimes	Rarely	Never
Watching TV			U	A	
Using a computer, stereo, MP3/CD/DVD player, radio			U	A	

were performed using a speech-weighted signal where NH verified that 65-dB-SPL input was "comfortable," 50-dB-SPL input was "soft," and 80-dB-SPL input was "loud, but OK."

The Washington University Hearing Aid Self-Assessment Scale is an internally generated questionnaire that was administered to NH at the hearing aid fitting and unaided (marked as "U" in ▶ Fig. 41.4) baseline information was obtained. It was noted that hearing difficulty was present in most situations (i.e., "sometimes") despite the minimal hearing loss. The unaided QuickSIN was also administered in sound field with the sentences presented at 40 dB HL at 0 degrees with a four-talker babble presented at 180 degrees. The noise level was increased along with each sentence that was presented by 5-dB increments per sentence. Therefore, for the first sentence, noise was presented at 15 dB HL (+25-dB SNR) and the last sentence was presented with 40 dB HL of noise (0-dB SNR). Three lists were presented and averaged and an unaided SNRHL of 18.17 dB was obtained indicating significant difficulty hearing in noise. Care and maintenance of the hearing aids were discussed as well as proper insertion and removal of the hearing aids and batteries. Her hearing aids were paired with her iPhone and NH was instructed on the use of the manufacturer application on her iPhone.

NH returned for a 2-week follow-up. NH stated she is doing well with her hearing aids and is satisfied with the overall results. NH reported she is doing significantly better in noise than she had previously. The Washington University questionnaire was administered demonstrating improvement in all categories (marked with the "A" in ▶ Fig. 41.4). The aided QuickSIN was also administered and significant improvement was noted with an SNRHL of 2.98-dB SNRHL. Therefore, a significant aided improvement of 15.19 dB was noted. According to the QuickSIN evaluation prior to being fitted with her hearing aids, she had a severe SNRHL (i.e., 18.17-dB SNRHL). With hearing aids, NH obtained significant improvement by reducing her unaided performance from 18.17-dB SNRHL to a mild (i.e., 2.98-dB SNRHL). NH was advised that further improvement may be obtained through the use of remote microphones; however, she did not feel that further intervention was warranted.

41.6 Key Points

- It is important to listen to patient concerns when determining hearing aid candidacy and not simply rely on audiometric data.
- There are many tools available to ensure a successful hearing aid fitting. Verification measures are valuable in assuring that sufficient gain/output is provided by hearing aids to meet hearing loss targets.
- Both subjective (e.g., questionnaires) and objective (e.g., QuickSIN) tools need to be incorporated for best practice and can be useful to measure the outcome of hearing aid fitting.

References

[1] Mueller G, Picou E. Survey examines popularity of real-ear probe-microphone measures. Hear J. 2010; 63:27–28, 30, 32

[2] Aazh H, Moore BC, Prasher D. The accuracy of matching target insertion gains with open-fit hearing aids. Am J Audiol. 2012; 21(2):175–180

[3] Sanders J, Stoody T, Weber J, Mueller G. Manufacturers' NAL-NL2 fittings fail real-ear verification. Hear Rev.. 2015; 21(3):24

[4] Valente M, Abrams H, Benson D, et al. Guidelines for the audiologic management of adult hearing impairment. Audiol Today.. 2006; 18(5):32–37

[5] Valente M, Bentler R, Kaplan HS, Seewald R. Guidelines for hearing aid fitting for adults. Am J Audiol. 1998; 7(1):5–13

[6] Dillon H, James A, Ginis J. Client Oriented Scale of Improvement (COSI) and its relationship to several other measures of benefit and satisfaction provided by hearing aids. J Am Acad Audiol. 1997; 8(1):27–43

[7] Sandridge SA, Newman CW. Improving the efficiency and accountability of the hearing aid selection process: use of the COAT. AudiologyOnline; 2006, Article 1541. Available at: http://www.audiologyonline.com/articles/improving-efficiency-and-accountability-hearing-995

[8] Clutterbuk N. It's the stigma, stupid–not! Hear J. 2008; 61(10):36–38

[9] Killion MC, Niquette PA, Gudmundsen GI, Revit LJ, Banerjee S. Development of a quick speech-in-noise test for measuring signal-to-noise ratio loss in normal-hearing and hearing-impaired listeners. J Acoust Soc Am. 2004; 116(4, Pt 1):2395–2405

[10] Dillon H, Katsch R, Byrne D, Ching T, Keidser G, Brewer S. The NAL-NL1 Prescription Procedure for Non-linear Hearing Aids. National Acoustics Laboratories Research and Development Annual Report. Macquarie Park, NSW: National Acoustics Laboratories; 1998:4–7

Suggested Readings

[1] Abrams HB, Chisolm TH, McManus M, McArdle R. Initial-fit approach versus verified prescription: comparing self-perceived hearing aid benefit. J Am Acad Audiol. 2012; 23(10):768–778

[2] Duncan KR, Aarts NL. A comparison of the HINT and QuickSIN tests. J Speech Lang Pathol Audiol. 2006; 30(2):86–93

42 Patient Decision to Purchase Hearing Aids: Bundling or Unbundling

Diane Duddy and Michael Valente

42.1 Clinical History and Description

AJ is a 62-year-old male who is the Business Manager of the Division of Biology at a major medical school. AJ has a long-standing history of a mixed hearing loss in his right ear and Sensorineural Hearing Loss (SNHL) in the left ear. AJ had middle ear surgeries in 1993 and 1997 to replace part of the ossicular chain and over the years AJ has experienced drainage from the ear canal and external otitis. At subsequent otology visits, AJ was advised to no longer consider surgery for his right ear and instead pursue amplification. AJ is a long-term user of several pairs of bilateral hearing aids purchased over the past 12 years where the adult audiology clinic used a bundling dispensing model providing care for the "life" of the hearing aids. Recently, the medical school had open enrollment for health care benefits and AJ learned that one health care plan offered the possibility of purchasing hearing aids through a buying group. The second author is responsible for negotiating insurance contracts and was not aware the medical school offered this. Thus, the authors investigated the buying group so the first author could effectively counsel AJ on the advantages and disadvantages of obtaining hearing aids through a buying group as well as learn more about the buying group to determine if the buying group could be a program the clinic could offer its patients. Up to this point, the audiology clinic had an agreement with only one insurance plan and that plan allowed balanced billing. Because hearing aids purchased through a buying group are considerably less expensive than what AJ had paid for his most recent pair of hearing aids, AJ was interested to investigate how the buying group program could be used to replace his current hearing aids.

42.2 Audiologic Evaluation

▶ Fig. 42.1 reports the most recent audiologic examination. AJ denied dizziness, otalgia, tinnitus, or aural fullness, and pure-tone audiometry for the right ear revealed a severe mixed hearing loss at 250 Hz rising to a moderately severe mixed hearing loss to 3,000 Hz and then falling to a profound mixed hearing loss at 8,000 Hz. Results for the left ear revealed normal hearing at 250 Hz falling to a slight to severe SNHL at 8,000 Hz. Speech Recognition Thresholds (SRT) revealed a moderately severe loss in the ability to receive speech in the right ear and a mild loss in the left ear. Word Recognition Scores (WRS) revealed normal ability to recognize speech in the right and left ears using the recorded version of a female talker of the Northwestern University Auditory Test Number 1 (NU-1) word lists.

42.2.1 Bundled, Hybrid, and Unbundled Models

The buying group provides hearing aids at a reduced cost to the patient. Hearing aids purchased through the buying group provide an audiologic examination (practice paid $75), 3-year warranty, 48 batteries, 45-day trial period, and **three visits during the first year**. These visits include fitting of the hearing aids plus two additional visits (i.e., bundled). After the third visit, the audiologist would charge for any provided services (i.e., unbundled). For these fitting services, the buying group pays the practice $325 to 600/aid depending upon the hearing aids that are ordered. For the three initial visits, services not covered by the buying group (i.e., coupler, validation [e.g., questionnaires such as the Client Oriented Scale of Improvement (COSI), Abbreviated Profile of Hearing Aid Benefit (APHAB), etc.,] and verification [e.g., Real Ear Measures (REM), Quick Speech-in-Noise (QuickSIN)]) can be charged if the patient elects to have those services performed. At the authors' audiology clinics, provision of best practices demands the inclusion of these measures. Our belief is that the inclusion of these "additional" services requires excellent counseling skills to explain to AJ the importance and the role of each measure and why it is in AJ's best interest to have those services provided. Ultimately, it is the patient's decision to select which measure he or she is willing to pay, but at the authors' clinics there is no compromise on performing REM and coupler measures.

To implement the buying group, AJ would call the buying group toll-free number. The buying group would refer AJ to a buying group provider for the audiometric evaluation and the provider would bill the buying group for the audiometric examination. After the audiometric evaluation, the provider orders the hearing aids and the aids are delivered with no invoice cost to the provider who fits the hearing aids. AJ pays the buying group and then the buying group later pays the provider the amount for the professional component of what the patient paid to the buying group.

AJ desired to replace his current traditional hearing aids with a current pair of premium hearing aids with a wireless remote multi-microphone and other accessories. With the 15% discount provided for all medical school employees, the charge would be $6,477 using a bundled model for the duration of the three warranties and convert to a unbundled model after the warranty expired (i.e., charge each visit based upon the duration of the visit). In the author's clinic, using an unbundled model for the duration of the warranty and then converting to a unbundled model at the termination of the warranty is termed a "hybrid" model. If AJ elected to purchase his hearing aids using the buying group, the cost would be $4,000 or a difference of $2,477 using an unbundled model. Most would consider this a considerable savings and would be very attractive to any patient.

At this point, the authors created a spreadsheet outlining the difference in procedures and charges using their existing bundled/hybrid model versus the buying group unbundled model. After counseling AJ about the differences, AJ decided which dispensing model he would elect to purchase his new hearing aids.

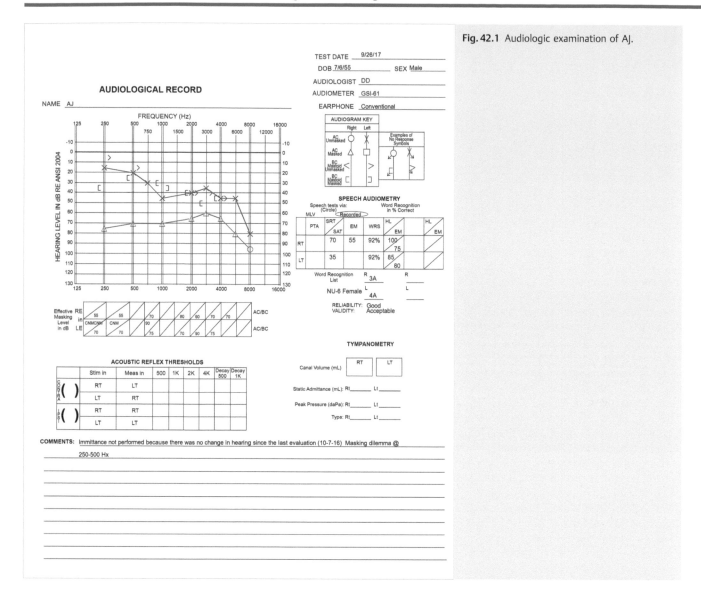

Fig. 42.1 Audiologic examination of AJ.

42.2.2 Using the Bundled and Unbundled Model (e.g., Hybrids) and Associated Charges for AJ

▶ Table 42.1 reviews the spreadsheet used to counsel AJ using the bundled (left column) and unbundled (right column) models. Using the bundled model, AJ would be charged $6,477 for a bilateral pair of premium hearing aids and wireless remote microphone, $24 for 48 batteries, and $200 for bilateral custom earmolds. AJ would receive the wireless remote microphone at no charge. The $6,477 includes a 15% discount that is applied to patients working at the university. The $6,477 charge would cover the cost of the following:

- **Hearing Aid Evaluation (HAE)**, which includes counseling on the impact of AJ's hearing loss on communication, differences in levels of technology (bands, channels, years of warranty, number of available programs, number of available automatic scenes, etc.), measuring the unaided QuickSIN and outcome measure (COSI). Also, AJ's audiometric thresholds would be entered into Noah and a pair of hearing aids and remote microphone would be programmed using the manufacturer

algorithm and demoed to AJ so he could experience what the hearing aids and remote microphone might offer in terms of benefit. On occasion, the audiologist will permit patients to use the hearing aids over a weekend.

- **Coupler measures** (ANSI-S3.22–2009 and verification of directional microphone performance) when the hearing aids arrive to be certain the aids adhere to manufacturer specification and the directional microphones are performing as expected.

- **Hearing Aid Fitting (HAF),** which includes REM to National Acoustic Laboratories' Nonlinear fitting procedure, version 1 (NAL-NL1) at 50, 65, and 80 dB sound pressure level (SPL); aided loudness discomfort levels (LDL) for a modulated speech weighted noise at 50, 65, and 80 dB SPL; counseling on use and care of hearing aids, earmolds, remote microphone, and the telecoil for use with telephones and looping. In addition, AJ's hearing aids would be paired to his cellphone and to the manufacturer App. AJ would be counseled on the use of his cellphone with his hearing aids and the various functions of the App. He is also provided one pack of batteries/hearing aid. AJ would be scheduled for a **Hearing**

Table 42.1 Differences in charges for a hearing aid (3-year warranty) using bundled and unbundled models

	Bundled ($)	Unbundled ($)
Hearing aid	6,477	4,000
Multi-microphone	NC[a]	390
Program accessories	0	115
Unaided outcome + QuickSIN	0	115
Batteries (48)	24	0
Fitting[b]	0	230
Pairing to Bluetooth	0	115
F/U to fitting	0	0
Aided outcome + QuickSIN	0	115
Dry/store	0	100
Sanitizer	0	10
F/U visits under warranty[c]	0	690
Earmolds	200	200
Total	6,701	6,080

Abbreviations: F/U, follow-up; QuickSIN, Quick Speech-in-Noise; REM, Real Ear Measure.
[a]NC during warranty for bundled.
[b]REM and coupler.
[c]$115/0.5 hour and assumes six visits during the 3 years.

Aid Assessment (HAA) at 4 to 6 weeks, but counseled to schedule an appointment sooner if any issues arise.

- **HAA** included fine-tuning the hearing aids if required; aided QuickSIN and COSI; provided a Dry and Store and counseled on its use; and coupler measure at user setting to act as a reference for future visits. Finally, at this visit, AJ would have the option to return at 3, 4, or 6 months where AJ's hearing aids would be dehumidified, earmolds cleaned, filters or ear hooks replaced, the battery compartments cleaned, and coupler measures completed and compared to the reference coupler measure. In addition, if the hearing aids were Receiver-In-the-Canals (RICs), the receivers would be replaced at no charge. If AJ elects to schedule these interval appointments, the services are provided at no charge during the duration of the warranty.
- During the 3-year warranty, AJ could schedule as many appointments as desired and all visits would be provided at no charge.
- At the expiration of the warranty, AJ would be counseled that he has the option to extend the warranty. If AJ elects to extend the warranty, then services for each hearing aid would be provided at no charge through the extended warranty. If AJ elected not to extend the warranty, then the dispensing model converts to an unbundled model where each visit would be charged at $55/15-minute visit or $115/30-minute visit. AJ would also be charged for any supplies (receiver, ear hook, filters, etc.). If AJ decided to drop off his hearing aids without an appointment, there would be an additional charge of $50 for this service.

42.2.3 Buying Group as an Unbundled Model and Associated Charges

If the Adult Division had elected to be a buying group provider, AJ would be counseled that the hearing aids would be serviced using an unbundled model (▶ Table 42.1, right column). This required significant counseling because AJ had purchased four sets of hearing aids using the "bundled for life" model.

As mentioned earlier, using the buying group unbundled model, AJ would receive the same hearing aids for $4,000. The hearing aids would have a 3-year warranty, 48 batteries, and a 45-day trial period. AJ's audiometric evaluation would be billed to the buying group and he is entitled to three visits during the first year. One of those visits would be for fitting the hearing aids. After the third visit, AJ would be charged $55/15 minute and $115/30 minute per visit. AJ would also be charged $200 for his earmolds and be required to pay for REM and coupler measures ($230) because our division will not dispense hearing aids without performing REM and coupler performance. Performing REM and coupler measures is not part of the buying group program and can be charged to the patient as "extra" services by the provider. In addition, AJ would be charged $390 if he elected to purchase the remote microphone; $115 to program any accessory and counsel on its' use; $115 for the unaided QuickSIN and outcome measure; $115 to pair his hearing aids to his cellphone, download the manufacturer App, pair his hearing aids to the App, and counsel AJ on the various features of the App; $100 for the Dry/Store at the HAA; and $115 for the aided QuickSIN and outcome measure. In addition, AJ was counseled that it is assumed that during the first year after using his third visit and assuming six visits for the remaining 2 years, he could be charged an additional $690 (i.e., six visits at $115/visit) over the course of the 3 years. His cost would be less if he had less than six visits, but more if he had greater than six visits.

At the medical school, audiology has the option not to join the buying group or any third-party payer for hearing aids. The second author carefully reviewed the buying group website and the requirements for being a provider. He recommended that the medical school not be a provider for the buying group program. The persons responsible within the medical school for contracting with third-party payers agreed with the recommendation. This information was shared with AJ, but the authors agreed to follow through on this exercise of explaining to AJ the difference between both models because of the long relationship AJ had with the first author and our interest in learning if given the opportunity to counsel AJ on the differences between dispensing models, which model AJ would eventually select.

42.3 Questions to the Reader

1. **In using the unbundled model, it is important to know the cost/hour to operate the clinic. How is cost/hour calculated?**
2. **In using the unbundled model, it is important to know the time/office visit type. How is time/office visit type determined?**
3. **The calculation of cost/hour assumes 0% profit. How should audiologists use that value to calculate the cost/hour to charge for services in order to be profitable at the conclusion of the fiscal year?**
4. **What other variables should audiologists consider when facing the question of whether to adopt a bundled, unbundled or hybrid model?**

42.4 Discussion of Questions

1. **In using the unbundled model, it is important to know the cost/hour to operate the clinic. How is cost/hour calculated?**

Cost/hour = total expenses (–) expenses for goods (hearing aids, earmolds, batteries, etc.) that are dispensed per **billable hours**. At the clinics used in this case report, calculating cost/hour required the skills of the second author and the Director of the Department Business Office. Using the skills and knowledge of these two working together, it was determined that the **direct and indirect costs** for the previous fiscal year was $3,022,584. It was also determined that of these costs, $890,514 was for items used for dispensing. Thus, costs were $3,022,584 to $890,514 or $2,132,070. Using several spreadsheets, it was calculated that there were 14,580 billable hours for nine audiologists. Thus, cost/hour was calculated to be $146.23/hour or $37/15-minute visit and $74/30-minute visit at 0% profit. *As an aside, it is important to remember that direct and indirect costs are fluid and thus calculation of cost/hour must be revisited on at least an annual basis.*

2. **In using the unbundled model, it is important to know the time/office visit type. How is time/office visit type determined?**

To accurately obtain this information, it is necessary to complete a time/motion analysis of the operation of the clinic. Several years ago, the department hired an outside consultant to obtain these data. As a result, each visit type was divided into 15-minute increments. For example, an audiometric examination is 45 minutes or three 15-minute increments, HAE is four increments, HAF is six increments, coupler measures is one 15-minute increment, etc. It is important when documenting the duration of visit types that the total time is the **sum of the time directly spent with the patient as well as the time required by the audiologist to prepare for the patient and complete any reports or associated paperwork.** Often, audiologists only count direct patient contact as the measure of calculating the time required for each visit type. Using this approach will grossly underestimate the duration required for each patient visit and the resulting charge to the patient.

3. **The calculation of cost/hour assumes 0% profit. How should audiologists use that value to calculate the cost/hour to charge for services in order to be profitable at the conclusion of the fiscal year?**

The $146.23/hour is the amount it costs to operate the clinic so that at the end of the year the clinic has covered its expenses, but left no margin for known and unknown expenses (i.e., loss) as well as a profit. Using the $143.23/hour charge for patient visits is not recommended because expenses mount during a fiscal year for repairs, new equipment, replacing equipment, salaries, fringe benefits, etc. Thus, an amount is added to the base cost/hour ($146.23) to achieve a desired profit margin (i.e., 10, 20, 30%, etc.). This additional amount must be added to the base. Thus, 10% calculation would convert the cost/hour to $161/hour, 20% to $175/hour, 30% to $190/hour, and 40% to $204/hour. The audiologist could also use a dollar amount that is desired to be present at the end of the fiscal year. In this case, a goal of a $50,000 profit would require the hourly rate to be $150/hour, $100,000 would require $153/hour, and $150,000 would require $156/hour, and so on.

4. **What other variables should audiologists consider when facing the question of whether to adopt a bundled, unbundled, or hybrid model?**

In the view of the authors, in order for the unbundling model to be successful, the following variables must be considered:

- There must be in place audiologists who charge the appropriate fee to patients for each visit. In the experience of the authors, numerous audiologists are hesitant to charge for services and are more comfortable with providing services at no charge. This is especially true if the audiologist has previous experience using a bundled "service-for-life" approach.
- Patients must fully understand the policy and charges. In addition, patients must sign a form verifying they understand the policy and associated charges. Legal counsel must be consulted to approve this form.
- It may be difficult to convert to an unbundled model for patients previously seen using a bundled model. Be prepared to answer many questions.
- If the clinic uses the hybrid model, a system must be present to **track the expiration of the warranty.** Prior to expiration, patients should be counseled that he or she has the option to extend the warranty and still be under the "bundled" model or let the warranty expire and he or she will be charged for each office visit using the charges present at the time of expiration and these charges are subject to change. As for extending the warranty, some manufacturers have a limit on the number of times the warranty can be extended, while others do not as long as the aid(s) is in good working condition.
- Because patients will be charged for each visit, it is a concern that patients might not make an appointment with his or her audiologist. There is a significant concern by the authors of the impact of this on optimum performance with hearing aids.
- If there is a hesitancy for patients to schedule appointments due to cost, this will impact the number of patient visits. This in turn will impact the need for as many staff. On the other hand, such hesitancy could be advantageous by reducing the number of frivolous visits audiologists often encounter.
- It is essential to have a director/supervisor who can interact with a competent business manager to accurately provide **all costs** associated with operating the practice. It is also imperative to know which costs are directly related to the dispensing side of the practice (i.e., those items that will be sold).
- It is essential that the director/supervisor have documentation of the time audiologists are providing *direct* patient care (i.e., **billable hours**). This task is not as straightforward as it may seem. It is easy to count the number of hours audiologists are not available to see patients due to vacations, holidays, and sick time. It is, however, not easy to accurately document time away from billing (i.e., **unbillable hours**) for services due to no-shows, cancellations too late to fill a patient visit slot, funerals, continuing education unit (CEU) events, jury duty, maternity leave, parties, meetings,

travel time between meetings, chart time, research, writing, program, and procedure development, etc.

- It is essential for a director/supervisor to complete a **time/motion analysis** to provide an accurate assessment of the average time it takes a staff member to complete every procedure provided by the clinic. This time/motion analysis *must* include the direct and indirect contact time required to complete each procedure.

- Finally, it is essential that the director/supervisor have a "business sense" and have knowledge of past profit/loss (P/L) reports to determine the **amount that needs to be added to the basic hourly charge** in order for the clinic to remain profitable at the conclusion of the fiscal year. The significant advantage of why it is imperative for a clinic to be profitable at the end of a fiscal year is beyond the scope of this case report.

42.5 Outcome

After detailing the differences between the cost and services between the unbundled and bundled model, AJ elected to purchase his new hearing aids using the bundled model. AJ had been using this dispensing model for the past 20 years and was accustomed to having the "freedom" to schedule an appointment at any time to resolve a problem. In reviewing AJ's medical record since 2003, it became very clear that AJ had far more than three visits per year. AJ quickly realized that if he elected the buying group unbundled model, his costs at the end of the 3 years would far exceed what he would have paid using the bundled model. Also, AJ was concerned that if he used the unbundled model he would need to "think twice" before making an appointment. This lack of "freedom" was a very significant concern for AJ. In addition, AJ mentioned he was so pleased with the care he received from the first author over the past 20 years that it did not make sense to "shop around for a better deal" in order to save less than $600 if he made no visits after the third visit. Finally, in reviewing and counseling AJ concerning the process described in this case report, it pointed out the knowledge AJ gained in appreciating the value of the services provided by his audiologist.

In January 2018, AJ was fitted with bilateral premium RIC hearing aids with a wireless remote microphone, wireless television streamer, wireless phone clip, and encased custom earmolds (number 2 ear wire; clear; faceplate beige; select-a-vent [SAV] for the left and pressure vent for the right; Cerustop wax trap at tip; removal cords; ultra power [UP] receiver for the right ear, and medium power [MP] receiver for the left ear). Prior to the fitting, both hearing aids demonstrated adherence to the manufacturer specification re: ANSI-S3.22–2009 and the directional microphones performed as expected. The hearing aids were programmed to NAL-NL1 for input levels of 50, 65, and 80 dB SPL, and the targets were corrected for bilateral and channel summation. AJ signed our form informing AJ that all services are provided at no charge for the 3-year warranty and he would be charged for each visit past the warranty if he elected not to extend the warranty. Aided QuickSIN re: unaided QuickSIN (sentences at 40 dB HL 0 degrees and competing sentences at 180 degrees) revealed significant improvement in

aided performance (i.e., –3.5 dB Signal-to-Noise Ratio Hearing Loss [SNRHL]). LDLs at 50, 65, and 80 dB SPL using a speech-weighted signal revealed 50 dB SPL was judged as "soft," 65 dB SPL signal was judged as "comfortably loud," and 80 dB SPL signal was judged as "loud, but OK." His various accessories were paired to his hearing aids and his hearing aids were paired to his smartphone and the manufacturer App. AJ was counseled on the use/care of the hearing aids and earmolds as well as use of the various accessories and the manufacturer App. The aided COSI revealed AJ felt his new hearing aids addressed his desire for aided performance in noise to be better than previous hearing aids (i.e., "much better" and "most of the time").

42.6 Key Points

- It is very important for a director/supervisor of an audiology practice to carefully review all the policies/procedures for proposals to dispense hearing aids through insurance plans or buying groups. The decision to join or not to join an insurance plan or buying group should be the sole decision of audiology and not a business manager or physician.
- If a practice decides to adopt an unbundling dispensing model, it is critical to know the cost/hour to operate the practice as well as the time it takes to perform each clinical procedure.
- It is important to include direct and indirect patient contact time when determining the average time required for each procedure.
- The audiology staff must become very competent in counseling patients on the costs per each procedure required to dispense hearing aids. A patient must understand and appreciate all the steps involved in the dispensing process.
- A goal of a clinic must be to provide high-quality patient care using evidence-based best practice (i.e., level 1 and 2 evidence in peer reviewed journals + patient preference + clinician experience) and be profitable at the end of the fiscal year.

Suggested Readings

[1] American Academy of Audiology. A guide to itemizing your professional services. Available at: http//www.audiology.org/sites/default/files/20141001_AAA_-Guide2ItemizingUrProfeServices.pdf. Accessed March 1, 2016

[2] Amlani AM, Taylor B, Weinberg T. Increasing hearing aid adoption rates through value-based advertising and price unbundling. Hear Rev.. 2011; 18 (13):10–17

[3] Amlani AM. How patient demand impacts pricing and revenue: understanding the concept of price elasticity. Hear Rev. 2008; 15(3):34–36

[4] Nemes J. To bundle or not to bundle? That is the question. Hear J. 2004; 57 (4):19–20, 22, 24

[5] Shaw G. Unbundling hearing healthcare pricing: up-front work pays off. Hear J. 2015; 68(9):28–, 30, 32

[6] Sjoblad S, Warren B. Can you unbundle and stay in business? Audiol Today. 2011; 23(5):37–45

[7] Wallhagen MI. Access to care for hearing loss: policies and stakeholders. J Gerontol Nurs. 2014; 40(3):15–19

[8] Windmill IM, Bishop C, Elkins A, Johnson MF, Sturdivant G. Patient complexity charge matrix for audiology services: a new perspective on unbundling. Semin Hear. 2016; 37(2):148–160

[9] Zeigler J. The cost of avoiding change. Hear J. 2016; 69(7):6

Part V

Cochlear Implants

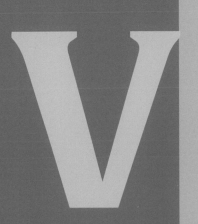

43 Cochlear Implantation in Meningitis Caused by *Streptococcus suis*

H.C. Yu, Vanessa Chan, Eddie Wong, and Lena L.N. Wong

43.1 Clinical History and Description

Streptococcus suis is a swine pathogen that may cause meningitis in humans via direct contact. Meningitis, in turn, may cause hearing loss of any magnitude. If patients have bilateral profound hearing loss, he or she may be a candidate for cochlear implant (CI), but cochlear ossification as a direct consequence of bacterial meningitis must be taken into careful consideration.

KF, a 66-year-old female, has been a bilateral CI user (Advanced Bionics HiRes 90K Advantage HiFocus Mid-Scala) for 3 years. She experienced sudden profound bilateral Sensorineural Hearing Loss (SNHL) due to bacterial meningitis caused by *S. suis*. KF was initially seen at the emergency room 3 years ago at the age of 63 years, presented with myalgia (i.e., muscle pain),

headache, fever, and general malaise. Acute onset of bilateral SNHL followed shortly afterward. Given that fever, headache, and muscle pain are hallmark symptoms of meningitis, a lumbar puncture was completed for cerebrospinal fluid collection and investigation. The cerebrospinal fluid culture and sensitivity test confirmed *S. suis* meningitis. KF was then placed on a course of antibiotic treatment of ceftriaxone, linezolid, and dexamethasone via intravenous infusion for 1 week. While her fever and headache improved post antibiotic treatment, only slight improvement in hearing was noted.

Ear, nose, and throat (ENT) consultation was scheduled 1 month later when bilateral profound SNHL was confirmed (▶ Fig. 43.1). Bilateral amplification was trialed, but provided insufficient aided benefit (▶ Fig. 43.2). At this point, the option of CI was introduced. Upon counseling, KF and her family

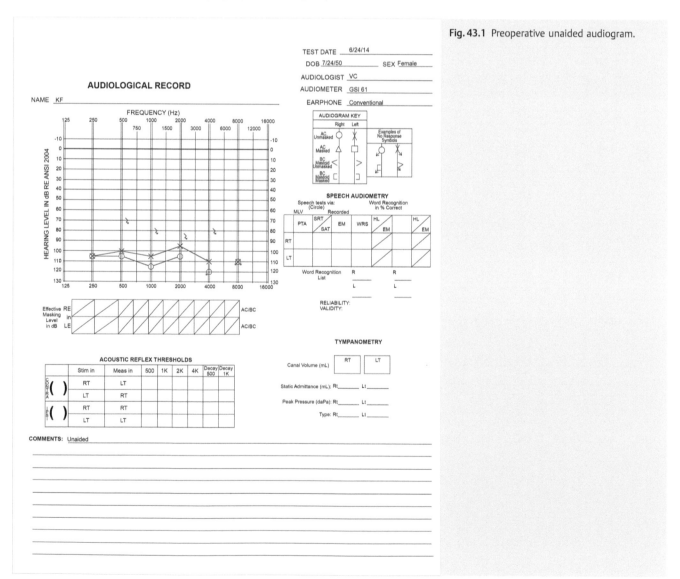

Fig. 43.1 Preoperative unaided audiogram.

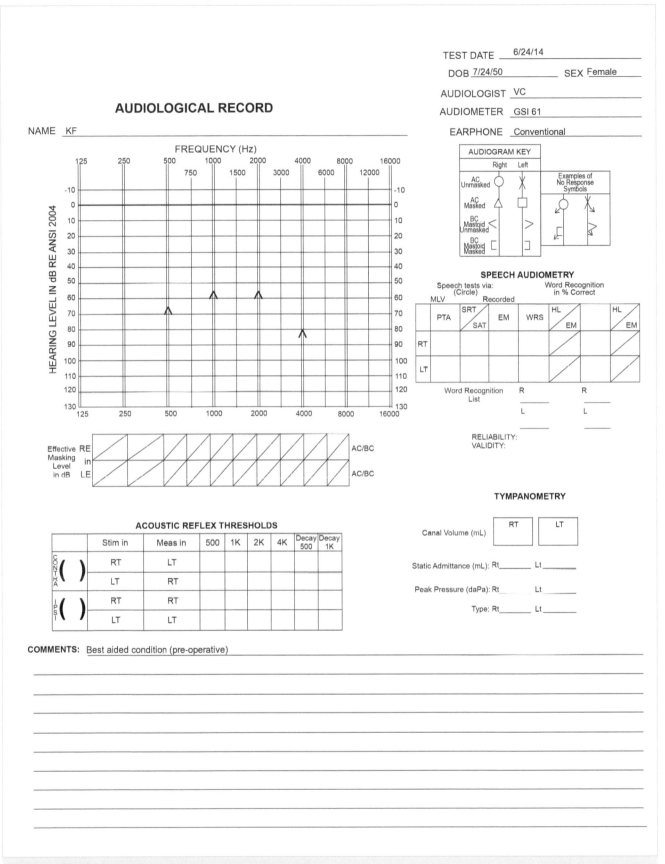

agreed to have the surgery as soon as possible to rehabilitate her hearing. Thorough audiologic and medical assessments were conducted. These included pure-tone audiometry, aided response in the sound field, aided speech perception test, temporal CT scan, and medical consultation. Subsequently, simultaneous bilateral cochlear implantation (Advanced Bionics HiRes 90K Advantage HiFocus Mid-Scala) was performed 2 months after onset of meningitis.

43.2 Clinical Testing

The preoperative pure-tone audiometric thresholds were obtained with good reliability as shown in ▶ Fig. 43.1, suggesting a bilateral profound SNHL. KF declined immittance testing as she could not tolerate probe insertion and pressure change.

KF was fitted with bilateral high-power hearing aids (Phonak Una SP AZ), which were adjusted to provide maximum gain and output. Real Ear Measures (REM) could not be performed as KF resisted probe insertion. Assessment of outcomes consisted of aided sound-field audiometric thresholds and the Hong Kong Speech Perception Test. Both tests were conducted in an acoustically treated sound booth. Aided sound-field audiometric thresholds were obtained by presenting warble tones across the octave frequencies from 500 to 4,000 Hz via a loudspeaker placed at 45-degree azimuth at a distance of 1 m on the left.

Aided sound-field thresholds at 500 to 4,000 Hz were essentially all at the lower edge of the "speech banana" (55–65 dB HL) across the frequency range. Aided response could not be obtained at 4,000 Hz at the limits of the equipment at 80 dB HL.

Speech reception was measured using the Hong Kong Speech Perception Test, which was developed by three CI centers in Hong Kong with the goal of providing a set of standardized materials to assess CI candidates and users. The test manual consists of 12 subtests as follows, with each subtest containing five test lists:

- Environmental Sound Identification.
- Number of Syllable Discrimination.
- Number of Syllable Identification.
- Tone Discrimination.
- Tone Identification.
- Vowel Identification.
- Consonant Identification.
- Word Identification.
- Word Recognition.
- Everyday Sentence Recognition.
- Open-Set Sentence Recognition.
- Passage Comprehension.

To ensure consistent results could be obtained using any of the test lists within a subtest, all lists are syntactically balanced. That is, the lists were constructed so that they have similar syntactic structure and levels of complexity.

Two of the subtests, the Everyday Sentence Recognition Test and the Open-Set Sentence Recognition Test, were administered to assess speech reception. The Everyday Sentence Recognition Test assesses the ability to recognize Cantonese sentences used in daily life. Each test consists of 10 Cantonese sentences with high probability of occurrence in daily conversations. These include common phrases such as greetings,

requests, acknowledgments, and comments (e.g., good morning). Each sentence contains seven or fewer syllables, which is within the auditory memory span. The test is scored according to the number of Chinese characters (syllables) repeated correctly in each of the 10 sentences in auditory-only and auditory + visual (lipreading) modes.

The Open-Set Sentence Recognition Test assesses the ability to recognize keywords and syllables in sentences of various structures and length. Each list contains 10 sentences comprising noun phrases, simple (subject) verb–object sentences, negative sentences, embedded sentences, compound sentences, passive sentences, and questions. Low-predictability sentences were used to construct the test so that a listener could not easily predict the rest of the sentence if parts of the sentence are heard. There are two to five keywords in each sentence. The length of each sentence ranges from three to eight syllables, which is within the auditory memory span. The Open-Set Sentence Recognition Test is scored according to the number of keywords and syllables repeated correctly for each of the 10 sentences in auditory-only and auditory + visual modes.

The Everyday Sentence Recognition Test and the Open-Set Sentence Recognition Test were presented via Monitored Live Voice (MLV) at 50 dB HL at 0-degree azimuth at a distance of 1 m from the center of the head of the patient in auditory-only and auditory + visual modes. KF's preoperative aided speech perception scores are reported in ▶ Table 43.1.

Although REM could not be performed, aided sound-field audiometric thresholds and speech perception tests confirmed bilateral amplification provided insufficient gain and were of limited benefit as reported by KF.

43.3 Questions to the Reader

1. **What is the relationship between meningitis and hearing loss?**
2. **What are the challenges in the rehabilitation of patients with bilateral profound SNHL as a sequela of meningitis?**
3. **What are the potential issues in pre- and postimplantation management in view of this history?**

43.4 Discussion of Questions

1. **What is the relationship between meningitis and hearing loss?**

Bacterial infection in the subarachnoid space may reach the cochlea via the cochlear aqueduct or the lateral end of the

Table 43.1 Preoperative speech perception test results obtained on the Hong Kong Speech Perception Test with hearing aids

List I	Auditory-only mode (%)	Audio + visual mode (%)
Everyday Sentence Recognition Test (syllable scoring)	0	41
Open-set Sentence Recognition Test (keyword scoring)	3	18
Open-Set Sentence Recognition Test (syllable scoring)	2	14

internal auditory meatus resulting in various magnitudes and configurations of hearing loss.

2. What are the challenges in the rehabilitation of patients with bilateral profound SNHL as a sequela of meningitis?

The timing of surgery is critical due to progression of cochlear ossification. Appropriate counseling is essential to prepare the patient and family regarding realistic expectations because outcomes vary across postmeningitis CI users ranging from sound detection only to open-set sentence recognition. Besides successful surgery and optimized mapping, a patient's motivation is critical in determining outcomes with CI.

3. What are the potential issues in pre- and postimplantation management in view of this history?

Preoperatively, it is essential that postmeningitis patients be assessed promptly, and suitable candidates should be implanted without delay to reduce the effects of osteoneogenesis (cochlear ossification) on outcomes with CI. Osteoneogenesis is well documented in cases of hearing loss caused by meningitis. Early radiologic evaluation to assess the degree of osteoneogenesis is essential in determining whether the CI electrode array can at least be partially inserted. Candidates should be implanted promptly to reduce the effects of osteoneogenesis on CI outcomes and optimize the benefits of CI in these patients. The patient and family should also be counseled regarding realistic expectations with CI. Postoperatively, patients should be encouraged to use CI consistently and be motivated to communicate with others.

43.5 Diagnosis and Recommended Treatment

S. suis is an important swine pathogen, primarily transmitted to humans by cutaneous contact with infected pigs or raw pork, especially when the skin has cuts and abrasions. While the incubation period of *S. suis* ranges from 3 hours to 14 days (median 2.2 days), a much shorter incubation time is expected with direct entry of *S. suis* into the blood via skin wounds. There was no direct evidence as to the cause of *S. suis* in this case, except that KF reported having wounds on her hands when she handled raw pork in preparation of a family meal a few days before the first symptoms surfaced. KF's case was reported to the Centre of Health Protection (Department of Health, the Government of Hong Kong Special Administrative Region), and the public was notified.

Infection in the subarachnoid space may reach the cochlea via the cochlear aqueduct or the lateral end of the internal auditory meatus. Any infection impacting the cochlea is likely to occur during the early course of meningitis. Permanent SNHL is observed in 11% of bacterial meningitis patients; the hearing loss could be unilateral or bilateral and the magnitude varies from mild to profound with no consistent audiometric pattern.

As mentioned earlier, *S. suis* was confirmed via lumbar puncture, cerebrospinal fluid culture, and sensitivity test. Antibiotic treatment consisting of ceftriaxone, linezolid, and dexamethasone was initiated immediately. Symptoms such as fever and headache improved after the initial treatment. KF was then placed on an additional 3-week course of antibiotic Rocephin to reduce the risk of meningitis recurrence.

Prompt ENT consultation was scheduled because of the persistent bilateral hearing loss once KF was ambulatory, a month after the onset of symptoms. Although KF reported slight improvement in hearing after the initial antibiotic treatment, audiologic evaluation confirmed bilateral profound SNHL (▶ Fig. 43.1) with insufficient benefit from bilateral amplification under the best aided condition (▶ Fig. 43.2). As mentioned earlier, aided thresholds were less than optimal (poorer than 55 dB from 500 to 4,000 Hz) and speech reception was not measureable. Urgent referral was made to the CI team as cochlear osteoneogenesis is observed in 35% of patients with meningitis. Ossification has been noted in these patients via high-resolution CT scans as early as 4 weeks postmeningitis. Although ossification is typically bilateral, involvement of the two ears is predominantly asymmetrical. The infective process may produce a reaction in the endosteum of the cochlea with a resultant overgrowth of new bone.

While cochlear implantation is not possible in an ossified cochlea, early implantation ensures that the CI electrode array could at least be partially inserted. Audiologic outcomes of postmeningitis CI users are difficult to predict, especially in the presence of cochlear ossification. Therefore, appropriate counseling is essential to prepare the patient and family regarding the realistic expectations of cochlear implantation. The ability to perceive speech without visual cues in quiet and noisy environments, to communicate on mobile phones, and watch TV cannot be guaranteed. Despite successful implantation, benefit from a CI largely depends on the patient's motivation and family support.

For this particular case, radiologic evaluation performed 1 month postmeningitis revealed no significant cochlear abnormality. Simultaneous bilateral cochlear implantation was completed 2 months postmeningitis without medical contraindications.

43.6 Outcome

Simultaneous bilateral CI surgery was uneventful. Implant electrodes of each CI (Advanced Bionics HiRes 90K Advantage HiFocus Mid-Scala) were fully inserted. The two devices were switched on 4 weeks postsurgery. The sound-field thresholds were obtained after CI programming was optimized (▶ Fig. 43.3). The CI sound-field thresholds were obtained in the sound-treated booth with KF using her right and left CI alternatively. Warble tones from 500 to 4,000 Hz were presented via the right and left loudspeakers placed at 45-degree azimuth at a distance of 1 m from the center of the head of the patient. The aided sound-field thresholds for both right and left CI were within the speech banana after optimal programming of the CI (▶ Fig. 43.3). While attempts were made to program the CI such that the thresholds are optimal, environmental and cultural differences must be considered. Hong Kong is a compact and densely populated metropolis with severe noise pollution, in particular from traffic, construction, commercial, and industrial sources. Attempts were made to improve KF's aided thresholds, but she felt extremely overwhelmed and could not tolerate the loud sound levels. After several mapping trials, the levels reported in ▶ Fig. 43.3 were reported by KF to be the most comfortable for daily usage. KF's speech perception scores at 3 years postoperation are reported in ▶ Table 43.2.

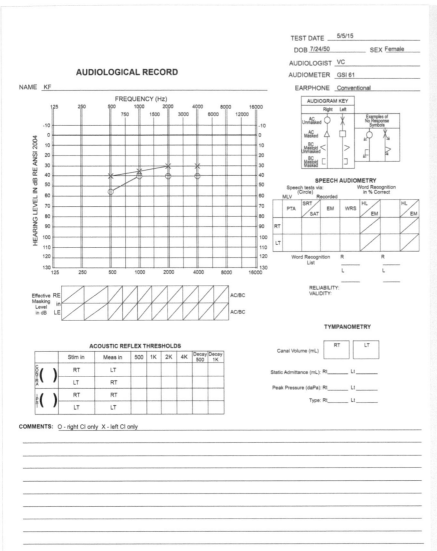

Fig. 43.3 Audiogram obtained with bilateral cochlear implants.

Table 43.2 Speech perception test results obtained on the Hong Kong Speech Perception Test at 3 years after cochlear implantation

List I	Auditory-only mode (%)
Everyday Sentence Recognition Test (syllable scoring)	100
Open-set Sentence Recognition Test (keyword scoring)	67
Open-Set Sentence Recognition Test (syllable scoring)	79

KF is now able to perceive open-set sentences without visual cues in the clinic and communicate verbally in quiet and in most daily noisy situations. KF and her family were grateful that meningitis caused by *S. suis* was promptly identified, appropriately treated, and bilateral cochlear implantation were completed without delay to enable her journey to recovery.

43.7 Key Points

- If hearing loss is reported in patients confirmed with meningitis, audiologic assessment and intervention should be provided promptly.
- If the severity of hearing loss warrants cochlear implantation, thorough evaluations should be done to determine extent of cochlear osteoneogenesis.
- The extent of electrode insertion due to cochlear osteoneogenesis and its effect on postoperative speech perception should be taken into account when considering cochlear implantation.
- Simultaneous bilateral cochlear implantation should be completed as soon as possible, when there are no contraindications.
- The patient and the family should be counseled regarding realistic expectations from cochlear implantation, as outcomes with CI vary and could not be predicted.

Suggested Readings

[1] Berlow SJ, Caldarelli DD, Matz GJ, Meyer DH, Harsch GG. Bacterial meningitis and sensorineural hearing loss: a prospective investigation. Laryngoscope. 1980; 90(9):1445–1452

[2] Caye-Thomasen P, Dam MS, Omland SH, Mantoni M. Cochlear ossification in patients with profound hearing loss following bacterial meningitis. Acta Otolaryngol. 2012; 132(7):720–725

[3] Cochlear Implant Working Group HK. Hong Kong Speech Perception Test Manual (HKSPT). Hong Kong, HK: Hospital Authority; 2000

[4] Dodds A, Tyszkiewicz E, Ramsden R. Cochlear implantation after bacterial meningitis: the dangers of delay. Arch Dis Child. 1997; 76(2):139–140

[5] Durisin M, Bartling S, Arnoldner C, et al. Cochlear osteoneogenesis after meningitis in cochlear implant patients: a retrospective analysis. Otol Neurotol. 2010; 31(7):1072–1078

[6] Nichani J, Green K, Hans P, Bruce I, Henderson L, Ramsden R. Cochlear implantation after bacterial meningitis in children: outcomes in ossified and nonossified cochleas. Otol Neurotol. 2011; 32(5):784–789

[7] Zalas-Wiecek P, Michalska A, Grabczewska E, Olczak A, Pawlowska M, Gospodarek E. Human meningitis caused by Streptococcus suis. J Med Microbiol. 2013; 62(Pt 3):483–485

[8] Yu H, Jing H, Chen Z, et al. Streptococcus suis study groups. Human Streptococcus suis outbreak, Sichuan, China. Emerg Infect Dis. 2006; 12(6):914–920

44 Cochlear Implantation in Chronic Suppurative Otitis Media with Cholesteatoma

H.C. Yu, Vanessa Chan, Eddie Wong, and Lena L.N. Wong

44.1 Clinical History and Description

Some patients may experience profound hearing loss as a result of chronic suppurative otitis media (CSOM). Although these patients may be candidates for cochlear implantation, there are specific challenges associated with active CSOM and the status of the mastoid cavity following cholesteatoma surgery.

CY, a 39-year-old female, regularly attended our ear, nose, and throat (ENT) clinic since childhood. She presented with repaired cleft lip and palate (CLP) and CSOM. In addition, left ear tuberculosis with left facial palsy was diagnosed and a cortical mastoidectomy was performed when she was 6 years old.

CY's hearing gradually deteriorated from a bilateral moderate to a bilateral profound Sensorineural Hearing Loss (SNHL;

▶ Fig. 44.1) when she was 30 years old. CY had a 50% central perforation on the left tympanic membrane and a myringotomy with grommet insertion was completed in the right ear to drain the middle ear fluid.

Because previous treatment procedures such as myringotomy and grommet insertion did not obliterate the disease process, CY underwent bilateral myringoplasty when she was 36 years old. By that time, CY's hearing had deteriorated to an extent that she was no longer able to communicate in daily situations (▶ Fig. 44.2). Cochlear implantation was performed in the right ear 1 year later when the ear was cleared after a myringoplasty. A myringoplasty was performed again in the left ear the following year and bilateral cochlear implantation will be considered if the left ear becomes clear in the future.

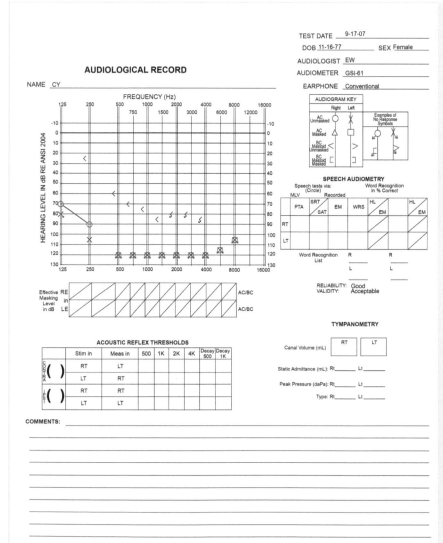

Fig. 44.1 Unaided audiogram when CY was 30 years old.

44.2 Clinical Testing

Audiologic evaluation was obtained with good reliability in 2007 when the patient was 30 years old (▶ Fig. 44.1). Tympanometry was not completed due to CY's persistent conductive pathologies in both ears (myringotomy and grommet insertion in the right ear and tympanic perforation in the left ear), which was closely monitored by ENT specialists every 3 to 4 months.

The Hong Kong Speech Perception Test Manual was used to assess CY's speech perception abilities. The test manual was developed by audiologists and speech therapists from the three main cochlear implant (CI) centers in Hong Kong to form a unified protocol to assess speech perception abilities of CI candidates. The test consists of 12 subtests, each containing five test lists. These subtests include the following:

- Environmental Sound Identification.
- Number of Syllable Discrimination.
- Number of Syllable Identification.
- Tone Discrimination.
- Tone Identification.
- Vowel Identification.
- Consonant Identification.
- Word Identification.
- Word Recognition.
- Everyday Sentence Recognition.
- Open-Set Sentence Recognition.
- Passage Comprehension.

All lists are syntactically balanced. That is, the syntactic structure used and the levels of complexity are the same across the five lists.

The Everyday Sentence Recognition Test and the Open-Set Sentence Recognition Test were administered. These tests were selected because they are more likely to reflect daily listening ability. The Everyday Sentence Recognition Test assessed CY's ability to recognize common everyday Cantonese sentences. This test consists of 10 open-set Cantonese sentences with a high frequency of occurrence in daily conversation (e.g., "good morning"). Common phrases include greetings, requests, acknowledgments, and comments. All sentences contain fewer than seven syllables in order to stay within a patient's auditory memory span. The test is scored according to the number of Chinese syllables repeated correctly in each of the 10 sentences in auditory-only and auditory + visual (lipreading) modes.

The Open-Set Sentence Recognition Test assessed CY's ability to recognize keywords and syllables in sentences of various structures and lengths. The test consists of 10 open-set Cantonese sentences. The sentences have different syntactic structures, such as noun phrases, simple (subject) verb–object sentences, negative sentences, embedded sentences, compound sentences, passive sentences, and questions. The sentences were constructed to minimize the chance that a listener could predict the content of the sentences. The number of keywords in each sentence ranged from two to five. The number of syllables in each sentence ranged from three to eight, which is again within the normal auditory memory span. The Open-Set Sentence Recognition Test is scored according to the number of keywords and syllables repeated correctly in each of the 10 sentences in auditory-only and auditory + visual modes.

Table 44.1 Speech perception test results obtained on the Hong Kong Speech Perception Test in 2007 with hearing aids adjusted to maximum gain and output

List I	Auditory only (%)	Auditory + visual (%)
Everyday sentence (syllable scoring)	21	100
Open-set sentence (syllable scoring)	18	85
Open-set sentence (keyword scoring)	16	88

Test materials of the Everyday Sentence Recognition Test and the Open-Set Sentence Recognition Test were presented via Monitored Live Voice (MLV) at 65 dB (A) at 0-degree azimuth at a distance of 1 m from the center of the head of the patient in auditory-only and auditory + visual modes. The test was completed in a sound-treated booth with CY fitted with bilateral high gain/output hearing aids (Phonak SuperFront PP-C-L 4 +) at maximum gain and output settings. Real Ear Measures (REM) could not be performed due to persistent conductive conditions in both ears. The scores obtained in 2007 when CY was 30 years old are reported in ▶ Table 44.1.

Open-Set Sentence Recognition scores were very low in quiet with auditory-only presentation at 16% (syllable) and 18% (keyword), but improved to 88 and 85%, respectively, with the addition of lipreading. In 2013 at age 36 years, CY's hearing deteriorated to a bilateral profound SNHL, even after bilateral myringoplasty that obliterated the CSOM (▶ Fig. 44.2). CY was not able to repeat any sentences with hearing aids (Phonak SuperFront PP-C-L 4 +) at maximum setting in auditory-only mode. Further testing in combined auditory + visual mode of presentation could not be performed due to patient fatigue and frustration.

44.3 Questions to the Reader

1. **What is the relationship between CLP and otitis media?**
2. **What is middle ear tuberculosis and its relationship with common otologic disorders?**
3. **While suppurative otitis media normally leads to a conductive hearing impairment, what is the mechanism involved when it results in a sensorineural component?**
4. **Given CY's medical history and audiologic findings, what are possible options for management of her communication problems?**
5. **What are the considerations and challenges when considering these options?**
6. **What are the potential issues in post implantation management?**

44.4 Discussion of Questions

1. **What is the relationship between CLP and otitis media?**

Otitis media is common among patients with CLP due to eustachian tube dysfunction and the palate not fusing during fetal development. The tensor veli palatini and the levator veli palatini, which are responsible for opening the eustachian tube,

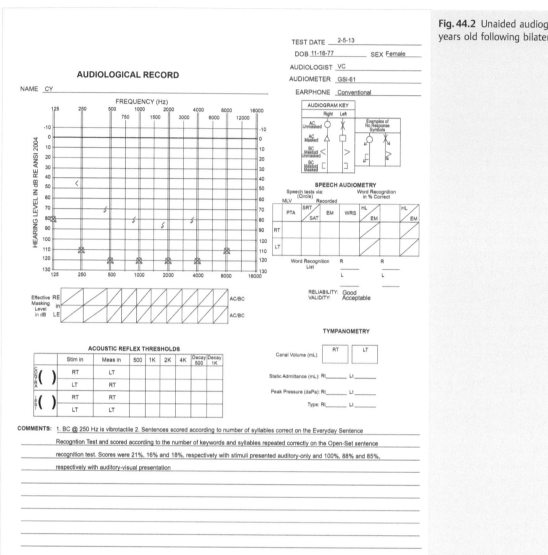

Fig. 44.2 Unaided audiogram when CY was 36 years old following bilateral myringoplasty.

exhibit an abnormal point of insertion. This lateral point of insertion causes a lack of anchorage, so the eustachian tube does not open properly. Because the middle ear cavity is not properly ventilated, a negative pressure is formed resulting in a retracted tympanic membrane. Finally, osmosis of mucous from surrounding tissues into the middle ear cavity leads to otitis media.

2. What is middle ear tuberculosis and its relationship with common otologic disorders?

Middle ear tuberculosis results in multiple perforations of the tympanic membrane, ear discharge, preauricular adenopathy, and progressive hearing loss that do not respond to routine treatment for fungal external otitis or bacterial otitis media. Facial paralysis has also been reported. Tuberculosis of the ear is a rare cause of CSOM and mastoiditis, accounting for 0.04% of all cases of CSOM and is mostly unilateral.

3. While suppurative otitis media normally leads to a conductive hearing impairment, what is the mechanism involved when it results in a sensorineural component?

The association between CSOM and SNHL is well documented. High exposure of the inner ear sensory cells to the inflamed middle ear due to its proximity makes the inner ear vulnerable against CSOM. It has been hypothesized that the inflammation may make the round window membrane more permeable, allowing bacteria such as endotoxins, to cause inner ear dysfunction.

4. Given CY's medical history and audiologic findings, what are possible options for management of her communication problems?

CY had bilateral profound hearing loss by 2013. She had no usable hearing in either ear; thus, hearing aids could no longer support her communication needs. Rehabilitation options include cochlear implantation, and/or use of sign language for daily communication.

5. What are the considerations and challenges when considering these options?

The choice would depend on the patient's otologic status and preference as well as support from significant others. Medical clearance from ENT must be obtained prior to implantation. Potential risks as stated below should be considered. Beside otologic findings, CY's communication needs and lifestyle should be taken into consideration. Verbal communication is an essential component of CY's work and daily life; thus, CY did not consider signing a feasible option.

6. **What are the potential issues in postimplantation management?**

Potential issues in postimplantation management in this particular case include possible spread of infection to the cochlear and the subarachnoid spaces with consequent meningitis, risk of electrode array extrusion, and possible recurrence of CSOM. Among the surgical techniques surgeons may prefer, securing an infection-free ear before implantation and creating a strong and healthy protective layer to cover the implant are of utmost importance. Routine telemetry should be done for impedance monitoring, as increased impedance and nonauditory stimulation in the basal channels are indications for electrode migration. Significant changes in impedance audition, mapping levels, and report of nonauditory stimulation warrant prompt ENT consultation for postoperative imaging to confirm or rule out electrode migration.

44.5 Diagnosis and Recommended Treatment

CLP is associated with CSOM, particularly in young children. The prevalence of CSOM in adults with CLP reduces, but the impact on hearing at a younger age could be permanent. The hearing loss is initially conductive, but many patients may develop a sensorineural component (i.e., mixed hearing loss). It has been hypothesized that persistent inflammation may make the round window membrane more permeable, allowing passage of toxins to cause inner ear dysfunction. Advancing age further increases this vulnerability. Thus, close monitoring of otologic and audiologic status (i.e., annual or as frequent as deemed necessary by ENT specialist) is necessary among those who have active CSOM.

Tuberculosis is a rare cause of CSOM. Patients typically present multiple perforations of the tympanic membrane, ear discharge, and progressive hearing loss. Tuberculosis of the ear was later diagnosed when CY did not respond to routine treatment for fungal external otitis or bacterial otitis media.

Hearing loss is normally unilateral, but in this case bilateral progressive hearing loss was noted. CY could suffice everyday life with hearing aids until 2007 when she was 30 years old.

As the sensorineural component became apparent, bilateral profound hearing impairment resulted. By 2013, when CY was 36 years old, she had bilateral profound hearing loss. CY could no longer benefit from hearing aids. Cochlear implantation was thus the only alternative for audiologic intervention. Cochlear implantation, however, in an ear with CSOM may lead to possible spread of infection to the cochlea and subarachnoid space with subsequent electrode array extrusion or meningitis.

As noted earlier, CY had a left central perforation with extensive tympanosclerosis of the posterior mesotympanum and posterosuperior area and right subtotal perforation with no rim inferiorly and anteriorly. No ossicles were identified in either ear. Finally, bilateral myringoplasty was performed by inserting temporalis fascia graft, underlying the membrane perforation. The myringoplasty finally cleared the right middle ear space of fluids when previous myringotomies and pressure equalization (PE) tube insertion could not. Cochlear implantation was performed in the right ear 1 year later when the right middle ear was confirmed to be cleared.

44.6 Outcome

Implantation of the Advanced Bionics HiRes 90K Advantage CI with the HiFocus Mid-Scala Electrode in the right ear was uneventful. The Advanced Bionics Naida CI sound processor was switched on 4 weeks later. The aided sound-field thresholds were obtained after CI programming was optimized. Aided sound-field thresholds were obtained in a sound-treated booth with CY using her right CI. Warble tones at 500 to 4,000 Hz in octave intervals were presented via the right loudspeaker at 45-degree azimuth situated 1 m from the center of the head of the patient. Aided sound-field thresholds obtained with the CI were within the speech banana after optimal programming of the CI (▶ Fig. 44.3). While the speech processor could be programmed such that CY's aided thresholds are at the upper range of the speech banana, effects of culture and listening environment must be taken into consideration when adjusting the CI. CY is living in Hong Kong, a compact and densely populated metropolis with noise pollution being a major issue. The Environmental Protection Department reported median daytime indoor L_{eq} noise levels in individual homes ranging from 60 to 70 dB(A) and more than 13.6% of the population is being exposed to traffic noise exceeding 70 dB(A) for 10% of the time on a daily basis. Attempts were made to improve CY's thresholds with CI, but the levels shown in ▶ Fig. 44.3 were reported by CY to be most comfortable.

CY's speech perception scores at 3 years postoperation are reported in ▶ Table 44.2, suggesting excellent speech perception ability (auditory only) with the CI.

CY's road to hearing rehabilitation was full of challenges due to persistent middle ear pathology. The CI team and CY persevered until the right ear finally became suitable for cochlear implantation. CY commented that her lipreading skills, which she once depended heavily on, have deteriorated as she now mostly relies on hearing for daily communication. A second implant is being planned for CY in the left ear when the otologic condition allows.

44.7 Key Points

- Although CSOM is commonly noted in CLP patients, further diagnostic considerations should be made when the hearing loss exceeds expectations and the CSOM does not respond to usual treatment.

Table 44.2 Speech perception test results obtained on the Hong Kong Speech Perception Test at 3 years postoperation

List II	Auditory only (%)
Everyday Sentence (syllable scoring)	100
Open-Set Sentence (syllable scoring)	98
Open-Set Sentence (keyword scoring)	97

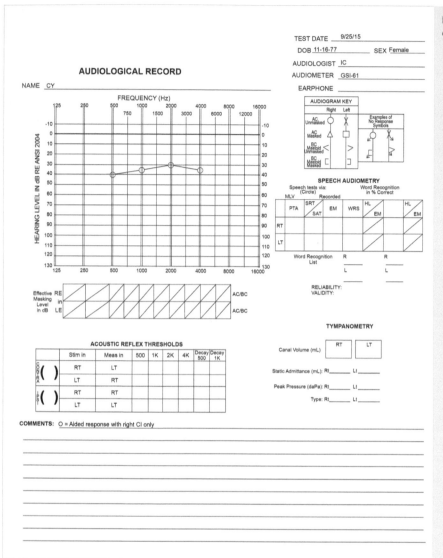

Fig. 44.3 Aided sound-field thresholds with a cochlear implant in the right ear.

- For patients with CSOM, a CI may lead to meningitis or intracranial complications by inserting the implant electrode through an infected mastoid or middle ear cavity.
- For patients with a history of CSOM, a profound hearing impairment, and a tympanic perforation, a CI may be considered 6 to 12 months after a myringoplasty if the ear remains consistently clear.
- CSOM is no longer a contraindication to CI if an effective procedure is used to adequately protect the electrode array.
- A CI is probably the only option to improve communication skills and quality of life for patients with bilateral profound hearing loss regardless of whether the hearing loss originates from disorders that typically result in sensorineural hearing loss.

Suggested Readings

[1] Adhikari P. Tuberculous otitis media: a review of literature. Internet J Otorhinolaryngol. 2008; 9(1):7

[2] Cochlear Implant Working Group HK. Hong Kong Speech Perception Test Manual (HKSPT). Hong Kong, HK: Hospital Authority; 2000

[3] de Azevedo AF, Pinto DCG, de Souza NJA, Greco DB, Gonçalves DU. Sensorineural hearing loss in chronic suppurative otitis media with and without cholesteatoma. Rev Bras Otorrinolaringol (Engl Ed). 2007; 73(5): 671–674

[4] Dietz A, Wennström M, Lehtimäki A, Löppönen H, Valtonen H. Electrode migration after cochlear implant surgery: more common than expected? Eur Arch Otorhinolaryngol. 2016; 273(6):1411–1418

[5] Environmental Protection Department, The Government of the Hong Kong Special Administrative Region. Population Exposed to Traffic Noise. 2010. Available at: http://www.epd.gov.hk/epd/misc/noisemodel1/CDROM_L10/images/exposure2010.htm. Accessed October 13, 2017

[6] Narayanan DS, Pandian SS, Murugesan S, Kumar R. The incidence of secretory otitis media in cases of cleft palate. J Clin Diagn Res. 2013; 7(7):1383–1386

[7] Papp Z, Rezes S, Jókay I, Sziklai I. Sensorineural hearing loss in chronic otitis media. Otol Neurotol. 2003; 24(2):141–144

[8] Sens PM, Almeida CI, Valle LO, Costa LH, Angeli ML. Tuberculosis of the ear, a professional disease? Rev Bras Otorrinolaringol (Engl Ed). 2008; 74 (4):621–627

[9] Vincenti V, Pasanisi E, Bacciu A, Bacciu S, Zini C. Cochlear implantation in chronic otitis media and previous middle ear surgery: 20 years of experience. Acta Otorhinolaryngol Ital. 2014; 34(4):272–277

Part VI

Hearing Assistive Technology

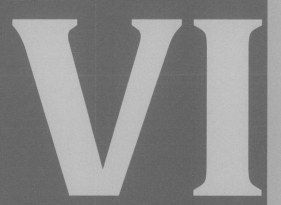

45 Hearing Assistive Technology: A Viable Alternative to Hearing Aids

Trent Westrick

45.1 Clinical History and Description

LN is an 88-year-old female who was seen for a hearing aid evaluation and consultation. LN attended the initial appointment alone. She reported having lost at least three pairs of hearing aids within the past 2 years (two sets of behind the ear [BTE], one pair of receiver in the canal [RIC]), all of which were acquired from other local facilities. LN reported she is unsure how she lost her hearing aids. While LN reportedly derived some benefit from her hearing aids, she had become frustrated with repeatedly losing or misplacing the devices.

Further discussions revealed that LN lives alone, but her daughter helps with daily activities including food shopping and house cleaning. Her lifestyle is self-described as "quiet," with much of her time spent gardening and reading. Her social activities are limited to family members visiting her at home and monthly small group meetings at her church.

LN's reporting was very vague and she had difficulty identifying specific listening situations in which she struggled to hear. She mentioned complaints from her daughters about the volume of her television being too loud. LN also reported having had some recent issues with her bank due to misunderstanding a voice message on her home landline telephone. Throughout the case history, LN would occasionally repeat herself or stray from the topic of conversation.

45.2 Audiological Testing

An audiologic examination (▸ Fig. 45.1) was administered. Pure-tone thresholds using insert earphones revealed a bilateral symmetrical gradually sloping mild to severe sensorineural hearing loss. Speech Recognition Thresholds (SRT) revealed a mild loss in the ability to receive speech bilaterally. Word Recognition Scores (WRS) using full-list recording of the Northwestern University Auditory Test No. 6 (NU-6) word lists were 96% in each ear, revealing normal ability to recognize speech. Tympanograms revealed normal ear canal volume, middle ear pressure, and static admittance bilaterally. Acoustic Reflex Thresholds (ART) were obtained at expected sensation levels for ipsilateral and contralateral stimulation bilaterally.

45.3 Questions to the Reader

1. **What additional tools are available to further investigate LN's communication needs?**
2. **What additional case history information might be required before making treatment recommendations and how could this information be obtained?**
3. **Given LN's long history of losing BTE hearing aids, what could be done to help prevent future loss?**
4. **Are hearing aids the best option for LN?**

45.4 Discussion of Questions

1. **What additional tools are available to further investigate LN's communication needs?**

While a case history can provide significant insight into a patient's communication needs, other factors such as listening lifestyle and perceived hearing handicap can be assessed by using any number of standardized questionnaires. One frequently used questionnaire for determining the degree of perceived hearing handicap is the Hearing Handicap Inventory for the Elderly (HHIE),[1] which is designed to explore the perceived emotional and the social impact of hearing loss.

For assisting with identification of specific listening situations in which a patient would desire improved communication, the open-ended Client Oriented Scale of Improvement (COSI)[2] can be a useful tool. The COSI is especially helpful to use with patients in which the recommendation for hearing aids is a possibility. The COSI allows the patient to identify specific situations in which he or she would like to improve hearing and communication. Up to five situations can be identified and ranked by the patient in order of significance. The COSI is then re-administered following the hearing aid trial to assess degree of perceived change.

Best practice guidelines for management of hearing loss in adults include validation (i.e., questionnaire) of outcomes associated with established treatment goals.[3] Several questionnaires, including the COSI, allow for the comparison of pre- and posttreatment subjective perceptions of hearing handicap, activity limitation, and quality of life. Moreover, administration of these questionnaires may help obtain greater information from a patient who may be a less than ideal historian. In this case, the HHIE and COSI were administered and the results are discussed later in this case report.

2. **What additional case history information might be required before making treatment recommendations and how could this information be obtained?**

Although questionnaires were helpful in obtaining more information regarding the patient's hearing and communication needs by identifying problematic listening situations and emotional reactions to communication difficulties, the audiologist felt additional information was needed regarding LN's previous history with hearing aids. Given LN's inability to clearly articulate the specific issues resulting in lost hearing aids, more information was felt to be required. Prior to moving forward with making specific recommendations regarding hearing aids, the audiologist suggested that LN schedule another appointment to continue the consultation and bring her daughter with her. Although LN made it clear her daughter does not assist her with making medical or financial decisions, it was explained that having a family member present would help in making the best recommendations for addressing her communication needs.

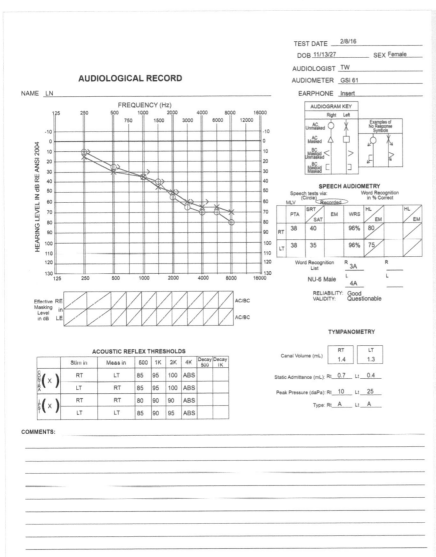

AUDIOLOGICAL RECORD

NAME LN

TEST DATE 2/8/16

DOB 11/13/27 SEX Female

AUDIOLOGIST TW

AUDIOMETER GSI 61

EARPHONE Insert

Fig. 45.1 LN's audiological examination results. Note the absence of contralateral masking stimuli used during Word Recognition Scores (WRS) testing. Although insert earphones were used during testing, minimal cross-hearing in the non–test ear is possible in the low frequencies at the selected presentation levels. In retrospect, contralateral effective masking levels of 50 and 45 dB HL would have been appropriate during WRS testing of the right and left ears, respectively.

Family-centered hearing health care, in which family members are actively engaged in the auditory rehabilitation process along with the patient, is gaining greater attention in the audiology community.[4] In some cases, however, family involvement does not necessarily result in successful outcomes. It is also important to be sensitive to cultural differences in which the traditional roles of family members result in varying levels of involvement. The role of LN's daughter and the influence of cultural norms are discussed later in this case report.

3. Given LN's long history of losing BTE hearing aids, what could be done to help prevent future loss?

For adult patients who frequently lose or misplace their hearing aids, it is important to determine the root cause of the repeated loss. Hearing aids have been known to fall out of pockets, fall behind furniture, or accidently get thrown away along with a tissue. Hearing aids that have a poor physical fit or that are not inserted properly are also prone to loss.

In cases of hearing aids being misplaced, consideration should be given to helping the patient establish a routine for storage. Using a small box or case every time the devices are removed can help prevent loss. Further investigation of why the hearing aids are being removed is also necessary, as the devices may be removed if sounds in certain environments are uncomfortably loud or if perceived benefit is limited. This issue may be addressed with hearing aid reprogramming.

When hearing aids are ill fitting, it is important for the clinician to investigate means of improving fit and retention. Ordering custom earmolds instead of using domes for fitting RIC hearing aids would be beneficial. Another suggestion is ordering of a canal lock. A tether and clip may be useful to prevent devices with poor retention from getting lost when they fall out. It is also important, however, to consider the patient's ability to properly insert the device or earmold. Even an appropriately made custom hearing aid or earmold will not stay in place in the ear if it is not inserted correctly. If the patient has a smartphone, it is helpful to use his or her phone to record the correct method for insertion and removal of earmolds and hearing aids. When the patient leaves the clinic, the patient or family member can retrieve the video to serve as a reminder for

APPENDIX Hearing handicap inventory for the elderly

Instructions:
The purpose of this scale is to identify the problems your hearing loss may be causing you. Answer YES, SOMETIMES, or NO for each question. Do not skip a question if you avoid a situation because of your hearing problem. If you use a hearing aid, please answer the way you hear without the aid.

		YES (4)	SOME-TIMES (2)	NO (0)
S-1.	Does a hearing problem cause you to use the phone less often than you would like?	X		
E-2.	Does a hearing problem cause you to feel embarrased when meeting new people?		X	
S-3.	Does a hearing problem cause you to avoid groups of people?		X	
E-4.	Does a hearing problem make you irritable?			X
E-5	Does a hearing problem cause you to feel frustrated when talking to members of your family?		X	
S-6.	Does a hearing problem cause you difficulty when attending a party?			X
E-7.	Does a hearing problem cause you to feel "stupid" or "dumb"?			X
S-8.	Do you have difficulty hearing when someone speaks in a whisper?		X	X
E-9.	Do you feel handicapped by a hearing problem?		X	X
S-10.	Does a hearing problem cause you difficulty when visiting friends, relatives, or neighbors?		X	
S-11.	Does a hearing problem cause you to attend religious services less often than you would like?			X
E-12.	Does a hearing problem cause you to be nervous?			X
S-13.	Does a hearing problem cause you to visit friends, relatives, or neighbors less often than you would like?			X
E-14.	Does a hearing problem cause you to have arguments with family members?			X
S-15.	Does a hearing problem cause you difficulty when listening to TV or radio?		X	
S-16.	Does a hearing problem cause you to go shopping less often than you would like?			X
E-17.	Does any problem or difficulty with your hearing upset you at all?			X
E-18.	Does a hearing problem cause you to want to be by yourself?			X
S-19.	Does a hearing problem cause you to talk to family members less often than you would like?			X
E-20.	Do you feel that any difficulty with your hearing limits or hampers your personal or social life?		X	
S-21.	Does a hearing problem cause you difficulty when in a restaurant with relatives or friends?		X	
E-22.	Does a hearing problem cause you to feel depressed?			X
S-23.	Does a hearing problem cause you to listen to TV or radio less often than you would like?			X
E-24.	Does a hearing problem cause you to feel uncomfortable when talking to friends?			X
E-25.	Does a hearing problem cause you to feel left out when you are with a group of people?		X	

FOR CLINICIAN'S USE ONLY: Total Score: _22_
Subtotal E: _8_
Subtotal S: _14_

Fig. 45.2 LN's responses on the HHIE (Hearing Handicap Inventory for the Elderly) administered at the initial visit. Questions relating to the emotional (E) impact of hearing loss were scored low compared to questions designed to identify difficult communication situations (S). A total score of 22 is interpreted as a mild perceived hearing handicap. (Reprinted from Ventry and Weinstein.[1])

the correct method for insertion and removal. This is also helpful for reminding patients how to insert and remove batteries and wax guards.

Recent advances in wireless technology in hearing aids allow for direct connectivity with smartphones and smartphone applications (i.e., Apps). In addition to allowing the user to stream music, change programs, and adjust volume settings within the App, some Apps have a "find your hearing aid" function. This feature allows the user to locate his or her misplaced hearing aids with relative accuracy. While not all hearing aid users own smartphones, including LN, this technology may be useful for patients who frequently misplace their hearing aids.

4. Are hearing aids the best option for LN?

In some cases, hearing aids may not be the best option. It is important to closely assess the patient's listening and communication needs as well as other patient factors before recommending hearing aids. The patient's cognitive status, available support system, and overall motivation play a significant role in identifying a potentially successful hearing aid candidate or conversely, patients who may derive greater benefit from Hearing Assistive Technology (HAT). Tools such as the Mini-Mental State Exam (MMSE)[5] and the Characteristics of Amplification Tool[6] may be used to further assess patient cognitive status and motivation regarding hearing aids, respectively. The MMSE, which is a screening tool for cognitive impairment, should not be used by audiologists for diagnosing cognitive impairment. It may, however, provide valuable information regarding treatment recommendations for hearing loss. When potential cognitive impairments are identified, audiologists should make appropriate physician referrals.

45.5 Diagnosis and Recommended Treatment

Following the completion of the case history, the audiologist did not have a clear indication of LN's specific listening needs and previous hearing aid history. The HHIE, which was completed with the audiologist's assistance (▶ Fig. 45.2), was administered. A score of 18 or greater is considered suggestive of a self-perceived hearing handicap.[1] LN's score of 22 suggests that LN believes she has a "mild" degree of hearing handicap. Of note is the score of 8 on the questions related to the emotional impact of hearing loss. This contributes to a lower perceived hearing handicap than would be expected based on LN's audiometric examination.

Completion of the first part of the COSI, which was administered by the audiologist, was used to identify specific listening situations for which LN desired to improve communication. She identified talking on the telephone, hearing her television, and hearing conversations at home as the listening situations she would most like to improve (▶ Fig. 45.3) and ranked these in order of significance. The second portion of the COSI, which measures degree of change, was completed following the implementation of treatment and is discussed later in this case report.

The HHIE and COSI questionnaires identified situations that would likely be improved by hearing aids. Based on LN's audiometric examination, information gathered from the initial case history, medical clearance, and communication needs identified by the HHIE and COSI, LN was identified as a potential candidate for hearing aids. A follow-up visit was scheduled during a time when LN's daughter could attend.

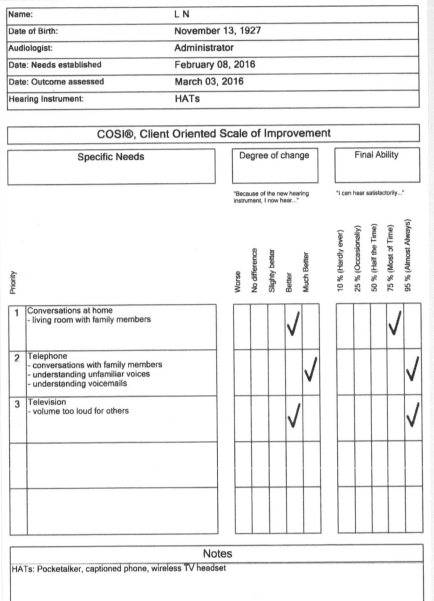

Fig. 45.3 LN's responses on the COSI (Client-Oriented Scale of Improvement). Specific listening situations were identified and ranked in order of significance. Following treatment, each situation was rated based on perceived degree of change.

At the follow-up visit, LN was accompanied by her daughter. In further discussing LN's history of lost hearing aids, the daughter was unable to provide significant insight beyond demanding her mother be fitted with new hearing aids. Throughout the visit, the daughter seemed uninterested and remained unengaged in the specific details of LN's communication needs. It became clear that LN's daughter was unlikely to provide significant support in the auditory rehabilitation process. It was, however, ultimately agreed that LN could potentially benefit from hearing aids and steps were taken to begin a hearing aid trial.

Based on the lack of information regarding LN's history of lost hearing aids, as well as positively identifying her limited vision and manual dexterity, the clinician recommended full-shell custom in-the-ear (ITE) hearing aids with a 2.5-mm vent, volume control wheel, program button, and telecoil. The patient was fitted with mid-level ITE hearing aids 2 weeks later. The volume control and program button deactivated, and the telecoil was set to automatically activate in the presence of a telephone's magnetic signal. These controls were deactivated in order to facilitate acclimatization to a new hearing aid style with the intention of activating the controls at a later appointment. The fitting was successfully verified using real ear measures (REM). As a group, the decision was made to include a grommet and tether clip to be attached to the hearing aids in an attempt to prevent loss. LN and her daughter were counseled on hearing aid insertion, use, and care, and were provided with customized user instructions. Effective communication strategies were also discussed.

45.6 Outcome

LN returned for a follow-up visit 2 weeks following the hearing aid fitting, again accompanied by her daughter. LN reported a lack of benefit with her new hearing aids in all listening situations and indicated the hearing aids had fallen out of her ears several times due to poor retention. The tether was disconnected from both hearing aids. The daughter expressed frustration with her mother's lack of hearing benefit. Further inspection revealed that the hearing aids were not properly inserted and number 312 batteries were in the devices instead of the required number 13 batteries. Data logging revealed a total usage time of 4 hours. LN was quizzed on the functionality of her hearing aids and was not able to answer basic questions about her devices. LN was able to report she had misplaced the hearing aids for about 4 days during the previous 2 weeks.

LN's daughter revealed she had not assisted her mother with her hearing aids during the past 2 weeks. As previously mentioned, cultural norms may have an impact on the role various family members play in the auditory rehabilitation process. LN's daughter displayed a significant amount of respect toward her mother, allowing her mother to speak without interjecting or contributing to the conversation unless prompted by LN to do so. Although the daughter assists LN with some daily household activities, it was apparent the daughter wished for her mother to maintain her independence as much as possible, particularly with more personal aspects of her life. The relationship between LN and her daughter was perceived by the audiologist as consistent with typical family roles observed in some Eastern cultures. It is the belief of the audiologist that the daughter's lack of involvement with assisting LN with her hearing aids was in alignment with the family's cultural identity and was done out of respect for her mother and not out of apathy as the audiologist initially believed.

At this point, it became clear to the audiologist that hearing aids may not be the best course of treatment. It was recommended that LN consider using HAT in place of traditional hearing aids to better address her communication needs. In revisiting the listening situations most important to LN, several solutions were suggested.

To assist with hearing conversations at home, a Pocketalker personal amplifier with supra-aural headphones was recommended. These devices are simple to operate and are big enough to reduce the risk of loss. The AA batteries need to be replaced infrequently. For watching television, in addition to using the Pocketalker, a wireless radio frequency headset system was suggested. Once connected to the television, the user can control the volume of the headset without disrupting the sound for others. To address ME's difficulties communicating on the telephone, an internet-based captioning telephone was recommended. Many states, including LN's home state of Oregon, have programs that provide captioning telephones at no cost to the patient.

LN and her daughter indicated interest in moving forward with these HAT recommendations in lieu of hearing aids and expressed relief in no longer needing to be concerned about losing expensive hearing aids. The hearing aids were returned for credit and LN and her daughter were instructed on the use and functionality of the recommended devices.

Upon her return to the clinic 2 weeks later, LN indicated improved understanding of conversation at home and in her church group while using the Pocketalker personal amplifier. She reported being able to enjoy television much more with the use of the wireless headset without having the volume of the television bothersome to others. LN and her daughter both reported improvement in conversation on the telephone with use of the captioning phone, especially the feature that transcribes voicemail messages. Although specific verification of these HAT devices was not performed, ratings on LN's COSI indicated perceived improvement in all identified areas. It was clear LN's communication needs were being better met based on subjective reports from the patient and her daughter.

45.7 Key Points

- Hearing aids may not always be the best option to adequately address patient communication needs. Not all patients have the same communication needs. Recommendations for rehabilitation are unique for each patient.
- For patients with limited familial support, potential cognitive decline, limited technical knowledge, lack of motivation, or many other patient factors, HAT can provide viable, efficient, and cost-effective solutions to address communication difficulties in place of, or in conjunction with, traditional hearing aids.
- Audiologists have an opportunity to distinguish themselves from other hearing health care providers by being well versed in all available HAT devices and recommending these options when appropriate. HAT includes devices and other technologies to augment hearing aids such as direct and indirect streaming of audio, wired and wireless remote microphones, and TV adaptor. The use of over-the-counter (OTC) "hearables" or Personal Sound Amplification Products (PSAPs), while controversial, will likely play a significant role in hearing health care in coming years, especially in the elderly population. Audiologists have an opportunity to add these solutions to their "audiologist's toolbox."

References

[1] Ventry IM, Weinstein BE. The hearing handicap inventory for the elderly: a new tool. Ear Hear. 1982; 3(3):128–134

[2] Dillon H, James A, Ginis J. Client oriented scale of improvement (COSI) and its relationship to several other measures of benefit and satisfaction provided by hearing aids. J Am Acad Audiol. 1997; 8(1):27–43

[3] Valente M, Abrams H, Benson D, et al. American Academy of Audiology guidelines for the audiologic management of adult hearing loss. Audiol Today. 2006; 18:32–36

[4] Hickson L, Lind C, Preminger J, Brose B, Hauff R, Montano J. Family-centered audiology care: making decisions and setting goals together. Hear Rev. 2016; 23(11):14–19

[5] Folstein MF, Folstein SE, McHugh PR. "Mini-mental state." A practical method for grading the cognitive state of patients for the clinician. J Psychiatr Res. 1975; 12(3):189–198

[6] Sandridge SA, Newman CW. Improving the efficiency and accountability of the hearing aid selection process. Audiology Online. http://www.audiologyonline.com/articles/article_detail.asp?article_id=1541. Published April 6, 2006. Accessed January 12, 2017

Suggested Reading

[1] Atcherson SR, Franklin CA, Smith-Olinde L. Hearing Assistive and Access Technology. San Diego, CA: Plural; 2015

[2] Blum H. Add PSAPs to your practice? ASHA Lead. 2016; 21(1):40–45

46 Coping with Hearing Challenges at Work

Mary Beth Jennings and Christine Meston

46.1 Clinical History and Description

Communicating effectively in the workplace with hearing loss can be challenging. The following case study provides an example of some of these challenges and how these challenges can be addressed when the patient and his or her audiologist interact collaboratively.

LD is a 50-year-old female. She was identified with hearing loss approximately 10 years ago and has been wearing bilateral hearing aids for the past 6 years. Her last hearing assessment was 1 year ago at which time she was fitted with more current bilateral hearing aids. At that time, LD reported the previous hearing aids were not meeting her listening needs. At the initial evaluation, LD presented with no other medical concerns and did not take any medications. There was no report of tinnitus, dizziness, vertigo, or history of ear infections. LD reports she continues to experience difficulty hearing in groups and in noisy situations. Of most concern, LD reports her hearing loss is beginning to impact her performance at work. LD currently works full-time with the same employer for 25 years and has been in a new position there for the last year. Her immediate supervisor has questioned LD's ability to cope with the listening challenges of her new position. She reports she is very concerned about the impact her hearing loss may be having on her work.

46.2 Audiologic Assessment

LD was recently seen for an audiologic assessment. Otoscopic examination was unremarkable bilaterally. Pure-tone audiometry (▶ Fig. 46.1) was conducted with good reliability using insert earphones coupled with foam tips. Results revealed a bilateral symmetrical mild to severe Sensorineural Hearing Loss (SNHL) that is gradually sloping in configuration. Speech Recognition Thresholds (SRT) were in good agreement with the pure-tone averages (PTA) and revealed a moderate loss in the ability to receive speech in each ear. Word Recognition Scores (WRS) revealed slight difficulty in the ability to recognize speech in each ear and tympanometry revealed normal middle ear function bilaterally.

46.3 Amplification

LD is wearing bilateral Behind-The-Ear (BTE) hearing instruments with custom molds she purchased within the past year. No additional accessories besides an amplified telephone are being used at this time. Real ear measures verified that LD's hearing aids met prescriptive targets (DSL v5.0 adult targets) for soft (55 dB Sound Pressure Level [SPL]), average (65 dB SPL), and loud (75 dB SPL) input levels and it is assumed the hearing aids are providing good audibility of amplified speech bilaterally. LD reports she wears her hearing aids most of the day and uses an amplified telephone in her workplace. She purchased

the new hearing aids because, as reported earlier, her previous hearing aids were no longer meeting her needs, particularly at work and she was counseled that new hearing aids may better meet her listening needs and the demands of her new position.

46.4 Questions for the Reader

1. **LD's audiologist identified the need for LD to gather more detailed information about her workplace, specifically wondering what were the challenges LD was facing and how she was coping with these new challenges. How could her audiologist gather this additional information?**
2. **How would the audiologist describe LD's challenges and strengths based on her case history and answers to a questionnaire?**
3. **Based on what is gained from a comprehensive case history and questionnaire, how would an audiologist proceed?**

46.5 Discussion of the Questions

1. **LD's audiologist identified the need for LD to gather more detailed information about her workplace, specifically wondering what were the challenges LD was facing and how she was coping with these new challenges. How could her audiologist gather this additional information?**

LD's audiologist would like to have greater details regarding LD's workplace and the challenges LD faces. Her audiologist elected to expand upon her initial case history with additional questions gathered from **The Amsterdam Checklist for Hearing and Work**.[1] The purpose of the Amsterdam Checklist for Hearing and Work[1] is to provide information on the relationship between hearing and work for the respondent. The checklist is organized into three sections that include closed- and open-ended items. The first section is composed of questions about the characteristics of the respondent's job and the features of the workplace. Five questions ask about the respondent's job title, hours of work, whether or not the job is temporary (scored as 0) or permanent (scored as 1), sick leave taken (0 = no; 1 = yes and number of days), and the reason for taking these (which is an open-ended question and the administrator codes the reasons into one of two categories: mental distress = 1; other reasons = 0) over the past month; a variety of activities performed on the job (e.g., using the telephone, meetings with more than three persons, desk activities, working with heavy machinery) are listed and the respondent is asked to identify up to three of these that they need to do during a regular work day. Two questions ask the respondent to indicate the amount of environmental noise and reverberation in the workplace (none = 1; a little = 2; much = 3; or very much = 4). The second section is composed of five types of hearing activities (e.g., speech communication in noise, localization of sounds) and the respondent is asked to identify the frequency (almost never = 0; sometimes = 1; often = 2; almost always = 3)

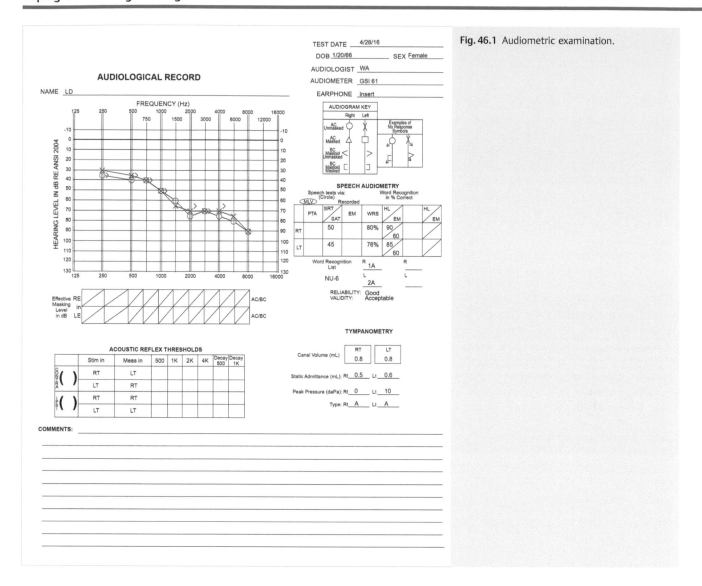

Fig. 46.1 Audiometric examination.

and effort experienced (no effort = 0; a little effort = 1; much effort = 2; very much effort = 3) for each activity. An overall effort score is calculated by averaging the effort scores for the five hearing activities. The third section asks the respondent to report on demand (four questions) and control (four questions) in their job, support provided on the job (four questions) and their satisfaction with their career (four questions). Each question within the factors has four possible responses: almost never = 0; sometimes = 1; often = 2; and almost always = 3. Average scores for each of the factors are calculated.

This checklist helped gather information regarding LD's workplace, her job description, the importance of hearing on her job performance, work conditions (specifically how LD experiences the demands of her job), how much control LD has in the work setting, how supported is LD in her workplace, and her satisfaction with her current position. Based on LD's answers to this questionnaire, the audiologist learned that LD is an administrative assistant within an academic degree–granting department at a college and she works 35 hours per week. Although LD reported she is satisfied with her current position, during the past 12 months she has taken 10 sick days that were

taken due to the stress level she is experiencing related to her work. Within her new position, LD reported she has the following job expectations:

- Make and receive telephone calls.
- Make inquiries regarding payroll, hiring, managing scheduling for senior administrators, and scheduling rooms for classes.
- Scheduling and booking rooms for examinations requiring communication with faculty and persons within the department responsible for scheduling rooms.
- Communication with visiting scholars for making travel arrangements, lodging, transportation, scheduling meetings and dinners, and liaison with internal university administration/faculty.
- Taking minutes at committee and department meetings with as few as 3 to as many as 20 persons.

LD reported there is "much" perceived environmental noise and "a little" perceived reverberation in her workplace. LD reported that speech communication in quiet and noise is very important for her job performance and trying to follow conversation in noisy environments is very challenging and effortful. LD reported, on average, her position is quite mentally demanding and is more demanding on her than her normal hearing colleagues. She reports less time to get her job done and she "often" feels worn out by the end of the workday. LD reported that she has limited control on scheduling her own activities at work. Further, LD reported it is not always possible to interrupt what she is doing, determine the content of, or organize her activities at work, or determine the timing of her workday and/ or breaks. LD stated that her supervisors and colleagues are very supportive of her at work.

2. How would an audiologist describe LD's challenges and strengths based on her case history and answers to a questionnaire?

LD has been employed with her employer for 25 years and 1 year ago, she accepted a new position. She is concerned that her hearing loss is beginning to impact her performance at work. Her immediate supervisor has expressed concerns regarding her ability to cope with the challenges of the new position and LD is concerned that if she cannot improve her communication it might jeopardize her ability to maintain the position.

LD reports only occasional difficulties with telephone communication and specifically with callers who she is unfamiliar with. She reports the amplified telephone at her desk is very helpful. One-on-one meetings are typically less of a problem, but larger meetings create challenges for following the flow of conversation and for minute taking. Within these meetings, there tends to be a free flow of conversation with limited turn taking, which creates challenges for her.

LD's primary challenge is understanding speech communication in noisy environments, including meetings. These challenges occur "almost always" and cause "much effort" for her in the workplace. LD reported high levels of job demand and low levels of job control. She also reported high levels of support from supervisors and colleagues on the job.

As reported earlier, LD's current hearing instruments were purchased within the past year and they are a good fit to prescriptive targets for average, loud, and soft speech, and should be able to provide good audibility of amplified speech bilaterally. LD feels comfortable using all methods of technology and she reported feeling comfortable working with her employer to investigate possible solutions, beyond her hearing aids, to her workplace challenges.

3. Based on what is gained from a comprehensive case history and questionnaire, how would an audiologist proceed?

Based on what the audiologist now knows about the patient's strengths and workplace challenges, the next step is to work collaboratively with LD to identify the specific communication challenges LD would like to target for intervention and determine if there could be improvement following intervention. To accomplish this, the audiologist decided to administer the Client Oriented Scale of Improvement (COSI).[2] The COSI involves working with LD to identify very specific listening situations that LD would like to have improved in the workplace following intervention and indicate their order of importance or significance. LD identified two specific listening situations where she

would like to see improvement following intervention. These included the ability to follow the flow of conversation more easily at the monthly department meetings and to increase her accuracy of minute taking. LD mentioned there are usually as many as 20 persons attending these meetings that are held in a standard classroom with seating in a "horseshoe configuration." LD also included the ability to follow the flow of conversation more easily at the three monthly committee meetings to increase the accuracy of minute taking. Each of these meetings has about five attendees and is held in a small boardroom with seating on both sides of a rectangular table that is approximately 8 feet in length.

46.6 Additional Questions to the Reader

1. **Now that LD has identified the communication challenges because of the COSI and the Amsterdam Checklist for Hearing and Work, she would like to learn more about her options to provide improved communication in her workplace. What should her audiologist do next?**
2. **After implementation of the intervention, how would an audiologist assess outcomes?**

46.7 Discussion of the Additional Questions

1. **Now that LD has identified the communication challenges because of the COSI and the Amsterdam Checklist for Hearing and Work, she would like to learn more about her options to provide improved communication in her workplace. What should her audiologist do next?**

LD and the audiologist identified two general intervention options. One is to make changes within the meeting room environment and the other is to use assistive listening devices (ALDs) in the meetings. Potential changes to the environment to facilitate communication include the use of sound dampening materials such as installing carpeting and draperies, providing better lighting or natural lighting to ensure faces of speakers are well lit at all times, and rearranging furniture to ensure optimal sightlines for the listener. Upon further discussion, LD expressed the opinion that it would be a challenge to make changes to the meeting rooms in which the meetings are held as meetings may not always be held in the same room, may change location at the last minute, and often classrooms are used as makeshift meeting rooms not allowing for great flexibility in changing furnishes, flooring, or drapery. As a result, LD decided to pursue the use of an ALD.

Now that LD decided to pursue ALDs, a decision aid was introduced to compare and weigh the advantages and disadvantages of each technology recommended to address her goals.[3] The **Ottawa Personal Decision Guide**[4] was chosen as a framework for comparing ALD options. This guide helps individuals explore decision options, identify their decision-making needs, plan next steps, and share their views regarding their decision. An individual is asked to list three decision options; in this case, it would be three levels of ALDs and assess the benefits and risks for each option. Each benefit and risk is rated to reveal how much each one "matters" to the individual on a scale of 0 to 5 stars (0: "not at all"; 5: "a great deal"). Individuals are instructed to choose the option with the benefits that matter most to them, while avoiding the options with the risks that matter most.

LD completed the Ottawa Personal Decision Guide. The three options in ALDs were as follows:

- **Option 1**: continued use of her current hearing aids alone.
- **Option 2**: hearing aids wirelessly connected to a conference or table microphone. This option would include a tabletop

conference microphone that would sit in the center of the meeting table or several microphones could be used for greater coverage in larger meeting spaces. The microphone(s) would connect wirelessly to LD's hearing aids via integrated receivers (▶ Fig. 46.2a).

- **Option 3**: hearing aids wirelessly connected to a microphone passed from speaker to speaker. This option could use various styles of microphone (clip-on, handheld, or lanyard) that could be passed around to speakers in the meeting room. The microphone would again connect wirelessly to LD's hearing aids via integrated receivers (▶ Fig. 46.2b).

In discussion with the audiologist, LD provided three reasons to select each option and three reasons to reject each option. How much each positive and negative response impact mattered to LD was ranked on a scale from "0" to "5." The results from her completed decision guide are presented in ▶ Table 46.1.

The **Ida Line Tool**[5] developed by the Ida Institute can be used in conjunction with the decision guide to further explore the individual's desire to make change. This tool consists of two questions. The first question identifies the goal; how important it is for the individual to improve his/her hearing at this time? The second question identifies the process and asks the individual to rank his or her ability to use the solution in question. Questions are ranked on a line from 0 (not at all) to 10 (very much). The Ida Line Tool was completed by LD. In this case, LD completed question 2 for each of the three technology options chosen in the decision guide. Results for the Line Tool are displayed in ▶ Table 46.2.

The use of the decision guide and Line Tool initiated further conversation with LD regarding her willingness to use the above-described technologies. Although LD realized that a pass-around microphone would provide the best listening situation of the three options, she was not certain she would consistently use this technology due to the engagement required by others attending the meetings and how she perceived the impact it would have on the flow of conversation during the meetings.

LD chose to try option 2 (hearing aids plus tabletop conference microphone). This option was implemented over 3 months and LD returned to meet with the clinician to assess the outcomes of the intervention.

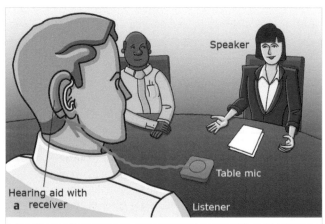

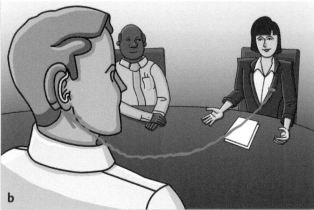

Fig. 46.2 Examples of **(a)** a table or conference microphone and **(b)** the speaker is using a clip-on microphone.

2. **After implementation of the intervention, how would an audiologist assess outcomes?**

Table 46.1 Results for the Ottawa Personal Decision Guide completed by LD

	Reasons to elect this option: benefits/advantages/pros	How much it matters to you: 0 not at all; 5 a great deal	Reasons to reject this option: risks/disadvantages/cons	How much it matters to you: 0 not at all; 5 a great deal
Option 1	No need for change	1	Does not work well	5
Hearing aids alone	No coworker participation required	5	Difficulty hearing in large meetings	5
	No additional cost	2	Limits job performance	5
Option 2	Easy to implement	5	Less discreet than hearing aids (HA) alone	3
HA + table mic	No coworker participation	5	Requires set-up	3
	Improves listening	5	May not solve all listening needs	4
Option 3	Optimal listening situation	4	Least discreet option	5
HA + pass-around mic	Reduces noise	5	Requires participation by others	5
	Seating arrangement not a factor	3	Can impact flow of meeting	5

Table 46.2 Results from Line Tool completed by LD

		Ranking (0 not at all; 10 very much)
Question 1	How important is it for you to improve your hearing right now?	10
Question 2	How much do you believe in your ability to use:	
	Option 1: hearing aids alone	10
	Option 2: hearing aids plus conference microphone	7
	Option 3: hearing aids plus pass-around microphone	4

The audiologist would re-administer the COSI.[2] The audiologist could also administer the International Outcome Inventory for Alternative Interventions (IOI-AI) for hearing difficulties[6] to specifically assess the outcomes of using the hearing aids plus the conference microphone at meetings in the workplace. The IOI-AI is an extension of the International Outcome Inventory for Hearing Aids (IOI-HA) that is designed to be used in addition to other outcome measures to assess the outcome of hearing aid provision. The IOI-AI consists of seven questions that assess the outcomes of interventions other than hearing aids. In this case, the audiologist would ask LD to complete the inventory to assess daily use (in hours on average over the past 2 weeks) of the hearing aids plus tabletop conference microphone and self-report:

- Benefit gained using the device.
- How much difficulty she still has in meetings when using the device (residual activity limitations).
- Her satisfaction with the device.
- How much what she is able to do is still affected even when using the device in meetings (residual participation restrictions).
- How much others are impacted by her hearing difficulties when she is using the device.
- How much using the devices has changed her enjoyment of life (quality of life).

46.8 Outcome

The aided segment of the COSI was completed. For the situations identified on the unaided COSI, LD rated the degree of change with the use of the ALD and her "final ability" (how well she could hear) with the ALD. LD rated the "degree of change" as "better" and she rated her "final ability to hear" as "most of the time."

For the IOI-AI, the questions were modified to ask LD about her use of the hearing aids in conjunction with the conference microphone. LD reported she used the device in meetings 100% of the time, that they "helped quite a lot," that she had "slight difficulty" in meetings, and using the devices was "quite a lot worth it." When asked how much her hearing affected the things she can do, LD reported she was "affected moderately," others were bothered "only slightly" by her hearing difficulties, and her quality of life was "quite a lot better" as a result of using the listening device at meetings in the workplace.

46.9 Key Points

- Expanding on a case history by gathering more information from the **Amsterdam Checklist for Hearing and Work** allowed the audiologist to collect additional patient information regarding listening challenges that was not captured in a typical case history and audiologic assessment. Audiologists could elect to administer the checklist in its entirety.
- Completion of the COSI allowed for LD's direct participation in identifying listening situations that were most important for her to receive intervention. This is also used as an outcome measure to rate the degree of change and her ability to hear with ALDs.
- Decision-making tools provide the opportunity for audiologists to work collaboratively with their patients and promote collaborative decision-making. By providing the opportunity for LD to develop the benefits and drawbacks of each option and rate each option allowed LD to develop a better understanding of each option and the impact each option might have on her daily life. The **Line Tool** provided an opportunity for the audiologist to gain a better understanding of LD's willingness to use the recommended ALDs in her workplace. Tools such as these assist in the decision-making process and can be a catalyst for further discussion with a patient regarding use of technology to augment his or her hearing aids.
- Assessment of outcomes postintervention (in this case, the addition of an ALD coupled with the individual's personal hearing aids) provided a measure of patient progress and help determine the efficacy of the intervention. LD continues to use ALDs during meetings.

References

[1] Kramer SE, Kapteyn TS, Houtgast T. Occupational performance: comparing normally-hearing and hearing-impaired employees using the Amsterdam Checklist for Hearing and Work. Int J Audiol. 2006; 45(9):503–512

[2] Dillon H, James A, Ginis J. Client Oriented Scale of Improvement (COSI) and its relationship to several other measures of benefit and satisfaction provided by hearing aids. J Am Acad Audiol. 1997; 8(1):27–43

[3] Laplante-Lévesque A, Hickson L, Worrall L. A qualitative study of shared decision making in rehabilitative audiology. J Acad Rehabil Audiol. 2010; 43:27–43

[4] O'Connor AM, Stacey D, Jacobsen M. Ottawa Personal Decision Guide. Ottawa Hospital Research Institute and University of Ottawa, Canada. Available at: https://decisionaid.ohri.ca/docs/das/OPDG.pdf. Accessed January 2017

[5] Ida Institute. The Motivational Tools: The Line, Box and Circle. 2009. Available at: www.idainstitute.com/fileadmin/user_upload/documents/Motivational_-Tools_final_nov13.pdf. Accessed January 2017

[6] Noble W. Extending the IOI to significant others and to non-hearing-aid-based interventions. Int J Audiol. 2002; 41(1):27–29

Suggested Readings

[1] Fok D, Shaw L, Jennings MB, Cheesman M. Towards a comprehensive approach for managing transitions of older workers with hearing loss. Work. 2009; 32(4):365–376

[2] Gussenhoven AHM, Jansma EP, Goverts ST, Festen JM, Anema JR, Kramer SE. Vocational rehabilitation services for people with hearing difficulties: a systematic review of the literature. Work. 2013; 46(2):151–164

[3] Laplante-Lévesque A, Hickson L, Worrall L. A qualitative study of shared decision making in rehabilitative audiology. J Acad Rehabil Audiol. 2010; 43:27–43

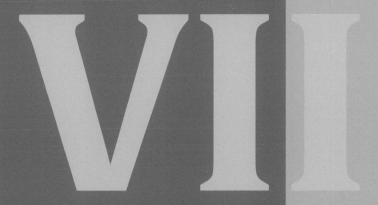

VII

47 Young Adult with Misophonia

Gemma Crundwell and David M. Baguley

47.1 Clinical History and Description

CW is a 19-year-old female referred by her ear, nose, and throat (ENT) consultant for misophonia. The experience of misophonia is of sound-evoked annoyance, irritation, or rage, usually associated with a specific sound (e.g., eating or sniffing),[1] and it has been suggested that there are three characteristic elements of misophonia (see Rouw and Erfanian,[2] for review):
- Disproportional aversive responses to the trigger sound(s).
- Awareness that this response is disproportionate.
- No clear physical feature (such as loudness of the sound) to explain the response on the part of the patient.

CW's sensitivity to sound was first noted when she was 14 years old, but she believes her symptoms were evident before that. She reported over 100 problematic sounds, with "wet or slapping sounds" such as eating and slurping being the most intrusive. Her response to these trigger sounds was disgust and rage. CW expressed that her sound tolerance had deteriorated over the course of 5 years prior to seeking support with a major change coinciding with her first major depressive bipolar episode. As well as having bipolar disorder, CW has diagnoses of social anxiety, panic disorder, agoraphobia, obsessive compulsive disorder, and attention deficit hyperactivity disorder. In addition, CW is currently being assessed to determine if she has autism. Although CW was under the active care of psychiatric colleagues, none of these clinicians felt sufficiently trained to explain or manage her aversion to sound.

The impact of the misophonia upon CW and her family was substantial. She was essentially a recluse, with the majority of her friendships having dissolved due to her friends and college colleagues being indifferent to her problems who actually teased her with trigger sounds. When exposed to trigger sounds, CW would become increasingly anxious and exhibit negative behaviors including screaming, self-harm, and aggression. Her negative behaviors were exacerbated when she felt trapped or out of control.

CW had used earplugs, but did not find these beneficial and instead choose to block sound using strident music. At home, every attempt was made to reduce sound, including having the heating, electricity, and all electronic devices turned off.

47.2 Clinical Testing

No abnormalities were detected on otoscopy. Pure-tone audiometry (air conduction) revealed hearing to be within normal limits bilaterally (▸ Fig. 47.1). Tympanometry was within normal limits bilaterally. No other otologic concerns were noted. There was no history of significant noise exposure, ear surgeries, or trauma.

47.3 Questions to the Reader

1. **Is misophonia essentially an audiologic or a psychological/psychiatric problem?**
2. **To what extent is this referral for audiologic counseling and management reasonable in the light of the context of significant psychiatric challenges?**

47.4 Discussion of Questions

1. **Is misophonia essentially an audiological or a psychological/psychiatric problem?**

Misophonia is a diagnosis that is attracting increasing attention in the audiology and psychology/psychiatry literature.[1] At best, this might lead to an integrated understanding of how misophonia involves the auditory system, neural systems of emotion, behavioral reaction, and learning. At worst, this might suggest that audiology, psychology, nor psychiatry fully understands or appreciates the challenges faced by a patient with misophonia and his/her family. The answer to the question then is that misophonia is generally considered an audiologic as well as psychological/psychiatric problem.

2. **To what extent is this referral for audiologic counseling and management reasonable in the light of the context of significant psychiatric challenges?**

Many audiologists could be forgiven for being daunted by the extent of the challenges facing CW, but there are several reasons why having audiologist involvement may be beneficial to such a patient. The first reason is pragmatic because no other health care colleagues have been able to explain or attempt to manage the sound intolerance issues. Unless this care is undertaken in an audiology clinic, in such a case it will not be done at all. Second, it may be that managing the psychological or psychiatric aspects of misophonia will be enabled by audiologic counseling and the initial management of the misophonia. Third, of all the indicated problems associated with misophonia, the sound intolerance leads to social isolation that reduces quality of life.

47.5 Description of the Disorder and Recommended Treatment

During the initial assessment, CW was offered informational counseling about misophonia and its involvement of the auditory and neural systems of emotion and reaction. She was dispensed bilateral Behind-The-Ear (BTE) GN ReSound I-Fit 71 TS combination device with nonoccluding slim tube fittings. The I-Fit 71 TS can be configured to provide amplification via standard hearing instrument technology and tinnitus sound

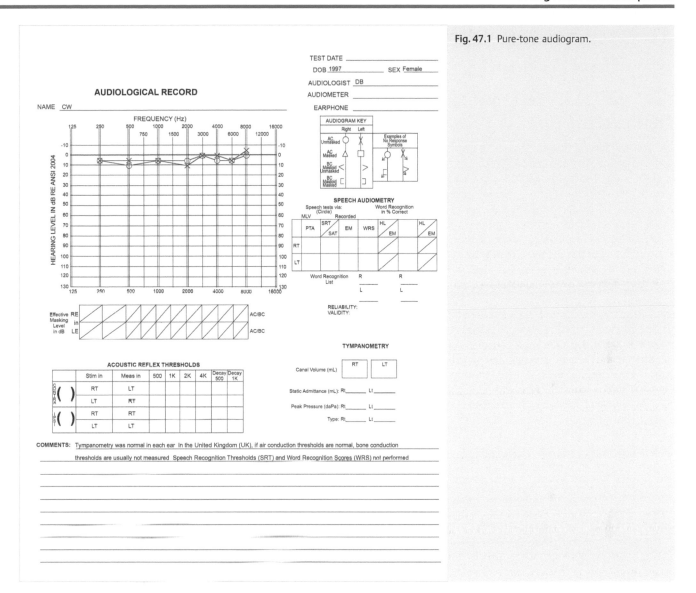

Fig. 47.1 Pure-tone audiogram.

generator features that aim to lower the perception of tinnitus. Given CW has normal hearing, the bilateral devices were programmed as ear level sound generators only, providing no amplification. CW was actively involved in fine-tuning the characteristics of the broadband signal. This was done to actively engage and empower CW in the treatment process so it would introduce a sense of control. Four sound programs (▶ Fig. 47.2) were created: (1) low cut programmed to manufacturer's minimum; high cut programmed at 2,000 Hz; (2) low-cut programmed to manufacturer's minimum; high cut programmed at 6,000 Hz; (3) low cut programmed at 2,000 Hz; high cut programmed at 6,000 Hz; (4) low cut programmed at 1,000 Hz; high cut programmed at 2,000 Hz. Amplitude modulation was not activated. The sound was programmed in the software to an output at 40 dB SPL on all four programs with a +6/−12 dB volume range. This level was selected by CW as being clear and comfortable level (▶ Fig. 47.2). CW was encouraged to use the devices instead of strident music to try and reduce the stridency of the trigger sounds and to partially mask the sounds. CW was advised to wear these devices when and where she prefers, in the hope of introducing some element of control. CW

was also issued Sound Oasis bedside sound generator for use at bedtime. The Sound Oasis features a variety of soothing natural sounds that CW could listen to via the integrated speaker or through speakers built into a pillow. The aim was to utilize sound with minimal emotional salience to attempt to reduce attention to the trigger sounds.

A follow-up appointment was arranged 2 weeks after the initial assessment and device fitting. The appointment was scheduled so CW could attend and leave the clinic before other patients arrived because CW became distressed and experienced panic resulting in self-harming in the waiting area when leaving the clinic previously. While CW had not yet used the bedside sound generator, she reported she had worn the ear level sound generators several times, primarily while on her own and found they were beneficial at masking her trigger sounds. CW was able to sit with her pets while using the sound generators. This was something she has not been able to do for many years. CW reports that her mood had improved with the sound generators by providing her with an alternative solution to her negative behaviors and providing her with a sense of control. The audiologist set the following goals for her next

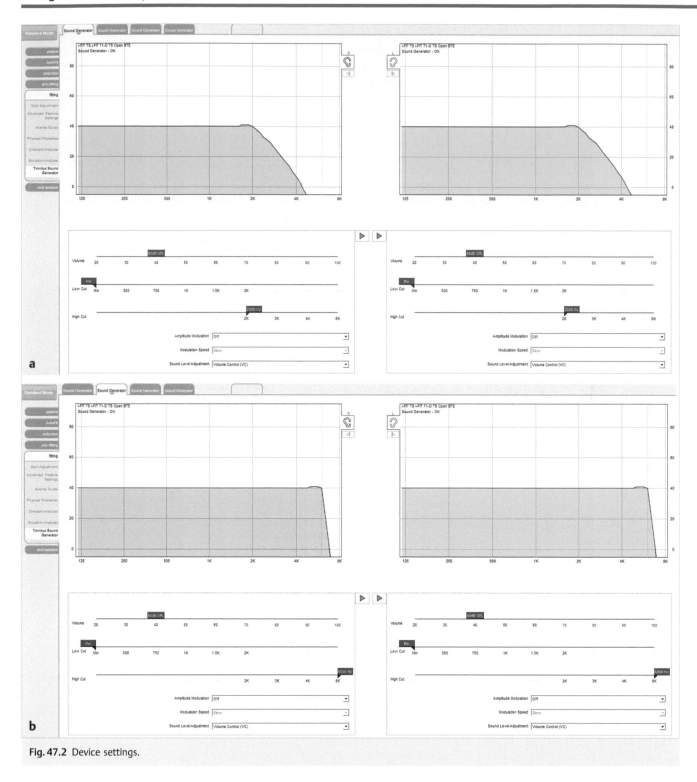

Fig. 47.2 Device settings.

appointment: increased use of the sound generators in a wider range of sound environments, gradual acclimatization to sounds that can be triggers, and finding a method for counseling significant others about triggers and the resulting mood state to prevent negative behaviors.

At a second follow-up appointment 6 weeks later, CW reported having recently been prescribed mood-stabilizing drugs, which she felt were having a beneficial effect on her sound sensitivity. She had been able to expose herself to sounds

she would previously have been unable to tolerate such as eating with a friend. She also has improved behavior with less self-harming and aggression in response to trigger sounds.

47.6 Outcome

CW had a final appointment 1 year after the initial visit. While she acknowledged there were still issues with sound tolerance,

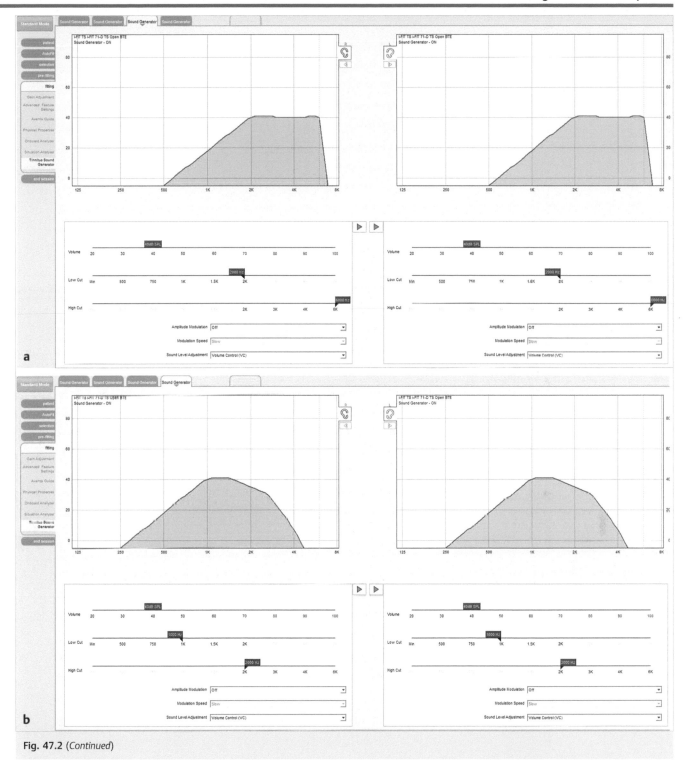

Fig. 47.2 (Continued)

she reported significant progress with her symptoms. She was able to participate in activities that she would not have been able to contemplate prior to her treatment. This included going to the supermarket and seeing her dentist, optician, and general practitioner during normal clinic hours. CW used the sound generators when necessary to manage these situations and gained a sense of control over the situation and they acted to mask sounds. CW reported satisfaction with the devices and did not have a preferred program choosing between the four based on her mood and situation.

47.7 Key Points

- In this case, counseling and management of misophonia contributed to a general improvement of social functioning.

- While significant psychological/psychiatric challenges were present, these did not prevent management of the misophonia.
- Small, but highly significant pragmatic actions contributed to the success of the management of misophonia. These included making appointments for CW before usual clinic hours to avoid anxiety at seeing other waiting patients and giving her the ability to shape and choose the therapeutic sound used.
- While this case report indicates contributions from empowerment, taking back a locus of control, and

potentially a placebo effect in the case of the sound generators, the relative contributions of each of these cannot be determined.

References

[1] McFerran D. Misophonia and phonophobia. In: Baguley DM, Fagelson M, eds. Tinnitus: Clinical and Research Perspectives. San Diego, CA: Plural; 2015:245–259

[2] Rouw R, Erfanian M. A large-scale study of misophonia. J Clin Psychol. 2018; 74(3):453–479

48 Tinnitus and Hyperacusis

Aniruddha K. Deshpande and Rich Tyler

48.1 Clinical History and Description

SS is a 66-year-old female originally seen in the otolaryngology clinic reporting ringing in her ears and being afraid to return to work because of the pain in her ears as a result of the noise level in the office where she works. SS reported the pain started 2 weeks ago when a caller unexpectedly yelled in her ears when she was wearing a telephone headset. SS reported she started experiencing bilateral tinnitus immediately after the incident. According to SS, whenever she hears a loud unexpected sound, she experiences pain, anxiety, and fear. Additional symptoms include a significant reduction in the ability to sleep, concentrate, and maintain a conversation. SS now has such a severe reaction to even moderately loud sounds that she locks herself in her room on some days.

SS also reports frequent pain, spasms, and aural fullness in both ears. She had seen her primary care physician and a pain specialist and was counseled that her symptoms were not related to temporomandibular joint (TMJ) disorder.

48.2 Audiologic Testing

48.2.1 Case History

As part of SS's clinical evaluation, she was asked about her job, which revealed the following:

- She worked in a call center and had to make approximately 70 calls per day.
- There were approximately 50 other call-center employees talking at the same time in the same room.

SS was asked about her hearing concerns at work. She reported she was fearful of the following situations:

- Any loud conversation.
- The overhead sound of music in the office.
- People speaking very loudly to her through her headset.
- Anyone talking loudly within a radius of 20 feet.
- Loud voices of other employees on nearby phones.
- Coworkers slamming their desks.
- The sound of chairs scraping against the floor.

48.2.2 Audiologic Examination

Pure-tone audiometry (▶ Fig. 48.1) revealed that SS has a mild bilateral symmetrical Sensorineural Hearing Loss (SNHL) that is essentially flat in configuration. Speech Awareness Thresholds (SATs) and Speech Recognition Thresholds (SRTs) revealed a mild loss in the ability to receive speech for each ear. Word Recognition Scores (WRS) were obtained for each ear at the most comfortable level (MCL; 65 dB HL) because the traditional presentation level of 40 dB sensation level (SL; ref: SRT) would have been 70 and 75 dB HL for the right and left ears, respectively, which was perceived to be uncomfortably loud by SS. Results revealed normal ability to recognize speech in the right ear and

slight difficulty in the left ear. Tympanometry revealed normal ear canal volume, static admittance, and middle ear pressure in each ear. Acoustic Reflex Thresholds (ARTs) could not be assessed because SS was concerned about the loud presentation level. Loudness Discomfort Levels (LDLs; ▶ Table 48.1) were measured for pure tones (PT) and narrowband noise (NBN) at 250 to 8,000 Hz and broadband noise (BBN) in each ear. LDLs hovered around 70 to 80 dB HL in each ear. These LDLs are lower than would be expected for someone with a mild hearing loss.

48.3 Questions to the Reader

1. **What could be the cause of the pain and spasms in SS's ears?**
2. **Based on the case history and audiologic information at the reader's disposal, what additional testing would the reader recommend?**

48.4 Discussion of Questions

1. **What could be the cause of the pain and spasms in SS's ears?**

SS has symptoms consistent with Tonic Tensor Tympani Syndrome (TTTS). This disorder was first investigated in the 1970s.[1,2] Patients with this syndrome may display one or more of the following symptoms: tinnitus, hyperacusis, aural fullness, otalgia, dull or sharp pain around the ears, numbness around the ear and cheek areas, tympanic flutter, frequent "ear popping," distorted speech, and mild vertigo.[3] TTTS is generally observed in patients with TMJ disorder; however, it can also follow acoustic trauma. It is believed to be caused by aberrant firing of the trigeminal nerve.[4]

2. **Based on the case history and audiologic information at the reader's disposal, what additional testing would the reader recommend?**

48.5 Additional Testing

48.5.1 Tinnitus Pitch Match

This tinnitus measure assists the clinician and the patient to know the approximate pitch of their tinnitus. The frequency of different auditory stimuli (i.e., PT, NBN, BBN, or speech noise) can be varied to estimate the pitch of the tinnitus perceived by the patient. Additional stimuli can also be used if the patient perceives more than one tinnitus sound. The result of this clinical procedure can be helpful during informational counseling as well as in management strategies such as the use of notched music. The premise of notched music therapy is to alter music such that it is presented at all frequencies except at frequencies around the tinnitus pitch of the patient. This approach has shown to reduce not only the loudness of tinnitus but also cortical activity corresponding to the tinnitus.[5] SS reported her

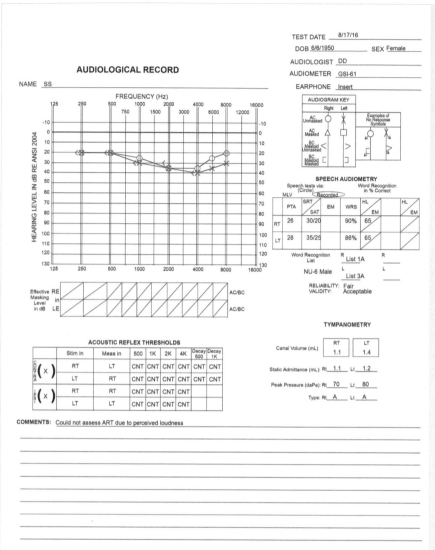

Fig. 48.1 Comprehensive audiologic evaluation of SS.

Table 48.1 SS's LDL (in dB HL) measured at the first visit using a 2-dB step size for PT and NBN across frequencies as well as for BBN for each ear

Stimulus	Frequency (Hz)											
	250		500		1,000		2,000		4,000		8,000	
	Right	Left	Right	Left	Right	Left	Right	Left	Right	Left	Right	Left
PT	76	78	72	74	72	74	72	72	74	76	78	78
NBN	72	74	70	72	70	72	70	72	70	70	74	76
BBN	70 (right); 74 (left)											

Abbreviations: BBN, broadband noise; LDL, Loudness Discomfort Level; NBN, narrowband noise; PT, pure tones.

tinnitus to be a high-pitched continuously ringing sound. Her tinnitus pitch was identified at 4,000 Hz in each ear.

48.5.2 Tinnitus Loudness Match

This tinnitus measure assists the clinician and the patient to know the approximate loudness of his or her primary tinnitus. It is usually performed at the pitch of the tinnitus identified during tinnitus pitch match as described earlier. Typically, a 2-dB step size involving multiple ascending or descending runs is recommended. The results of this clinical procedure can be

helpful in deciding the intensity of sounds presented via sound therapy as well as to monitor its effectiveness. Sound therapy refers to a form of tinnitus management wherein the tinnitus patient listens to auditory stimuli—either amplified ambient sounds via hearing aids or specialized sounds such as noises—in order to minimize the effects of tinnitus. Although there are no normative loudness-match data due to the heterogeneity of this disorder, values can be used to customize sound therapy options for an individual patient. SS's tinnitus loudness was measured at 56 and 60 dB HL in the right and left ears, respectively.

48.5.3 Minimum Masking Level

Minimum Masking Level (MML) is a tinnitus measure that helps identify the amount of masking noise required to completely mask tinnitus. Although studies[6,7,8,9,10] have shown that low-level background sounds may be effective at reducing the loudness of tinnitus, MMLs can be used as an efficacy measure to monitor progress of sound therapy. For SS, MMLs could not be identified because masking sounds were judged to be uncomfortably loud.

48.5.4 Loudness Discomfort Level

LDL in response to various stimuli such as NBN and BBN at different frequencies may help the clinician obtain a more accurate assessment of a patient's sound tolerance profile. An ascending procedure is followed and a smaller step size (typically 2 dB) is used so as not to accidently reach the patient's LDL. It is important to assure the patient that testing will never be performed at or above the patient's LDL and that testing will be immediately suspended if he or she feels uncomfortable. For SS, LDL were measured for each ear individually in response to PT, NBN, and BBN, and are reported in ▶ Table 48.1.

48.5.5 Tinnitus and Hyperacusis Questionnaires

Standardized and clinically validated questionnaires such as the Tinnitus Handicap Questionnaire (THQ),[11] Tinnitus Functional Index (TFI),[12] Tinnitus Primary Function Questionnaire (TPFQ),[13] and Hyperacusis Questionnaire[14] can be administered to assess the impact of tinnitus and hyperacusis on different aspects of the patient's life. Pre–post comparisons should focus not only on statistical significance but also on clinically significant changes. SS's TFI score was 60 on a scale from 0 to 100 (a higher score indicates a greater impact of tinnitus on the patient's life).

48.6 Diagnosis and Recommended Treatment

SS has tinnitus as well as fear and pain hyperacusis—possibly resulting from acoustic trauma/TTTS. The diagnosis of acoustic shock (or acoustic shock disorder, if symptoms persist) is common among call center employees.[15,16,17] It is important to emphasize that although there may be no "cure" for tinnitus and hyperacusis, there are tools and techniques that will help with adaptation. The management plan for SS involved the following components:

- Management of tinnitus:
  - Informational counseling was provided to SS including information about how the normal auditory system works; causes of hearing loss, tinnitus, and hyperacusis; prevalence of tinnitus and hyperacusis; and brief overview of assessment and management strategies. She was provided brochures about these topics as well as access to resources for additional information such as websites and support forums.
  - After obtaining medical clearance from her physician, SS's audiologist fitted SS with bilateral receiver-in-the-canal (RIC) hearing aids (Widex Clear Fusion 440s) that were coupled to the ears via open domes. Real Ear Measures (REM) were performed to verify gain targets. During the first hearing aid fitting appointment, prescribed gain at all input levels (50, 65, and 80 dB SPL) was well below the target level (1–6 dB across frequencies). This was achieved by programming the acclimatization level at two out of four. The audiologist performed Real Ear Saturation Response to a 90-dB SPL input sound (RESR$_{90}$) to verify the output did not exceed the patient's LDL. Additionally, SS's audiologist reviewed hearing aid data logging at each follow-up visit to ensure appropriate gain levels across programs (universal and tinnitus programs). This was possible because SS's hearing aids logged the average volume control reduction and the corresponding environments in which she surrounded herself.
  - Sound generators:
    - SS's audiologist demonstrated the use of various external sound generators (such as the Sleep Pillow, Neuromonics Oasis, HoMedics Sound Machine) including those that can be presented through smartphone applications.[18] SS chose to use the Widex Zen tinnitus program through her hearing aids, which presents fractal tones at different pitch-loudness-tempo combinations.[6,19] SS was presented all five available Zen options and instructed to choose those she would find acceptable after listening all day at a "soft, but comfortable level," input level. After completing this task, SS chose "Zen Aqua."
- Management of reaction to tinnitus:
  - It is vital for individuals with tinnitus to understand that the symptoms of tinnitus are different from a patient's reaction to the tinnitus. The Tinnitus Activities Treatment (TAT)[20] contains pictorial examples to emphasize that a neutral stimulus (e.g., a doorbell) can evoke both positive and negative reactions depending on the association a patient makes with the stimuli. Analogies were drawn between these examples and tinnitus to assist SS understand the distinction between tinnitus and her reaction to it.
- Management of hyperacusis:
  - The goal of hyperacusis management is habituation.[21,22] The following strategies were used to assist SS deal with her hyperacusis:
    - **Counseling:** SS was counseled that although moderately loud sounds may seem annoying they were unlikely to damage her hearing. She was provided information about the relationship between auditory, emotional, and fear centers in the brain, which helped SS understand the fear component of hyperacusis.
    - **Sound enrichment and desensitization**: It was emphasized that the use of earplugs was counterintuitive as it may increase central gain ("compensatory increase in the central auditory activity in response to the loss of sensory input"[23]), thereby making hyperacusis worse. SS was asked to begin desensitization by listening to bothersome sounds (e.g., multiple people talking at once) at very soft input levels for 15 minutes at least 4 to 5 day/week. SS was asked to increase her exposure to the loudness of the

Table 48.2 SS's LDL (in dB HL) measured at the 6-month follow-up visit using a 2-dB step size for PT and NBN across frequencies as well as for BBN for each ear

Stimulus	Frequency (Hz)											
	250		500		1,000		2,000		4,000		8,000	
	Right	Left	Right	Left	Right	Left	Right	Left	Right	Left	Right	Left
PT	78	82	78	76	76	80	82	80	78	82	78	80
NBN	78	80	76	76	74	78	78	80	76	80	76	78
BBN	78 (right); 80 (left)											

Abbreviations: BBN, broadband noise; LDL, Loudness Discomfort Levels; NBN, narrowband noise; PT, pure tones.

sounds every week in increments that were comfortable to her. She was asked to continue auditory sessions even after sounds seemed comfortable, to maintain progress. Finally, SS journaled her observations in a sound diary and met with the audiologist once a month.

- Possible accommodations at work:
  - Request a separate room that would reduce unexpected loud noise.
  - Use of low-level background sounds/noise played through either wearable devices (e.g., via smartphone applications such as ReSound Relief, Hear-Tinnitus, Starkey Relax) or stand-alone sound generators.
  - Wear noise cancelling headphones while making calls.
  - Request a cushioned door that cannot be slammed shut.
  - Request colleagues to use rubber/plastic caps at the end of chair legs to minimize the scraping noise.

48.7 Outcome

After following the tinnitus and hyperacusis management plan for 6 months, SS reported significant improvements in the annoyance from her tinnitus and hyperacusis. She requested the audiologist to increase the acclimatization level of her hearing aids to target (level four out of four). SS's tinnitus loudness was measured at 46 and 50 dB HL in the right and left ears, respectively—a reduction of 10 dB in each ear. Furthermore, SS's TFI score was 30—a reduction of 30 points. A 13-point reduction is considered to be a meaningful reduction on the TFI.[7] SS reported she could now tolerate moderately loud sounds. The audiologist confirmed that SS's LDL had increased by 6 to 10 dB across frequencies (▶ Table 48.2). SS no longer feared moderately loud sounds although she preferred that people not talk too loudly around her. She used noise-canceling headphones at work and used ear protection while attending sporting events or other noisy events. Finally, whenever SS felt a caller was becoming agitated, she transferred the caller to her supervisor.

48.8 Key Points

- It is important to convey to individuals with tinnitus the distinction between tinnitus and the reaction to it.
- Audiologists should be vigilant concerning the presence of hyperacusis in patients experiencing tinnitus.
- Even after implementing a management plan, it may take months for patients to notice an improvement in their tinnitus and/or hyperacusis attributes.

References

[1] Klockhoff I. Tensor tympani syndrome: a source of vertigo. Barany Society Ordinary. Meeting in Uppsala, Sweden, June 1–3; 1978;31–32

[2] Klockhoff I. Impedance fluctuation and a tensor tympani syndrome. Proceedings of the 4th International Symposium on Acoustic Measurements. Lisbon; 1979;69–76

[3] Westcott M, Sanchez TG, Diges I, et al. Tonic tensor tympani syndrome in tinnitus and hyperacusis patients: a multi-clinic prevalence study. Noise Health. 2013; 15(63):117–128

[4] Ramirez LM, Ballesteros LE, Sandoval GP. Topical review: temporomandibular disorders in an integral otic symptom model. Int J Audiol. 2008; 47(4):215–227

[5] Okamoto H, Stracke H, Stoll W, Pantev C. Listening to tailor-made notched music reduces tinnitus loudness and tinnitus-related auditory cortex activity. Proc Natl Acad Sci U S A. 2010; 107(3):1207–1210

[6] Tyler RS, Deshpande AK, Lau CC, Kuk F. The effectiveness of the progression of Widex Zen tinnitus therapy: a pilot study. Am J Audiol. 2017; 26(3):283–292

[7] Mahboubi H, Haidar YM, Kiumehr S, Ziai K, Djalilian HR. Customized versus noncustomized sound therapy for treatment of tinnitus: a randomized crossover clinical trial. Ann Otol Rhinol Laryngol. 2017; 126(10):681–687

[8] Theodoroff SM, McMillan GP, Zaugg TL, Cheslock M, Roberts C, Henry JA. Randomized controlled trial of a novel device for tinnitus sound therapy during sleep. Am J Audiol. 2017; 26(4):543–554

[9] Shekhawat GS, Searchfield GD, Stinear CM. Role of hearing AIDS in tinnitus intervention: a scoping review. J Am Acad Audiol. 2013; 24(8):747–762

[10] Hoare DJ, Searchfield GD, El Refaie A, Henry JA. Sound therapy for tinnitus management: practicable options. J Am Acad Audiol. 2014; 25(1):62–75

[11] Kuk FK, Tyler RS, Russell D, Jordan H. The psychometric properties of a tinnitus handicap questionnaire. Ear Hear. 1990; 11(6):434–445

[12] Meikle MB, Henry JA, Griest SE, et al. The tinnitus functional index: development of a new clinical measure for chronic, intrusive tinnitus. Ear Hear. 2012; 33(2):153–176

[13] Tyler R, Ji H, Perreau A, Witt S, Noble W, Coelho C. Development and validation of the tinnitus primary function questionnaire. Am J Audiol. 2014; 23(3):260–272

[14] Khalfa S, Dubal S, Veuillet E, Perez-Diaz F, Jouvent R, Collet L. Psychometric normalization of a hyperacusis questionnaire. ORL J Otorhinolaryngol Relat Spec. 2002; 64(6):436–442

[15] Patuzzi R, Milhinch J, Doyle J. Acute aural trauma in users of telephone headsets and handsets. In Abstracts of XXVI International Congress of Audiology. (Spec ed). Melbourne, 17–21 March. Aust N Z J Audiol. 2002; 23:13:2

[16] Westcott M. Acoustic shock injury (ASI). Acta Otolaryngol Suppl. 2006; 126 556:54–58

[17] Westcott M. Acoustic shock disorder. Tinnitus discovery-Asia and pacific tinnitus symposium, Auckland, September 2009. N Z Med J. 2010; 123:25

[18] Deshpande AK, Chang J. A Preliminary Evaluation of Tinnitus Apps. Phoenix, AZ: AudiologyNow!; 2016

[19] Sweetow RW, Sabes JH. Effects of acoustical stimuli delivered through hearing aids on tinnitus. J Am Acad Audiol. 2010; 21(7):461–473

[20] Tyler RS, Gogel SA, Gehringer AK. Tinnitus activities treatment. Prog Brain Res. 2007; 166:425–434

[21] Tyler RS, Pienkowski M, Roncancio ER, et al. A review of hyperacusis and future directions: part I. Definitions and manifestations. Am J Audiol. 2014; 23(4):402–419

[22] Pienkowski M, Tyler RS, Roncancio ER, et al. A review of hyperacusis and future directions: part II. Measurement, mechanisms, and treatment. Am J Audiol. 2014; 23(4):420–436

[23] Auerbach BD, Rodrigues PV, Salvi RJ. Central gain control in tinnitus and hyperacusis. Front Neurol. 2014; 5:206

49 A Case of Extreme Misophonia and Hyperacusis

Emily Sharp and Suzanne Kimball

49.1 Clinical History and Description

JM is an 18-year-old male originally scheduled for an appointment at a university speech and hearing clinic with the primary report of extreme sensitivity to specific sounds and situations. It was reported that JM's only previous encounter with an audiologist was at age 4 and those test results were normal. JM was accompanied to the initial and all following appointments by a parent. A thorough case history revealed JM would often "get lost in his own complex creations" of toys and was able to remember over 200 "super-powers" associated with a popular brand of toy cars. It was also reported that JM was obsessively concerned with germs and would refuse to touch the hands of others and become angry if unable to wash his hands immediately. JM's family described him as very meticulous about the exact order, arrangement, and process of items and situations in his daily life.

The extreme nature of JM's sound sensitivity was reported to cause physical discomfort when JM was unable to remove himself from situations that triggered, or initiated, his emotional and physical reactions. Offending sounds included talking, chewing, eating, and the sounds of silverware scraping on dishes. These sounds were reported to be more bothersome when created by members of JM's family. These sounds were so offensive that JM resorted to self-mutilating behaviors including digging his fingernails into the backs of his hands and scratching the inside of his wrists with his fingernails. These injuries were noted during the initial appointment and a follow-up appointment, but JM denied knowing how the injuries occurred.

49.2 Audiologic Testing

A comprehensive audiologic examination (▶ Fig. 49.1) obtained with EARTone 3A insert earphones and Sennheiser HDA 200 circumaural headphones revealed normal hearing sensitivity

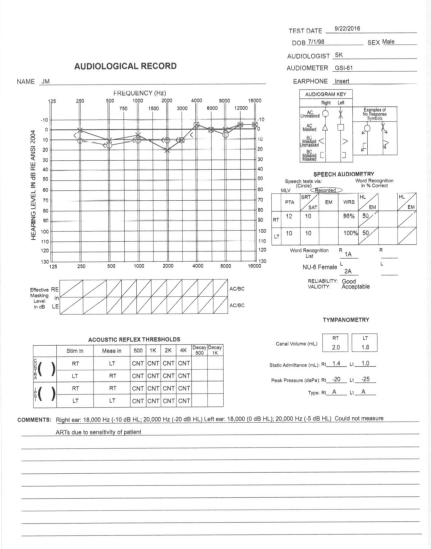

Fig. 49.1 Conventional audiologic testing conducted at the initial misophonia and hyperacusis evaluation.

from 250 to 20,000 Hz by air conduction with a pure-tone average (PTA) of 12 dB HL in each ear. Otoscopy results revealed clear external canals and normal appearance of tympanic membranes bilaterally. Bone conduction thresholds were consistent with air conduction thresholds at 500 to 4,000 Hz. The tympanometric results, including ear canal volume, static admittance, and peak pressure were all within normal range bilaterally. Acoustic Reflex Thresholds (ART) were unable to be assessed due to the patient's extreme sound hypersensitivity. A Speech Recognition Threshold (SRT) of 10 dB HL in each ear was consistent with the PTA, and the Word Recognition Scores (WRS) were 96% in the right ear and 100% in the left ear with a presentation level of 50 dB HL.

49.3 Questions to the Reader

1. **What additional case history information might be pertinent to this case?**
2. **What additional audiologic testing would be recommended?**
3. **What treatment options might be considered?**

49.4 Discussion of Questions

1. **What additional case history information might be pertinent to this case?**

It would be beneficial to determine (1) the approximate time of onset of the misophonia (abnormally strong autonomic and limbic system reactions in response to specific auditory stimuli) and hyperacusis (decreased loudness tolerance) symptoms; (2) whether there are any coexisting psychological conditions such as anxiety, depression, or obsessive compulsive disorder; and (3) how the current misophonia and hyperacusis symptoms are being managed, if at all.

2. **What additional audiologic testing would be recommended?**

Additional audiologic measures could include the following:

- High-frequency audiometry measured bilaterally from 9,000 to 20,000 Hz, per standard protocol at this clinic to determine the integrity of the entire peripheral auditory system.
- Loudness Discomfort Levels (LDL) measured for each ear at 500, 1,000, 2,000, and 4,000 Hz and speech.
- Use of the Tinnitus and Hyperacusis Initial Interview Form[1] to determine the effects of the sound sensitivity on the well-being of JM.
- Standardized subjective misophonia measurements such as the Misophonia Assessment Questionnaire (MAQ)[2] and the Amsterdam Misophonia Scale (A-MISO-S)[3] to measure and monitor the severity of the JM's misophonia and its impact on quality of life.

3. **What treatment options might be considered?**

Based on Jastreboff's protocol of Tinnitus Training Therapy (TRT),[4] hyperacusis and misophonia can be managed with a systematic program of sound therapy and counseling. The protocol recommends a gradual increase in sound exposure starting with full control given to JM and slowly transitioning control

Table 49.1 Loudness Discomfort Levels at the initial evaluation

	500 Hz	1,000 Hz	2,000 Hz	4,000 Hz	Speech
Right	70 dB HL	70 dB HL	60 dB HL	65 dB HL	75 dB HL
Left	80 dB HL	75 dB HL	70 dB HL	65 dB HL	75 dB HL

away from JM. Also, ear-level sound generators or other personal listening devices programmed with a designated sound therapy may be used in conjunction with the specific misophonia protocol exercises.

49.5 Additional Testing

Initial LDL (▶ Table 49.1) were obtained for each ear at 500, 1,000, 2,000, and 4,000 Hz as well as for live-voice speech stimuli. JM was instructed that this was not a test of endurance and that stimuli will cease immediately once judged by him to be "too loud to tolerate for 1 to 2 seconds." The LDL were measured between 60 and 80 dB HL for the pure-tone stimuli and at 75 dB HL for speech in each ear. Recent studies[5] indicate that LDL for adults with normal hearing average 100 dB HL, with a standard deviation ranging from 10.67 to 13.58 dB depending on frequency. JM's lower LDL indicate the presence of decreased sound tolerance.

The Tinnitus and Hyperacusis Initial Interview Form, including baseline subjective sound sensitivity ratings, was administered during the initial evaluation. JM was asked to rate the following three questions on a scale of 1 (not at all) to 10 (extremely): "How severe is your sound sensitivity?," "How annoying is your sound sensitivity?," and "How much does your sound sensitivity affect your quality of life?" This baseline can be used to evaluate JM's progress as treatment progresses. JM's responses were that the severity of his sound sensitivity was 9, its annoyance was 10, and its impact on his quality of life was between 9 and 10. These subjective ratings indicate that JM is extremely bothered by his sound sensitivities.

The MAQ was administered and JM's total score was 51 (▶ Fig. 49.2). The MAQ consists of 21 questions regarding the negative impact of misophonia rated on a scale of 0 (not at all) to 3 (almost all the time). The maximum score on the MAQ is 63. JM's score of 51 places him in the extreme misophonia category, indicating his misophonia has a significant negative impact on his activities, thoughts, and feelings.

The A-MISO-S was also administered to JM during the initial evaluation and a total score of 19 was obtained (▶ Fig. 49.3). The A-MISO-S includes six questions regarding the impact of and preoccupation with misophonic sounds scored from 0 (none) to 4 (extreme) as well as a final subjective free-response question. The highest possible score is 24 and indicates extreme misophonia. JM's score of 19 places him in the severe range of misophonic symptoms.

49.6 Additional Questions to the Reader

1. **What additional referrals may be appropriate for JM?**

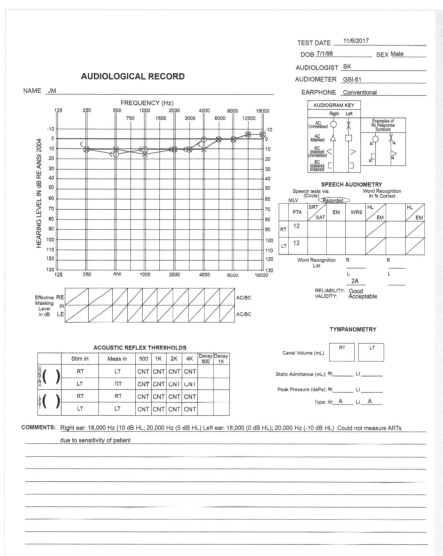

Fig. 49.2 Misophonia Assessment Questionnaire completed at the initial misophonia and hyperacusis evaluation.

49.7 Discussion of Additional Questions

1. What additional referrals may be appropriate for JM?

Taking into consideration JM's case history and interactions with him during the initial evaluation and follow-up appointments, it was strongly recommended JM be referred to a psychologist or psychiatrist for evaluation and intervention. This decision was made due to JM's parent-reported history of anger and rage, obsessive thoughts and actions, as well as the visible self-mutilation injuries noted during the initial evaluation. There are several mental health screenings that can be administered by an audiologist to determine if a referral should be considered, including the Beck Depression Inventory (BDI)[6] or the Hospital Anxiety and Depression Scale (HADS).[7] These screenings were not administered during the initial evaluation or any follow-up, as JM's parents were unwilling to seek referral to a mental health professional.

49.8 Diagnosis and Recommended Treatment

The diagnoses of misophonia and hyperacusis were made at the conclusion of the initial evaluation and were based on loudness tolerance measures and case history report. Realistic counseling concerning the management of misophonia and hyperacusis was included as part of the treatment plan. It was determined that JM would benefit from ear-level sound therapy devices and it was recommended that JM also be referred to a psychologist or psychiatrist for evaluation and possible intervention.

49.9 Outcome

JM was fitted with bilateral Resound LINX2 5 receiver-in-the-canal (RIC) hearing aids programmed with his "water creek" sound therapy and no prescribed amplification. JM was counseled regarding the consistent use of his selected sound therapy

Name: _____   Date: _____

Amsterdam Misophonia Scale (A-MISO-S)*

Rate the characteristics of each item during the prior week up until and including the time you fill out this survey. Scores should reflex the average (mean) occurrence of each item for the entire week. "Sounds" can mean any misophonic trigger (sound, sight, touch, motion, etc.)

1. How much of your time is occupied by misophonic sounds? (How frequently do the (thoughts about the) misophonic sounds occur?)

None	○	0
Mild, less than 1 hr/day,or occasionally (thoughts about) sounds (no more than 5 times a day)	○	1
Moderate, 1 to 3 hrs/day, or frequent (thoughts about) sounds (no more than 8 times a day, most of the hours are unaffected).	○	2
Severe, greater than 3 hrs and up to 8 hrs/day or very frequent (thoughts about) sounds.	●	3
Extreme, greater than 8 hrs/day or near constant (thoughts about) sounds.	○	4

2. How much do these misophonic sounds interfere with your social, work or role functioning? (Is there anything that you don't do because of them? If currently not working determine how much performance would be affected if you were employed.)

None	○	0
Mild, slight interference withi social or occupational/school activities, but overall performance not impaired.	○	1
Moderate, definite interference with social or occupational performance, but still manageable.	○	2
Severe, causes substantial impairment in social or occupational performance.	●	3
Extreme, incapacitating.	○	4

3. How much distress do the misophonic sounds cause you? (In most cases, distress is equated with irritation, anger, or disgust. Only rate the emotion that seems triggered by misophonic sounds, not generalized irritation or irritation associated with other conditions.)

None	○	0
Mild, occasional irritation/distress.	○	1
Moderate, disturbing irritation/anger/disgust, but still manageable.	○	2
Severe, very disturbing irritation/anger/disgust.	○	3
Extreme, near constant and disturbing anger/disgust.	●	4

*Amsterstam Misophonia Scale (A-MISO-S) from Schröder, A., Vulink, N., & Denys, S. (2013). Misophonia: Diagnostic criteria for a new psychiatric disorder. *PLoS ONE*, *8*(1), e54706. doi:10.1371/journal.pone.0054706

Fig. 49.3 Amsterdam Misophonia Scale questionnaire completed at the initial misophonia and hyperacusis evaluation.

and was instructed to increase the volume of his sound therapy when he was most bothered by offending sounds, and decrease the volume when he was less bothered. JM was seen on an as-needed basis following the initial fitting to ensure the sound therapy was used consistently and that the hearing aids remained in good working order. His parents reported JM had not seen a mental health professional because they were concerned of JM "being labeled." Therefore, JM was never prescribed medication or treatment plan for any possible mental health disorder.

JM was seen in clinic on three occasions for hearing aid repairs and maintenance following the initial evaluation and fitting. Approximately 1 year after his initial evaluation, JM was seen for a follow-up of pure-tone air conduction thresholds at 250 to 20,000 Hz (▶ Fig. 49.4) and speech and LDL at 500 to 4,000 Hz (▶ Table 49.2). Results from that appointment did not reveal any change in pure-tone air conduction thresholds, but

Table 49.2 Loudness Discomfort Levels at 1-year follow-up

	500 Hz	1,000 Hz	2,000 Hz	4,000 Hz	Speech
Right	35 dB HL	35 dB HL	40 dB HL	35 dB HL	45 dB HL
Left	50 dB HL	45 dB HL	45 dB HL	45 dB HL	40 dB HL

speech and pure-tone LDLs were markedly decreased to levels between 35 and 50 dB HL in each ear. It should be noted that upon arrival at the clinic, JM was removed from the waiting room due to his inability to tolerate his sound sensitivity. JM was visibly distressed during the evaluation and he was not utilizing his sound therapy. It was reported by his parent that JM "triggered" on the drive to the clinic and was only able to communicate by text message to his parent. These events leading to the appointment may have contributed to the significant decrease in LDL obtained during the evaluation. JM again completed the MAQ (▶ Fig. 49.5) and A-MISO-S (▶ Fig. 49.6), with

4. How much effort do you make to resist the (thoughts about the) misophonic sounds? (How often do you try to disregard or turn your attention away from these sounds? Only rate effort made to resist, not success or failure in actually controlling the thought or sound.)

Makes an effort to always resist, or symptoms so minimal, doesn't need to actively resist.	○ 0
Tries to resist most of the time.	● 1
Makes some effort to resist.	○ 2
Yields to all (thoughts about) misophonic sounds without attempting to control them, but does so with some reluctance.	○ 3
Completely and willing yields to all obsessions.	○ 4

5. How much control do you you have over your thoughts about the misophonic sounds? How successful are you in stopping or diverting your thinking about the misophonic sounds? Can you dismiss them?

Complete control.	○ 0
Much control, usually able to stop or divert thoughts about misophonic sounds.	○ 1
Moderate control, sometimes able to stop or divert thoughts about misophonic sounds.	○ 2
Little control, rarely successful in stopping or dismissing thoughts about misophonic sounds, can only divert attention with difficulty.	○ 3
No control, experience thoughts as completely involuntary, rarely able to alter thinking about misophonic sounds.	● 4

6. Have you been avoiding doing anything, going any place, or being with anyone because of your misophonia? (How much do you avoid, for example, by using other loud sounds, such as music?)

No deliberate avoidance.	○ 0
Mild, minimal avoidance, Less than an hr/day or occasional avoidance.	○ 1
Moderate, some avoidance. 1 to 3 hr/day or frequent avoidance	○ 2
Severe, much avoidance. Greater than 3 up to 8 hr/day. Very frequent avoidance.	○ 3
Extreme very extensive avoidance. Greater than 8 hr/day. Doing almost everything you can to avoid triggering symptoms.	● 4

19 - Severe

Finally:
What would be the worst thing that could happen (to you) if you were not able to avoid the misophonic sounds?
Describe

Loss of any relationship (friend or more than friend)

Fig. 49.3 (Continued)

scores of 60 and 21, respectively, placing JM in the extreme misophonia category.

At this time, and for unknown reasons, JM is not consistently utilizing his sound therapy and has not shown measurable improvement in managing his sound sensitivities. JM did express the belief that the sound therapy, when utilized, helped him function while with friends in noisy environments, but that little improvement had been noted when exposed to his trigger sounds around his family.

At the follow-up evaluation, it was discussed with JM and his parents that additional intervention be considered to address the possibility of underlying psychological disorders that may be contributing to the severity of his sound sensitivities. JM's parents inquired as to whether medication for anxiety could prove beneficial. She was told to discuss that with the physician, but likely medication could provide JM some relief of his symptoms. It was also noted that JM is interested in pursuing higher education and it was discussed at length with JM the challenges he may face in the academic, social, and communal living settings of a college campus. It was suggested that JM focus on consistently utilizing his sound therapy devices immediately so that he may be as prepared as possible to manage his sound sensitivities in the college environment.

Name: _____ Date: _____

MISOPHONIA ASSESSMENT QUESTIONNAIRE (MAQ)

If a parent or caregiver, please answer for the child as best you are able, or substitute the words, "I feel that my child's sound issues" for the words "my sound issues".

RATING SCALE: 0 = not at all, 1 = a little of the time, 2 = a good deal of the time, 3 = almost all the time	0	1	2	3
1. My sound issues currently make me unhappy	○	○	○	●
2. My sound issues currently create problems for me.	○	○	○	●
3. My sound issues have recently made me feel angry.	○	○	○	●
4. I feel that no one understands my problems with certain sounds.	○	○	○	●
5. My sound issues do not seem to have a known cause.	○	○	○	●
6. My sound issues currently make me feel helpless.	○	○	●	○
7. My sound issues currently interfere with my social life.	○	●	○	○
8. My sound issues currently make me feel isolated.	○	○	●	○
9. My sound issues have recently created problems for me in groups.	○	○	○	●
10. My sound issues negatively affect my work/school life (currently or recently).	○	○	○	●
11. My sound issues currently make me feel frustrated.	○	○	○	●
12. My sound issues currently impact my entire life negatively.	○	○	○	●
13. My sound issues have recently made me feel guilty.	○	○	○	●
14. My sound issues are classified as 'crazy'.	○	○	○	●
15. I feel that no one can help me with my sound issues.	○	●	○	○
16. My sound issues currently make me feel hopeless.	○	●	○	○
17. I feel that my sound issues will only get worse with time.	○	○	○	●
18. My sound issues currently impact my family relationships.	○	○	○	●
19. My sound issues have recently affected my ability to be with other people.	○	○	○	●
20. My sound issues have not been recognized as legitimate.	○	○	○	●
21. I am worried that my whole life will be affected by sound issues.	○	○	●	○

51 - Extreme

By Marsha Johnson, revised by Tom Dozier

Revised 07/20/13

Fig. 49.4 Pure-tone air conduction testing at 250 to 20,000 Hz at 1-year follow-up.

Name: _____   Date: _____

MISOPHONIA ASSESSMENT QUESTIONNAIRE (MAQ)

If a parent or caregiver, please answer for the child as best you are able, or substitute the words, "I feel that my child's sound issues" for the words "my sound issues".

RATING SCALE: 0 = not at all, 1 = a little of the time, 2 = a good deal of the time, 3 = almost all the time	0	1	2	3
1. My sound issues currently make me unhappy	○	○	○	●
2. My sound issues currently create problems for me.	○	○	○	●
3. My sound issues have recently made me feel angry.	○	○	○	●
4. I feel that no one understands my problems with certain sounds.	○	○	○	●
5. My sound issues do not seem to have a known cause.	○	○	●	○
6. My sound issues currently make me feel helpless.	○	○	○	●
7. My sound issues currently interfere with my social life.	○	○	○	●
8. My sound issues currently make me feel isolated.	○	○	○	●
9. My sound issues have recently created problems for me in groups.	○	○	○	●
10. My sound issues negatively affect my work/school life (currently or recently).	○	○	●	○
11. My sound issues currently make me feel frustrated.	○	○	○	●
12. My sound issues currently impact my entire life negatively.	○	○	○	●
13. My sound issues have recently made me feel guilty.	○	○	○	●
14. My sound issues are classified as 'crazy'.	○	○	○	●
15. I feel that no one can help me with my sound issues.	○	○	○	●
16. My sound issues currently make me feel hopeless.	○	○	○	●
17. I feel that my sound issues will only get worse with time.	○	○	○	●
18. My sound issues currently impact my family relationships.	○	○	○	●
19. My sound issues have recently affected my ability to be with other people.	○	○	○	●
20. My sound issues have not been recognized as legitimate.	○	○	●	○
21. I am worried that my whole life will be affected by sound issues.	○	○	○	●

60-Extreme

By Marsha Johnson, revised by Tom Dozier

Revised 07/20/13

Fig. 49.5 Misophonia Assessment Questionnaire at 1-year follow-up.

Name: _____ Date: _____

Amsterdam Misophonia Scale (A-MISO-S)*

Rate the characteristics of each item during the prior week up until and including the time you fill out this survey. Scores should reflex the average (mean) occurrence of each item for the entire week. "Sounds" can mean any misophonic trigger (sound, sight, touch, motion, etc.)

1. How much of your time is occupied by misophonic sounds? (How frequently do the (thoughts about the) misophonic sounds occur?)

None	○	0
Mild, less than 1 hr/day,or occasionally (thoughts about) sounds (no more than 5 times a day)	○	1
Moderate, 1 to 3 hrs/day, or frequent (thoughts about) sounds (no more than 8 times a day, most of the hours are unaffected).	○	2
Severe, greater than 3 hrs and up to 8 hrs/day or very frequent (thoughts about) sounds.	●	3
Extreme, greater than 8 hrs/day or near constant (thoughts about) sounds.	○	4

2. How much do these misophonic sounds interfere with your social, work or role functioning? (Is there anything that you don't do because of them? If currently not working determine how much performance would be affected if you were employed.)

None	○	0
Mild, slight interference withi social or occupational/school activities, but overall performance not impaired.	○	1
Moderate, definite interference with social or occupational performance, but still manageable.	○	2
Severe, causes substantial impairment in social or occupational performance.	○	3
Extreme, incapacitating.	●	4

3. How much distress do the misophonic sounds cause you? (In most cases, distress is equated with irritation, anger, or disgust. Only rate the emotion that seems triggered by misophonic sounds, not generalized irritation or irritation associated with other conditions.)

None	○	0
Mild, occasional irritation/distress.	○	1
Moderate, disturbing irritation/anger/disgust, but still manageable.	○	2
Severe, very disturbing irritation/anger/disgust.	○	3
Extreme, near constant and disturbing anger/disgust.	●	4

*Amsterstam Misophonia Scale (A-MISO-S) from Schröder, A., Vulink, N., & Denys, S. (2013). Misophonia: Diagnostic criteria for a new psychiatric disorder. *PLoS ONE, 8*(1), e54706. doi:10.1371/journal.pone.0054706

Fig. 49.6 Amsterdam Misophonia Scale questionnaire at 1-year follow-up.

Fig. 49.6 (Continued)

4. How much effort do you make to resist the (thoughts about the) misophonic sounds? (How often do you try to disregard or turn your attention away from these sounds? Only rate effort made to resist, not success or failure in actually controlling the thought or sound.)

Makes an effort to always resist, or symptoms so minimal, doesn't need to actively resist.	○	0
Tries to resist most of the time.	○	1
Makes some effort to resist.	●	2
Yields to all (thoughts about) misophonic sounds without attempting to control them, but does so with some reluctance.	○	3
Completely and willing yields to all obsessions.	○	4

5. How much control do you you have over your thoughts about the misophonic sounds? How successful are you in stopping or diverting your thinking about the misophonic sounds? Can you dismiss them?

Complete control.	○	0
Much control, usually able to stop or divert thoughts about misophonic sounds.	○	1
Moderate control, sometimes able to stop or divert thoughts about misophonic sounds.	○	2
Little control, rarely successful in stopping or dismissing thoughts about misophonic sounds, can only divert attention with difficulty.	○	3
No control, experience thoughts as completely involuntary, rarely able to alter thinking about misophonic sounds.	●	4

6. Have you been avoiding doing anything, going any place, or being with anyone because of your misophonia? (How much do you avoid, for example, by using other loud sounds, such as music?)

No deliberate avoidance.	○	0
Mild, minimal avoidance, Less than an hr/day or occasional avoidance.	○	1
Moderate, some avoidance. 1 to 3 hr/day or frequent avoidance	○	2
Severe, much avoidance. Greater than 3 up to 8 hr/day. Very frequent avoidance.	○	3
Extreme very extensive avoidance. Greater than 8 hr/day. Doing almost everything you can to avoid triggering symptoms.	●	4

21- Extreme

Finally:
What would be the worst thing that could happen (to you) if you were not able to avoid the misophonic sounds?
Describe

- Answer Not Provided -

49.10 Key Points

- Misophonia and hyperacusis may be successfully treated with sound therapy, but it must be utilized consistently for measurable improvements to be seen.
- If a patient is not illustrating improvement in symptoms after utilizing sound therapy, additional intervention may be needed in conjunction with sound therapy, and referral to a mental health professional should be considered.

References

[1] Tarnowska K, Ras K, Jastreboff PJ, et al. Decision Support System for Diagnosis and Treatment of Hearing Disorders: The Case of Tinnitus. Studies in Computational Intelligence 685. Berlin: Springer; 2017

[2] Johnson M. Misophonia Assessment Questionnaire (MAQ). Revised by Dozier T. Livermore, CA: Misophonia Institute; 2013

[3] Schröder A, Vulink N, Denys D. Misophonia: diagnostic criteria for a new psychiatric disorder. PLoS One. 2013; 8(1):e54706

[4] Jastreboff P. Tinnitus retraining therapy. In: Møller AR, Langguth B, De Ridder D, Kleinjung T, eds. Textbook of Tinnitus. New York, NY: Springer; 2011

[5] Sherlock LP, Formby C. Estimates of loudness, loudness discomfort, and the auditory dynamic range: normative estimates, comparison of procedures, and test-retest reliability. J Am Acad Audiol. 2005; 16(2):85–100

[6] Beck AT, Steer RA, Brown GK. Manual for the Beck Depression Inventory-II. San Antonio, TX: Psychological Corporation; 1996

[7] Zigmond AS, Snaith RP. The hospital anxiety and depression scale. Acta Psychiatr Scand. 1983; 67(6):361–370

Suggested Readings

[1] Edelstein M, Brang D, Rouw R, Ramachandran VS. Misophonia: physiological investigations and case descriptions. Front Hum Neurosci. 2013; 7: 296

[2] Jastreboff P, Jastreboff M. Decreased sound tolerance: hyperacusis, misophonia, diplacousis, and polyacousis. In: Aminoff MJ, Boller F, Swaab DF, eds. Handbook of Clinical Neurology. Vol. 129. Amsterdam: Elsevier; 2015:375–387

[3] Rouw R, Erfanian M. A large-scale study of misophonia. J Clin Psychol. 2018; 74(3):453–479

[4] Schröder A, Vulink N, Denys D. Misophonia: diagnostic criteria for a new psychiatric disorder. PLoS One. 2013; 8(1):e54706

[5] Schwartz P, Leyendecker J, Conlon M. Hyperacusis and misophonia: the lesser-known siblings of tinnitus. Minn Med. 2011; 94(11):42–43

50 Maximizing Tinnitus/Hyperacusis Sound Therapy with Real Ear Measures

D. Bradley Davis

50.1 Clinical History and Description

JW, a 70-year-old female, was seen for an audiometric evaluation with the primary complaint of severe bilateral hyperacusis and continuous tinnitus, but was more prominent and bothersome in the left ear. JW reported that in a recent motor vehicle accident the air bag deployed and impacted, with significant force, on the left side of her head. A Pressure Equalization (PE) tube was inserted into her left tympanic membrane following the accident to reportedly relieve a buildup of pressure behind her tympanic membrane secondary to the head trauma. JW arrived at the audiometric evaluation with a recently purchased left Receiver-In-the-Canal (RIC) hearing aid coupled to an open dome (i.e., maximum venting). JW's hearing aid included a tinnitus/hyperacusis sound therapy program that she reported provides "very little benefit in improving hearing or providing relief of my tinnitus/hyperacusis." The therapy sound in her hearing aid was a continuous broadband noise with a high-frequency emphasis that was not patient controllable. It was noted by JW that the hearing aid was not verified to meet a valid prescriptive target using Real Ear Measures (REM). Also, it was believed by the audiologist that due to the severity of the hearing in the low frequencies a more occluding dome should have been used. This concern, along with the reported lack of benefit for JW's hearing and relief from her tinnitus/hyperacusis, suggested the hearing aid may not have been appropriately fitted.

JW also reported that she almost always uses foam earplugs, even in relatively quiet environments, because any sudden noise caused distress. JW also reported that a box fan in her bedroom provides significant relief from her tinnitus and hyperacusis. It was not surprising that the broadband noise from a box fan provided relief for JW's tinnitus and hyperacusis because it likely provided some measure of masking of the tinnitus. Also, because the broadband noise emitted by the box fan is not dissimilar to the often recommended white noise for hyperacusis desensitization therapy, the resultant constant low-level stimulation is plausibly beneficial to JW for the same reason.

50.2 Clinical Testing

Pure-tone air and bone conduction audiometry (▶ Fig. 50.1) for the right ear revealed normal hearing at 250 to 1,000 Hz, followed by a slight to moderately severe sensorineural hearing loss at 1,500 to 8,000 Hz that is precipitously falling in configuration beyond 1,000 Hz. Results for the left ear revealed a moderate to moderately severe mixed hearing loss at 250 to 8,000 Hz that is flat in configuration. Significant air–bone gaps were present at 250 to 1,000 Hz. Speech Recognition Thresholds (SRTs) were in agreement with Pure-Tone Averages (PTA) and indicated normal ability to receive speech in the right ear and a moderate loss in the ability to receive speech in the left ear.

Word Recognition Scores (WRS) revealed slight difficulty recognizing speech in the right ear and moderate difficulty in the left ear. Immittance audiometry revealed normal physical volume in the right ear and a large physical volume in the left ear indicating patency of the PE tube. Static admittance was in the lower limits of normal for the right ear and unmeasurable in the left ear, again, indicating patency of the PE tube. Middle ear pressure in the right ear was negative, indicating a malfunctioning Eustachian tube, and unmeasurable in the left ear. Acoustic Reflex Thresholds (ARTs) and acoustic reflex decay were not tested due to the patient's reported distress to loud sound.

In addition to conventional audiometric tests, a tinnitus/hyperacusis test battery was completed including the following: (1) tinnitus pitch matching, (2) Minimum Masking Levels (MMLs), (3) residual inhibition, and (4) loudness discomfort levels (LDLs). All tinnitus/hyperacusis testing was performed using a calibrated two-channel clinical audiometer. Tinnitus pitch matching was accomplished using a bracketing technique. Beginning with a 1,000 Hz tone presented at a comfortable listening level, JW was asked, "Is the pitch of your tinnitus higher or lower than the pitch of the tone?" If the patient answers "higher," a 2,000 Hz tone is presented and so on. Once pitch matching has been bracketed to an octave band, pitch matching is measured to the closest half-octave. JW's tinnitus was judged to be close to 1,000 Hz. Next, a narrowband masking noise centered at 1,000 Hz was presented and JW was asked, "Is this noise more like your tinnitus than the tone?" JW reported that the narrowband masking noise at 1,000 Hz was more similar to her tinnitus than the 1,000 Hz pure-tone. Finally, a broadband speech noise was presented as a third choice as the closest match to her tinnitus. JW reported that the broadband speech noise was most similar to her tinnitus.

The tinnitus evaluation continued with tests using the broadband speech noise. Hearing threshold for speech noise was assessed and was measured as 17 dB hearing level (HL) for the right ear and 50 dB HL for the left ear. Using these thresholds for speech noise as a starting point and increasing in 1-dB steps binaurally, JW was asked to indicate the MML that completely masked her tinnitus. The MML was recorded as 30 dB HL for the right ear and 64 dB HL for the left ear. The MML is often included in the test battery for patients undergoing Tinnitus Retraining Therapy (TRT). A decrease in the MML has been reported to correlate with patient improvement.[1]

Residual inhibition of the tinnitus sound was assessed by increasing the MML of the broadband speech noise by 10 dB HL in each ear, to 40 dB HL in the right ear, and 74 dB HL in the left ear. The noise was presented at this level for 1 minute. At the cessation of the noise, JW was asked to rate any perceived change in the tinnitus. JW reported that immediately after the presentation of noise there was an approximately 80% reduction of the tinnitus within the first minute, 70% reduction in the tinnitus after 3 minutes, and 50% reduction of the sound at 4 minutes. The tinnitus sound reached a "normal" level within 7 to 10 minutes.

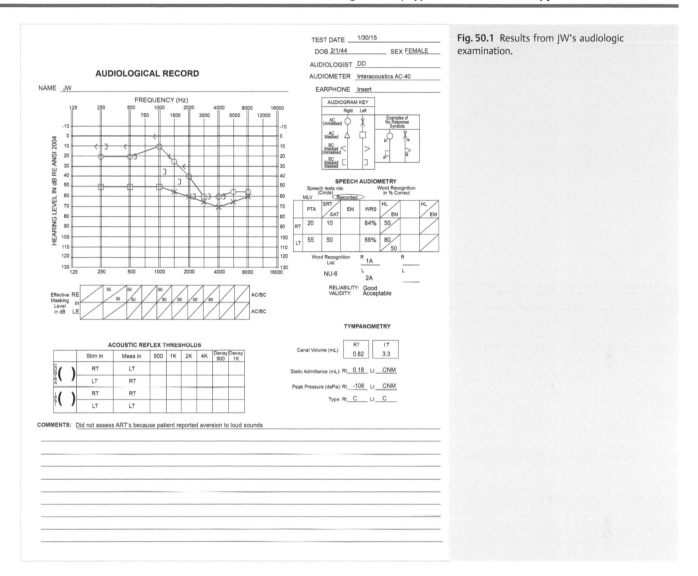

Fig. 50.1 Results from JW's audiologic examination.

Table 50.1 JW's loudness discomfort levels (dB HL) at 250 to 8,000 Hz

Frequency (Hz)	Right ear (dB HL)	Left ear (dB HL)
250	75	95
500	80	90
1,000	75	90
2,000	75	85
4,000	80	85
6,000	75	85
8,000	70	85

LDLs were then measured in each ear at the octave frequencies between 250 and 8,000 Hz and mid-octave 6,000 Hz[1] (► Table 50.1). Using an ascending method that increased in 5-dB steps, JW was asked to indicate the loudness level she would "not want to listen to the tone for more than a few seconds." Once the hearing threshold level (in dB HL) was indicated, the signal was quickly attenuated and the procedure repeated for the other test frequencies.

LDLs are an important consideration for any patient being fitted with hearing aids and are especially important for the hyperacusis patient. By including patient-specific LDLs during REM, the Output Saturation Sound Pressure Level (OSSPL in dB SPL) of hearing aids can be monitored and adjusted so that loud sounds do not exceed the LDLs. Caution should be exercised before decreasing the OSSPL excessively as this can severely restrict the dynamic range and negatively impact sound quality due to excessive output compression.

50.3 Questions to the Reader

1. **What is hyperacusis?**
2. **ARTs and reflex decay are important tests for diagnosing the seventh and eighth cranial nerve disorders. Is it acceptable not to include these tests due to patient distress?**
3. **What is residual inhibition and why is it an important test procedure in the tinnitus evaluation battery?**

50.4 Discussion of Questions

1. **What is hyperacusis?**

Hyperacusis is a hearing disorder that causes sounds that seem to be of normal loudness to most people to be distressingly loud. There is little reliable information on the number of people with bothersome hyperacusis. A conservative estimate suggests that approximately 2% of the adult population have some degree of hyperacusis.[2] Many persons with tinnitus report hyperacusis and almost all patients with hyperacusis report tinnitus. Sound desensitization is a common treatment for hyperacusis. There are many sound desensitization protocols, but all involve the introduction of sound into the ear. Sound desensitization therapies range from short-term moderately intense exposure to broadband noise to long-term low-level stimulation, to presenting a broadband noise for several hours per day for many months. These sound therapies endeavor to reset the increased gain within the central auditory nervous system. Other approaches to hyperacusis therapy include biofeedback and relaxation techniques.

2. **ARTs and reflex decay are important tests for diagnosing the seventh and eighth cranial nerve disorders. Is it acceptable not to include these tests due to patient distress?**

Patient distress should be considered of paramount importance during a tinnitus/hyperacusis evaluation. The patient is, after all, having an abnormal reaction to the perception of tinnitus or an abnormal reaction to normally loud sounds. Intentionally delivering a stimulus that is above the recorded LDLs should only be conducted if there is a suspicion of retrocochlear pathology. Because ART testing typically precedes LDL testing in the clinical test battery, if a patient expresses distress or alarm due to the high-level stimulus used to evoke the ART, the LDLs may have to be gathered first and ARTs revisited if retrocochlear involvement is suspected. Audiologists must be vigilant in identifying retrocochlear pathology. The audiologist is often the first health care professional to assess the patient with a primary complaint of tinnitus. Because tinnitus (especially unilateral tinnitus) is a "red flag" for retrocochlear pathology, if audiological findings suggest retrocochlear involvement (unexplained asymmetrical pure-tone thresholds, differences in WRS not explained by the audiogram, abnormally latent auditory evoked potential findings, etc.), the audiologist must consider conducting ARTs.

3. **What is residual inhibition and why is it an important test procedure in the tinnitus evaluation battery?**

Residual inhibition is the temporary suppression of tinnitus following auditory stimulation. Although there is conflicting research on the usefulness of the test protocol, it has been suggested that a change in the perception of the tinnitus following auditory stimulation is an indicator that sound therapy is a viable approach.[3]

50.5 Description of Disorder and Recommended Treatment

JW has a moderate high-frequency sensorineural hearing loss in the right ear and a moderate to severe mixed hearing loss in the left ear. She also reports bilateral continuous tinnitus and hyperacusis, but is more prominent in the left ear.

JW was fitted with bilateral Phonak Audeo Q70 RIC hearing instruments and a PilotOne remote control. Because of the differences in hearing thresholds in the low frequencies, the right hearing aid was coupled to an open dome and left aid was coupled to a closed power dome. The hearing aids are high-quality digital hearing instruments and provide tinnitus therapy sounds. There are many such devices available on the market today. The Audeo Q70 instrument includes a frequency and amplitude adjustable broadband noise as a therapy sound. The noise is highly adjustable using the available 16 bands of signal processing. The hearing aid fittings were verified using the Verifit Axiom real ear analyzer using desired sensation level (DSL) 5.0a prescriptive targets for input levels of 55 and 65 dB SPL with corrections for the bilateral fitting and air–bone gaps in the left ear.

The DSL 5.0a targets were verified using input levels of 55 and 65 dB SPL using standard speech. The OSSPL was verified to JW's individual LDL that was converted to dB SPL by the software within the Verifit analyzer.

Three programs were programed into JW's hearing instruments. After the verification procedure using REMs was performed on program 1 (▶ Fig. 50.2 and ▶ Fig. 50.3, for the right and left ears, respectively), the programmable parameters for program 1 were copied twice into programs 2 and 3 for three programs with the same programmable parameters for each ear. Program 1 provided amplification to correct for the hearing loss in each ear and contained no therapy sound. As can be seen in ▶ Fig. 50.1 and ▶ Fig. 50.2, the measured real ear aided response (REAR; i.e., smooth curves) closely matched the DSL 5.0a targets (i.e., crossed bar icon) for the 55 (green) and 65 (pink) dB SPL input levels. This was accomplished because it was felt there was a good chance that amplification alone would help relieve JW's tinnitus/hyperacusis. In tinnitus/hypersensitivity treatment, the final goal is to eliminate the need for a therapy sound and program 1 was included as the initial "start-up" program. The subsequent two programs utilized the sound therapy option and programming was monitored in real time using the REM probe microphone, but converted to a spectrum analyzer by turning off the signal from the loudspeaker within the analyzer. Program 2 used a combination of the previously verified acoustic program and Phonak's default therapy sound. The default therapy sound is a narrowband of noise starting at 1,500 Hz and rising to a peak of approximately 75 dB SPL in the 3,000 to 4,000 Hz region for the right ear (▶ Fig. 50.4), and a broader band of noise starting at 125 Hz and rising to approximately 80 dB SPL in the 2,000 to 3,000 Hz region for the left ear (▶ Fig. 50.5). Because JW reported that the box fan in her bedroom provides significant relief from her tinnitus and hyperacusis, program 3 utilized a therapy sound that attempted to replicate a box fan's frequency spectrum. With the assistance of a colleague and Google internet search engine, a box fan's frequency response was estimated to be broadband noise with energy in the 500 to 1,000 Hz frequency region and gently sloping thereafter. This is in essence similar to -3 dB per octave pink noise. Although it would have been ideal to measure JW's actual box fan, doing so would have been impractical and the estimated frequency response of a typical box fan was thought to be sufficient for the task. Along with JW's input, the final

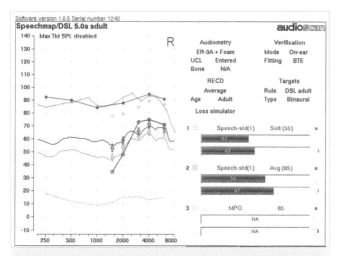

Fig. 50.2 Measured REAR (Real-Ear Aided Response) for the right ear for 55 and 65 dB Sound Pressure Level (SPL) to Desired Sensation Level (DSL) 5.0a using standard speech. Also displayed is an 85 dB SPL swept pure-tone to verify the output did not exceed the individually measured LDL (Loudness Discomfort Level).

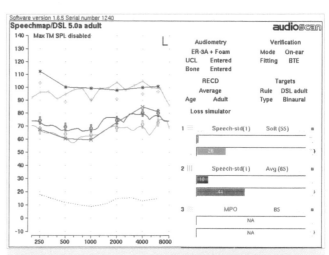

Fig. 50.3 Measured REAR (Real-Ear Aided Response) for the left ear for 55 dB Sound Pressure Level (SPL) and 65 dB SPL to Desired Sensation Level (DSL) 5.0a using standard speech. Also displayed is an 85 dB SPL swept pure-tone to verify the output did not exceed the individually measured LDL (Loudness Discomfort Level).

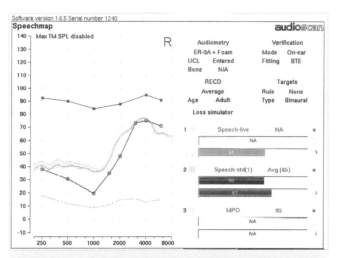

Fig. 50.4 Real Ear Measure (REM) of the default tinnitus signal for the right ear using the Verifit as a spectrum analyzer.

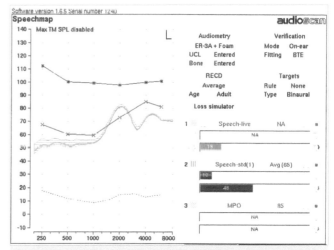

Fig. 50.5 Real Ear Measure (REM) of the default tinnitus signal for the left ear using the Verifit as a spectrum analyzer.

frequency spectrum of the "box fan" therapy sound at the eardrum was a relatively flat broadband noise with peak energy of approximately 70 dB SPL at 500 Hz for the left ear (▶ Fig. 50.6), a significant deviation from the default therapy sound for the left ear (▶ Fig. 50.5). The right ear therapy sound was left unchanged from Phonak's default settings at the patient's request (▶ Fig. 50.4).

50.6 Outcome

After two follow-up visits and a slight increase in the low-frequency output of the "box fan" noise in the left ear at approximately 300 Hz, JW reported that program 3 (hearing aid plus low-frequency emphasis "box fan" noise) was the most beneficial for both audibility and for tinnitus/hyperacusis relief.

Approximately 1 year after the patient's hearing aid fitting, in a phone conversation, JW reported continued benefit from the hearing aids. She reported that although she still carries earplugs in her purse, she uses them much less often than in the past. She reported that her consistent use of the tinnitus therapy sounds (i.e., programs 2 and 3) has decreased in the past year. JW reported that she rarely uses the tinnitus sound therapy programs and prefers the hearing instrument–only sound in program 1.

50.7 Key Points

- REMs were used for not only fitting the hearing instrument to DSL 5.0a targets, but also fine-tuning the therapy sound spectrum.

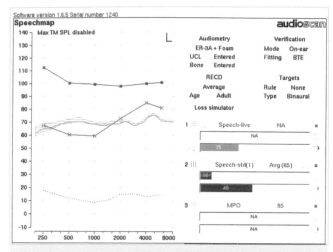

Fig. 50.6 Real Ear Measure (REM) of the customized "box fan" signal created as an approximation of the frequency spectrum of a commercially available "box fan." Note the difference in the REM between this customized therapy sound and the default setting for the left ear (i.e., ▶ Fig. 50.5).

- REM allows for real-time monitoring while adjusting the frequency and amplitude of the therapy sounds.
- These sounds can be tailored to match the results from a tinnitus/hyperacusis evaluation or for creating a custom therapy sound for maximum therapeutic impact.
- JW reported no benefit from the default setting of the therapy sounds generated by the hearing aid fitting software for the left ear, but did find the therapy sound created using real-time monitoring with the REM equipment beneficial.

References

[1] Henry J. Audiologic assessment. In: Snow J, ed. Tinnitus: Theory and Management. Hamilton, Ontario: BC Decker Inc.; 2004:220–236

[2] Baguley DM, McFerran D. Hyperacusis, and other forms of reduced sound tolerance. Tinnitus Network Web site. Available at: http://www.hyperacusis.net/media/1347/hyperacusis.pdf. Published August 2010. Accessed January 13, 2017

[3] Feldmann H. Homolateral and contralateral masking of tinnitus by noise-bands and by pure tones. Audiology. 1971; 10(3):138–144

Index

Note: Page numbers set **bold** or *italic* indicate headings or figures, respectively.